Ergogenic Aids and Muscular Performance

CONTRIBUTORS

Charles B. Corbin
David L. Costill
Harold B. Falls
B. Don Franks
Lawrence A. Golding
Donald H. Horstman
Leonard H. Kreit
Luigi F. Lucaccini
Robert M. Malina
Rainer Martens
William P. Morgan
Robert N. Singer
Jack H. Wilmore

Ergogenic Aids and Muscular Performance

Edited by

William P. Morgan

Department of Physical Education
University of Wisconsin
Madison, Wisconsin

ACADEMIC PRESS 1972 *New York and London*

ACADEMIC PRESS, INC.
111 Fifth Avenue, New York, New York 10003

United Kingdom Edition published by
ACADEMIC PRESS, INC. (LONDON) LTD.
24/28 Oval Road, London NW1

LIBRARY OF CONGRESS CATALOG CARD NUMBER: 72-82666

PRINTED IN THE UNITED STATES OF AMERICA

Contents

Chapter 3. Information Feedback

Robert M. Malina

Chapter 4. Mental Practice

Charles B. Corbin

Chapter 5. Heat and Cold Applications

Harold B. Falls

Chapter 6. Physical Warm-up

B. Don Franks

List of Contributors

Numbers in parentheses indicate the pages on which the authors' contributions begin.

CHARLES B. CORBIN, *Department of Physical Education, Kansas State University, Manhattan, Kansas* (93)

DAVID L. COSTILL, *Human Performance Laboratory, Division of Physical Education and Athletics, Ball State University, Muncie, Indiana* (293)

HAROLD B. FALLS, *Kinetoenergetics Laboratory, Department of Health and Physical Education, Southwest Missouri State University, Springfield, Missouri* (119)

B. DON FRANKS, *Biokinetics Research Laboratory, Department of Health, Physical Education, and Recreation, Temple University, Philadelphia, Pennsylvania* (159)

LAWRENCE A. GOLDING, *Applied Physiology Research Laboratory, School of Health, Physical Education, and Recreation, Kent State University, Kent, Ohio* (367)

DONALD H. HORSTMAN,* *Institute of Environmental Stress, University of California, Santa Barbara, California* (343)

LEONARD H. KREIT, *Professional Education Branch, Division of Dental Health, National Institute of Health, San Francisco, California* (235)

LUIGI F. LUCACCINI, *Professional Education Branch, Division of Dental Health, National Institute of Health, San Francisco, California* (235)

* Present address: United States Army Research Institute of Environmental Medicine, Natick, Massachusetts.

ROBERT M. MALINA, *Department of Anthropology, University of Texas, Austin, Texas* (67)

RAINER MARTENS, *Motor Performance and Play Research Laboratory, Children's Research Center, University of Illinois, Champaign, Illinois* (35)

WILLIAM P. MORGAN, *Ergopsychology Laboratory, Department of Physical Education, University of Wisconsin, Madison, Wisconsin* (3, 193)

ROBERT N. SINGER, *Department of Physical Education, Health and Recreation, Florida State University, Tallahassee, Florida* (263)

JACK H. WILMORE,* *Preventive Medicine Center, Palo Alto, California* (321)

* Present address: Department of Physical Education, University of California, Davis, California.

Preface

The facilitation of muscular performance has been of interest to investigators concerned with athletics, industry, and the military for many years. This is quite understandable since increases of several tenths of a second frequently make the difference between the runner-up and the world record performance in athletics; savings in the thousands of dollars may result in the industrial setting by increasing worker output by only one or two percent; and the ability of explorers and soldiers to function under hostile conditions is often governed by the availability of ergogenic aids. Ergogenic aids are defined in this volume as *substances* and *phenomena* which elevate performance above normal expectations.

The contributors to this volume are specialists in various areas of human performance such as experimental psychology, physical anthropology, social psychology, physical education, stress physiology, sport psychology, motor learning, and exercise physiology. The work represents an attempt to construct a multidisciplinary synthesis of the literature dealing with ergogenic aids and muscular performance. This is a departure from the traditional approach to this topic which has historically been limited to physiological, psychological, or medical orientations. This volume also differs from previous articles on this topic in at least two additional respects. Previous reviews have been limited entirely to *substances,* usually powerful drugs, hormones, and dietary supplements. The result has been that the mere mention of ergogenic aids has tended to evoke a negative atmosphere. This has indeed been unfortunate since a wide variety of substances and phenomena which apparently possess no after or side effects can be subsumed under the ergogenic rubric. For example, it is well documented that pure, unadulterated water facilitates the performance of man working in hot, humid environments, but most discussions of ergogenic aids do not even allude to this powerful substance. In addition to their being limited to selected substances, previous reviews have failed to evaluate the efficacy of phenomena such as mental practice, warm-up, hypnosis, music, social facilitation, information feedback, hot and cold applications, and anxiety states. The influence of these phenomena on muscular performance as well as substances are considered so that ergogenic aids are treated in a broadly conceived fashion.

The first section is limited to a single chapter which presents a conceptual framework for the volume and points out numerous methodological problems which must be considered when evaluating the efficacy of an ergogenic aid. The second section contains eight chapters dealing with anxiety, information feedback, mental practice, hot and cold applications, warm-up, hypnosis, music, and social facilitation. Four chapters dealing with water and electrolytes, drugs and hormones, oxygen, and nutrition are presented in the third section. An attempt is made in each chapter to present a thorough synthesis of the existing literature, and these reviews are followed by summary statements regarding the effectiveness of the substance or phenomenon. In most cases the summaries tend to raise more questions than they answer, and it is hoped that they will create a heuristic rather than serve as a source of frustration to the reader.

It should also be emphasized that the work is intended to be purely academic. No attempt has been made to consider the ethical, legal, and moral considerations which must be taken into account prior to the use of specific ergogenic aids. While such considerations are extremely important, they are far beyond the scope of this volume.

William P. Morgan

Part I

INTRODUCTION

Chapter 1

Basic Considerations

William P. Morgan

I. Introduction

A. Overview

Whether one is concerned with maximal physical performance in the athlete, astronaut, or factory worker, the concept of ergogenic aids assumes paramount importance. Ergogenic aids are defined as substances and phenomena that are work-producing aids, and these aids are thought to enhance performance above levels anticipated under normal conditions.

Concern over the value of ergogenic aids is readily appreciated when one considers that several tenths of a second often represents the difference between a mediocre and a championship performance in the athletic arena. Hence, an ergogenic aid that is capable of improving athletic performance by only a small percentage is of considerable practical importance. Likewise, if enhanced illumination or salt tablets increase the output of industrial workers by 1 or 2%, savings in the thousands of dollars may result. Many similar situations make it easy to see why ergogenic aids are of interest to anyone concerned with human performance.

B. Orientation

It is unfortunate that certain writers have discussed ergogenic aids in only a negative context. This topic has often been limited to substances such as powerful drugs, anabolic steroids, and highly questionable dietary supplements. The present work assumes a positive orientation and, as such, the ergogenic aid is treated in a broadly conceived fashion. It appears reasonably certain that unadulterated water possesses ergogenic benefits for individuals working in hot, humid environments. Water ingested immediately prior to work has been demonstrated to enhance physical performance (Londeree *et al.*, 1969), and there is considerable scientific evidence that withholding this ergogenic aid is both criminal and medically unsound. It is interesting to note, however, that most discussions of ergogenic aids do not refer to this most important substance.

C. Purpose

The primary purpose of this book is to present a synthesis of the literature dealing with ergogenic aids. It is not the authors' intention to answer the question of whether certain aids should be employed with the athlete or worker. The effort is purely academic. The ethical and legal considerations that must be taken into account prior to employment of certain ergogenic aids, while extremely important, are far beyond the scope of this work. However, a brief discussion of the importance of such considerations in experimental settings will be presented.

II. Typologies

A. Substances and Phenomena

Various substances such as drugs, hormones, oxygen, salts, caffeine, and vitamins have been discussed within the general framework of ergogenic models by a number of writers (Bartley, 1965; Blix, 1967; Bourne, 1968; de Vries, 1966; Fowler, 1969; Ganslen, 1968; Karpovich, 1965; Mathews *et al.*, 1964; Ricci, 1967; Van Itallie *et al.*, 1960). It seems reasonable to suggest, however, that the topic of ergogenic aids should be conceived in a much broader context to include work-producing phenomena such as hypnosis (Ikai and Steinhaus, 1961; Johnson, 1961), mental practice (Corbin, 1967; Richardson, 1967), physical warm-up (Massey *et al.*, 1961; Nelson and Lambert, 1965), hot and cold applications (Falls, 1969; Steinhaus and Wendhut, 1953), music (Ayres, 1911; Konz and McDougal, 1968), social facilitation (Martens, 1969; Singer, 1965), information feedback (Malina, 1969; Pierson and Rasch, 1964), and psychological states (Brown, 1961; Carron 1968). Therefore, ergogenic aids can be classified as being either substances or phenomena, and this will be the approach adopted in this work.*

B. Acute and Chronic Aids

Additional classification systems are readily apparent. For example, ergogenic aids are usually viewed in an "acute" context; that is, some substances and phenomena, such as drugs and hypnosis, affect today's performance. It should be pointed out, however, that the concept of ergogenic aids also includes important "chronic" components; that is, some substances and phenomena, such as vitamins and mental practice, affect long-term performance. It is important that both acute and chronic effects be examined when attempting to assess the appropriateness of a particular aid. This consideration should relate to harmful after and side effects, as well as performance per se.

* This does not mean that all ergogenic aids must fall into either the substance or phenomenon category. Indeed, a substance such as the placebo (Morgan, 1970) is not an ergogenic aid until its delivery is associated with suggestion, which would be a phenomenon in the proposed typology.

C. Task Specificity

In addition to viewing ergogenic aids as being either acute or chronic, one might view them within the context of "task specificity"; that is, a classification system can be arrived at on the basis of the nature of the physical performance. Indeed, such an approach is preferable in certain circumstances. Specifically, various ergogenic aids enhance endurance performances but have little or no effect on strength and power activities (de Vries, 1966; Karpovich, 1965). Conversely, certain ergogenic aids provide increments in strength (Ikai and Steinhaus, 1961) but have little or no effect on endurance activities (Massey *et al.*, 1961). For this reason, one must discuss the efficacy of a particular substance or phenomenon within the context of task specificity.

D. Paradoxical Distance Effects

Paradoxical distance effects are associated with certain ergogenic aids; that is, certain aids are work producing up to a point, and then further increases in dosage result in impairment of performance (Brown, 1961; Ganslen, 1968). To further complicate the issue, these paradoxical distance effects have been shown to vary considerably for different individuals.

E. The Consumer

The "consumer" of the substance or phenomenon is another important variable to be considered in the overall assessment of a particular ergogenic aid. It has been demonstrated that certain ergogenic aids appear to enhance the performance of the highly trained athlete but have little or no effect on the untrained individual (Blix, 1967). Conversely, certain aids enhance the performance of untrained subjects but have little or no effect on the highly trained individual (Ikai and Steinhaus, 1961). Finally, irrespective of training status, certain "types" of individuals respond negatively and others positively to the same ergogenic aids (Morgan, 1970). It appears to be quite clear that the value of a particular ergogenic aid is governed by the unique characteristics of the consumer.

III. Research Strategies

Human-performance investigators such as exercise physiologists, applied physiologists, engineering psychologists, and sport psychologists have assessed the effects of various substances and phenomena on muscular performance. They have attempted to determine if special substances, e.g., drugs, hormones, oxygen, water, salts, and various foods, or phenomena, e.g., mental practice, warm-up, hypnosis, music, social facilitation, information feedback, and anxiety states, enhance physical performance. Investigators have also been interested in whether certain of these substances and phenomena elicit harmful after or side effects. Such research has often yielded conclusive evidence regarding the efficacy of certain substances and phenomena. An equal number of investigations, however, have yielded inconclusive and contradictory findings. One of the reasons for this dilemma is that, with the exception of drug experimentation, very few of these investigations have attempted to control psychological variables. Invariably, however, these same investigators have discussed their findings to a certain point and then commented that the remainder is explained by "psychological factors." Such explanations are at best naïve and at worst grossly misleading.

Rather than dismissing an event as being partially psychological, an investigator should employ such an educated guess as a springboard to further inquiry. It would appear that a multivariate psychobiological model would be the most fruitful to adopt. Unfortunately, the writing of this work has been handicapped by the lack of evidence generated in such a fashion. In this regard it is hoped that our presentation will be heuristic.

IV. Methodological Considerations

A. Overview

The decision-making process regarding the efficacy of a particular aid may simply reflect the experimental protocol itself. Specifically, psychological factors such as the halo (Eysenck, 1958), Hawthorne (Roethlisberger and Dickson, 1939), and experimenter effects (Rosenthal, 1966) may be responsible for observed outcomes since such factors have been demonstrated to be experimental contaminants. The present section considers problems of bias inherent in given paradigms and offers recommendations for alternative designs. Of course, the scope of this chapter prevents an exhaustive discussion of such problems and, therefore, the reader is referred to "Artifact in Behavioral Research" (Rosenthal and Rosnow, 1969), which examines this matter in detail.

Various methodological considerations must be entertained in order to accurately evaluate the influence of a presumed ergogenic aid. Indeed, the alleged value of a particular substance or phenomenon often reflects statistical and design inelegancies related to the assessment process rather than an actual ergogenic influence. This viewpoint is reinforced in subsequent chapters.

While numerous investigations suggest that the outcomes of behavioral research are often influenced by various artifacts (Rosenthal and Rosnow, 1969), the extent to which these artifacts interact with muscular performance remains to be demonstrated for the most part (Martens, 1970). Furthermore, when a parameter such as the maximal oxygen uptake is regarded as the point at which an exercising S's oxygen consumption plateaus or begins to decrease, there is little reason to believe that such a physiologically defined event is subject to psychological artifacts. On the other hand, if this parameter is defined as the subjective point at which the S reports he cannot continue, one would intuitively expect experimental contamination due to behavioral cognitive phenomena such as demand characteristics, the "pact of ignorance," compliance, and experimenter expectancy effects (Evans, 1968; Orne, 1962).

Unfortunately, performance parameters are seldom defined in rigorous physiological terms. Historically, investigators concerned with the efficacy of a presumed ergogenic aid have employed dependent variables which are commonly thought to be influenced by subjective factors. For example, "all-out" exercise bouts performed on treadmills and bicycle ergometers are influenced in part by the S's "willingness" to continue; that is, while actual physical working capacity governs maximal performance, it is also clear that the S's decision to discontinue physical work is regulated to varying degrees by his subjective impressions of discomfort (Simonson, 1971). Hence, physical performance is dependent in part on both man's ability and willingness to tolerate pain. Furthermore, pain is associated with individual differences that are thought to reflect a wide variety of physiological, psychological, and sociological factors (Sternbach, 1968).

In addition to evaluating the facilitative effects of a particular substance or phenomenon, investigators are frequently concerned with the S's reaction to such treatment. For example, while high oxygen concentrations may or may not hasten recovery from anaerobic work, another consideration pertains to whether the S "thinks" and "feels" that it does. In short, even though a given "ergogenic" aid does not increase physical performance, the S's feeling that his performance was improved or that he "felt better" under such a condition is of practical significance. Also, the decision to make a substance (e.g., oxygen) or phenomenon (e.g., music) available in work settings might conceivably be based on the consumer's affect rather than actual increases in performance. A case in point is the widespread use of overload for purposes of increasing muscular performance; that is, overload has no effect on speed of movement, but it does result in a kinesthetic illusion of increased speed (Nelson and Lambert, 1965). Another example is the observation that, although music usually does not improve the output of industrial workers, it generally evokes positive attitudes in workers (Uhrbrock, 1961).

The pragmatist might argue that, even though a salt solution, oxygen breathing stations, or music do not improve assembly-line production, such "ergogenic" aids should be employed if the worker feels that they are beneficial. Similarly, even though the same "ergogenic" aids are not demonstrated to improve athletic performance, the pragmatist might argue that they be employed if the athlete believes that such aids improve his efficiency. Ultimately, the important question might not relate to the physiological effect of a presumed ergogenic aid, but rather to the effect that the consumer thinks such a substance or phenomenon has.

Historically, investigators have administered various substances and phenomena to Ss, informed them of the anticipated effect, and then measured their response to such treatments. This has often been done without a control group or placebo plot; it usually has involved a small number of "select" Ss; blind designs have seldom been employed (i.e., *E* has typically been cognizant of S's treatment); statistical analyses have frequently been descriptive; and these have often been followed by inferential conclusions. With the exception of research dealing with drugs, investigations dealing with ergogenic aids have often been characterized by serious design and statistical inadequacies.

The purpose of the present section is to review various methodological principles that should be employed in the evaluation of a particular ergogenic aid. In given instances, of course, only certain of these principles are applicable. It is hoped that this section will assist the reader in understanding the efficacy of ergogenic aids to be discussed in subsequent chapters. Also, since the decision to employ a presumed ergogenic aid is often based on not only its physiological efficacy, but "psychological" factors as well, it is imperative that one consider the many variables involved in such reports. The variables to be examined are capable of influencing both the decision to discontinue work, as well as the S's postwork affect.

B. Ethical and Legal Considerations

1. *Guidelines*

In order to minimize artifacts due to methodology it is frequently necessary for the investigator to deceive the S. On the other hand, deception paradigms run the risk of violating certain ethical and legal considerations. If one were interested in evaluating the effect of high oxygen concentrations on recovery from muscular exertion it might be appropriate to provide S with the oxygen mixture during one treatment and room air during another, and it would probably not be necessary to advise the S that different oxygen concentrations were being employed. If this were done in a double-blind setting most of the obvious experimental contaminants would be under control and a deception paradigm of this type would probably evoke little criticism. On the other hand, if one were interested in testing the influence of amphetamine sulfate on muscular performance it would be imperative that S understand that a drug was being employed.

Beecher (1958) has suggested that a prerequisite for experimentation on other men be the willingness on the part of the *E* to first experiment on himself. However, he emphasizes that self-experimentation might be impractical, as well as misleading. In this context, he cites the case of John Hunter, who, in 1767, inoculated himself with gonorrheal pus in order to demonstrate that the disease could be transmitted in this fashion. Unfortunately, he contracted not only gonorrhea, but syphilis as well, and this led to the erroneous conclusion ". . . that gonorrhea and syphilis were merely manifestations of the same disease!" (Beecher, 1958, p. 7). At any rate, Beecher's suggestion that the investigator demonstrate his willingness to submit to the experimental conditions is worth considering.

In addition, the judgments made by the Nuremberg Military Tribunal regarding experimentation with human Ss offer some positive guidelines. Most investigators concerned with the assessment of human performance would probably accept the 10 points outlined in the Nuremberg Code, and they might even suggest more rigorous controls. Indeed, many of these rules have had a profound influence on medical experimentation. A summary of the Nuremberg Code's ten points on human experimentation can be found in Beecher (1958).

Additional guidelines appear in the 1964 Declaration of Helsinki, which asserts the rights of human Ss who participate in experiments. Furthermore, since 1966 the U.S. Department of Health, Education, and Welfare has required "peer group" approval of human experimentation funded by the federal government. Also, ethical codes pertaining to experimentation have been developed by many professional associations. At the same time, investigations are frequently published which do not seem to meet these minimal standards. This has prompted the development of committees on human welfare and experimentation on most university campuses, and these committees are charged with the responsibility of reviewing proposed experiments involving human Ss. An excellent discussion of one university committee's experience involving human experimentation has been presented by Melmon *et al.* (1970). While this report reveals that ethical judgments of proposed experiments are difficult and far from perfect, they are possible. Although the scope of this section does not permit an extensive discussion of the matter, it is emphasized that investigators concerned with the assessment of ergogenic aids should pay careful attention to the ethical and legal dimensions of their work.

2. *Informed Consent*

The matter of informed consent appears to be rather straightforward. The S is informed of the nature and requirements of the investigation (presumably questions regarding any danger inherent in the experiment are thereby answered), and he then consents or declines to participate. The amount of information provided to the S varies widely from none at all when the experimental treatment is presumed to be innocuous, to rather thorough discussions when risk is envisioned.

Unfortunately, the complexity of modern-day medicine may simply preclude the possibility of the S understanding the full significance of the proposed treatment. Also, cultural factors can at times prohibit a meaningful informed consent policy. For example, Rimoin *et al.* (1969) reported on an investigation that dealt with the responsiveness of African pygmies to human growth hormones. In a subsequent issue of the same journal Asnes (1970), in a letter to the editor, raised several questions regarding the informed consent policies of Rimoin *et al.* (1969). In a rebuttal statement, Rimoin (1970) reported that ". . . with the use of Bantu interpreters, we obtained full consent from the pygmies after a detailed explanation of the procedures" (p. 634). On the other hand, a report titled "South Africa (I)," which was published in *Science* (News Comment section, 1970, p. 161), suggests that informed consent in such settings is simply meaningless. This article, the letter, and the rebuttal demonstrate one of several problems involved with obtaining a true informed consent under certain circumstances.

Obtaining valid "informed consent" is further complicated in situations where the after and side effects of a given substance are not known. For example, while Johnson and O'Shea (1969) apparently did not employ an informed consent policy in their experiment dealing with the effect of an anabolic steroid on muscular strength, they did report that volunteers were reluctant to take the steroid. Furthermore, they reported that many Ss were apprehensive about participating in the study ". . . because of the paucity of knowledge concerning side effects." (p. 957) These investigators attributed the apprehension of many Ss to the widespread rumor that steroid treatment reduces one's libido. At any rate, it would seem wise to employ informed consent paradigms when hormonal research is involved. Also, when widespread rumors prevail they should be discredited if, in fact, they are unfounded.

Another feature of informed consent that has not been given adequate attention relates to experimentation in children, and existing regulations are not well defined. For example, obtaining informed consent from the child's parents or guardian is possible when the research is defined as therapeutic. Minors may be employed in nontherapeutic research if they are ". . . 14 years of age or older and if intelligent and mature enough to give informed consent" (Curran and Beecher, 1969, p. 77). Investigators contemplating work with young children will find the report of Curran and Beecher (1969) to be of particular value. They have reexamined various legal and ethical principles associated with experimentation in children.

There seems to be a wide range of opinion regarding just what does qualify as being ethically sound experimentation. Dempster (1970) has suggested that one means of controlling the problem would be for editors to refuse ethically objectionable material.

3. *Compensation*

Even though an investigator may obtain valid informed consent from the S and take every conceivable precaution in safeguarding the S's welfare, it is possible that the S still might suffer harm. Such harm might be of an acute nature, with rapid and complete recovery, or it might be chronic, with little likelihood of recovery. Havighurst (1970) has proposed that ethical considerations must not stop at employment of adequate safeguards and obtaining informed consent but should also include compensatory arrangements for the injured S. A similar plea has been advanced by Beecher (1969). However, the realities of the situation clearly suggest a disproportionate treatment of the informed consent topic in our contemporary literature. Indeed, according to Havighurst (1970) only six of 386 pages of the Spring 1969 issue of *Daedalus*, which dealt with ethical aspects of experimentation, considered the matter of compensation. While this aspect of experimentation has been neglected, it is quite clear that such considerations warrant immediate attention.

The intention of the present section has been to alert the prospective investigator to certain ethical and legal considerations that should be considered in evaluating the efficacy of ergogenic aids. A good general guideline for the conduct of such research is that the investigator first demonstrate his willingness to experiment on himself and, second, employ "true" informed consent policies.

C. Volunteerism

1. *Overview*

A methodological problem closely related to the matter of informed consent can be subsumed under the rubric "volunteerism." By virtue of the fact that one employs an informed consent policy, potential Ss are free to accept (volunteer) or reject (nonvolunteer) the investigator's invitation to participate in an experiment. Also, of those Ss who accept such an invitation a certain number do not report for the experiment (pseudovolunteers). What are the characteristics of the volunteer S? Does the volunteer S differ in any respects from the nonvolunteer S? Does the pseudovolunteer differ in any way from the volunteer or nonvolunteer? While such questions have been examined within the context of volunteerism and the psychological experiment, there is almost a complete lack of such information for experiments involving muscular work.

It seems rather obvious that investigators should be concerned with the respects in which their Ss differ from the general population on the dependent or related variables. A striking illustration of this point can be found in a report by Rohles *et al.* (1967), who hypothesized that thermal stress tolerance is governed by the S's general anxiety level. To test this view they administered the Taylor Manifest Anxiety Scale to a large number of Ss. They identified 35 high-anxiety Ss and 35 low-anxiety Ss, who were then asked to volunteer for a thermal stress study. All of the low-anxiety Ss volunteered for the investigation while none of the high-anxiety Ss volunteered. Does this mean that findings from thermal stress physiology can be generalized only to that portion of the general population scoring low on trait anxiety? The significance of this point from a performance standpoint becomes more obvious in Chapter 2.

2. *External Validity*

External validity relates to the generalizability of findings. If one were interested in evaluating the efficacy of a particular ergogenic aid for high-level marathon runners, it would be imperative that the substance or phenomenon be tested on runners of such caliber, and hopefully the sample would be randomly selected.

For example, preexercise water feeding might have little or no effect on endurance treadmill runs for freshman college students, whereas the same treatment might evoke a significant increase in the performance of seasoned endurance runners. In short, the investigator's sample must be representative of the group to whom he plans to generalize the experimental observations. This principle holds true for numerous other independent variables such as age, sex, height, weight, percent body fat, I.Q., and personality type.

3. *Ecological Validity*

A given experiment may possess external validity and lack what has come to be known as "ecological validity"; that is, while the observed events might be perfectly generalizable to the targeted population, the constraints imposed by the experimental milieu may prohibit generalization to field settings. Orne (1962) defines ecological validity as ". . . appropriate generalization from the laboratory to nonexperimental situations" (p. 776). In the same context, Chapanis (1967) has stated that ". . . variables always change when they are brought into the laboratory" (p. 557). In his discussion of the relevance of laboratory studies to practical situations, Chapanis (1967) has concluded that investigators should employ extreme caution in generalizing from experimental observations in the laboratory to practical settings. This position has striking implications for the use of ergogenic aids in solving practical problems, since the majority of all such investigations have been performed in laboratory settings.

It might be argued, for example, that human-performance investigators who shave the S's chest for purposes of electrocardiogram (ECG) electrode placement, insert a rectal thermistor for monitoring core temperature, draw blood before, during, and following a treadmill run to complete exhaustion, block the flow of air through the nose and require the S to bite down on a mouthpiece in order to measure gas exchange, and require the S to report to the laboratory at 7:00 A.M. in the post-absorptive state might be dealing with Ss who differ in a number of ways from nonvolunteers as well as pseudovolunteers. Indeed, it would be rather surprising to learn that such Ss were not unique in a number of ways!

4. *Pseudovolunteerism*

Most investigators concerned with human performance have probably had Ss who volunteered to participate in experiments but did not report at the scheduled times. In the case of an experiment such as Johnson and O'Shea's (1969), which was discussed earlier, it is understandable that Ss might first volunteer and then change their minds after learning that anabolic steroids might have a harmful effect. On the other hand, it is not clear why certain Ss volunteer for experiments that are presumed to be completely harmless and then do not report for their appointment. It may be that pseudovolunteers differ from real volunteers in ways that restrict generalizability; that is, perhaps investigators should generalize their findings only to real volunteers.

Wrightsman (1966) reported that Ss who appeared and failed to appear for an experiment differed significantly ($P < 0.01$) on the Revised Social Responsibility Scale (RSRS); that is, those Ss with low RSRS scores were less likely to keep their appointment. It might be argued that social responsibility would not represent an interactive variable in the ergogenic aid experiment. On the other hand, Wrightsman has suggested that this S dimension is probably related to other important dimensions. At any rate, this raises a question regarding the matter of external validity, and it is suggested that human-performance investigators consider this matter when advancing generalizations.

An investigation by Williams *et al.* (1970) illustrates the potential problem of volunteerism when evaluating muscular performance. These investigators evaluated the personality characteristics of participants in the 1968 National Fencing Championships. Of the sixty females participating in the tournament, forty-five volunteered to complete a battery of psychological tests. Subsequently, fifteen of the Ss failed to return the tests; that is, there were thirty volunteers, fifteen pseudovolunteers, and fifteen nonvolunteers. Hence, the observed "fencer's profile" may represent a unique personality style, or it might simply reflect volunteerism.

5. *Summary*

While there is considerable evidence suggesting that volunteers for psychological experiments differ from nonvolunteers and pseudovolunteers on various personality measures, there is a lack of evidence as to the ways in which these S categories differ on muscular performance. At any rate, volunteers for behavioral research tend to be brighter and better educated, occupy higher status positions, possess higher approval need, are less authoritarian, more sociable, younger, more arousal-seeking, more unconventional, and more frequently firstborn than nonvolunteers.

The extent to which differences between volunteers and nonvolunteers in the behavioral research setting may be generalized to the muscular performance domain remains to be demonstrated. On the other hand, it seems reasonable to assume that muscular performance of volunteers and nonvolunteers would differ if such groups differed on certain psychological variables. For example, it appears that muscular performance is related to extroversion as measured by the Eysenck Personality Inventory (Morgan, 1972). Also, since many muscular performance studies involve stress tolerance, the report of Rohles *et al.* (1967) suggests that volunteerism is a potential contaminant in stress paradigms.

Rosnow *et al.* (1969) have concluded that ". . . volunteers may be more sensitive and accommodating than nonvolunteers to demand characteristics" (p. 843). This, of course, would increase the likelihood of committing Type I errors. Research is urgently needed on the psychological characteristics of volunteers for muscular performance studies. In the meantime it is recommended that psychometric assessment be incorporated into research designs directed toward understanding various ergogenic aids.

D. Controls

Rigorous methodological controls must be employed in the experimental evaluation of an ergogenic aid's potential to facilitate muscular performance. However, with the possible exception of drug-related investigations, rigorous controls have seldom been employed in this area of inquiry. For this reason, much of the research pertaining to the efficacy of particular ergogenic aids has been contradictory. The purpose of this section is to suggest several fundamental principles to consider in designing investigations concerning the value of various ergogenic aids.

1. *Sampling*

An investigator must first designate the population to whom he hopes to generalize his findings. Next, an appropriate sampling technique (Cochran, 1963) involving the random selection of Ss from the target population should be employed. For example, it would be incorrect to evaluate the influence of wheat germ oil on recovery curves for Olympic swimmers and then generalize the findings to middle-aged adults.

2. *Minimum Sample Size*

Another feature of sampling that deserves serious attention is minimum sample size. The actual number of Ss employed in an investigation should be governed by the degree of precision required. For most muscular performance variables there are published estimates of the population variance. With the estimate of population variance available the investigator can quickly compute the minimum sample size required to demonstrate "significance" for a given α level and power ($1-\beta$).

Assume that an investigator is interested in evaluating the influence of a particular substance or phenomenon on strength of grip. Further, assume that existing data reveal the mean for this parameter to be 48.35 kg and the standard deviation 12.68. Also, assume that the investigator elects to employ an α level of 0.05 and a power of 0.90. The investigator must ask himself what he would regard to be an increase of practical importance. Assume that he decides that an increase in strength of 10 kg will be regarded as significant. In such an experiment it would be appropriate to employ experimental, placebo, and control groups (i.e., $k = 3$). The minimum sample size required for such an experiment is computed to be 10 per group by the technique of Winer (1962).* In other words, for a given variance, α level, and power the minimum sample size required to demonstrate a significant difference between treatments if, in fact, such a difference actually exists is calculated to be 30. However, if the computed ϕ statistic of 0.78 were decreased to 0.60, 0.50, or 0.40, the minimum sample size would increase to about 42, 54, and 72, respectively.

The statistical power ($1-\beta$) would be less with fewer Ss and, hence, the likelihood of committing a Type I error would be greater. Actually, the investigator's decision regarding α and β levels should be determined in large part by the "payoff" function. Also, the feasibility of a given investigation might well be governed by the number of Ss required to demonstrate a significant treatment effect. It should be noted that the greater the variance for a given parameter, the higher the minimum sample size. Of course, if computed minimum sample size is regarded as prohibitive from a cost standpoint, one has the option of (a) not conducting the study or (b) employing a descriptive rather

* Another concern is that the number of Ss not be too large. In this case, attention should be paid to optimal sample size (Cohen, 1969).

than a statistical model. At any rate, computation of minimum sample size represents the logical first step in experimentation with ergogenic aids.

3. *Control Subjects*

It is imperative that control groups be employed when assessing the efficacy of an ergogenic aid. The sole exception is the situation in which Ss can legitimately serve as their own controls in a repeated measures schedule.

For example, an investigator might be concerned with the influence of water on man's ability to work in hot (110°F), humid (80%) environments. Experimental Ss might be required to consume a liter of water in 5 minutes and then cycle a bicycle ergometer at 600 kpm and 50 rpm for 60 minutes. Various physiological measurements such as heart rate, blood pressure, rectal temperature, oxygen uptake, carbon dioxide production, ventilation, and respiratory exchange ratio could be performed throughout this period for comparative as well as safety purposes. Control Ss could then be required to perform the same task without first receiving water. Differences between the two groups could then be compared.

The preferred approach to such a problem involves the posttest-only control group design outlined by Campbell and Stanley (1963). In this design Ss are randomly assigned to the two treatments, and observations are performed following the stress stimulus. Randomization of experimental units (Ss) generates groups that are thought to be initially comparable on the dependent variable(s). Hence, any observed differences are attributed to the respective treatments. This design is illustrated below.*

AFTER-ONLY DESIGN

$$R \cdots X \cdots O_1$$
$$R \cdots C \cdots O_1$$

An alternative approach, and one that has been widely employed in applied physiology, consists of pretesting Ss, randomly assigning them to treatments, and then posttesting for treatment effects. Investigators who prefer this design over the former usually argue that it insures initial equality of groups. However, this should not be a matter of concern if adequate sample size is employed. A thorough discussion of the "before–after" and "after-only" designs can be found in an article by Namboodiri (1970). The "before–after" design is illustrated below.

* In such schematics R stands for randomization, X for experimental treatment, C for control condition, and O for observation.

BEFORE–AFTER DESIGN

$R \cdots O_1 \cdots X \cdots O_2$
$R \cdots O_1 \cdots C \cdots O_2$

The disadvantage of employing pre- and posttests relates to the problem of pretest sensitization in which Ss at times regulate their pretest performances. For example, Shor (1964) has reported that prior to the induction of hypnosis, Ss who were later to be hypnotized selected lower criterion electric shock levels than Ss who later simulated hypnosis. Hence, such research is dependent on pretest sensitization effects as well as actual treatment effects. Other related examples of this methodological contaminant can be found in Rosenthal and Rosnow (1969).

Another approach, and one that is actually optimal, incorporates both of the preceding designs. Such a design is the Solomon four-group design illustrated below.

SOLOMON DESIGN

$R \cdots O_1 \cdots X \cdots O_2$
$R \cdots O_1 \cdots C \cdots O_2$
$R \cdots\cdots\cdots X \cdots O_1$
$R \cdots\cdots\cdots C \cdots O_1$

The Solomon design enables the investigator to assess the interactive effects of the pretest. Unfortunately, such an approach requires a large increase in total sample size and, therefore, it has not been popular in the experimental literature.

4. *Counterbalanced Designs*

As mentioned previously, it is sometimes appropriate to employ repeated measures designs in which the S serves as his own control. Indeed, in certain situations such a design is preferred. The inherent danger in such a design relates to the S becoming cognizant of the hypothesis being tested and attempting to respond in the manner he perceives as correct. This contaminant will be discussed in more detail in the later section dealing with demand characteristics.

One method of controlling for pretest sensitization, learning, and order effects is to counterbalance treatments. For example, if S is to serve as his own control as outlined in the previous section, the treatments should be rotated; that is, for each S receiving a water–control order another S should receive a control–water order. Also, it is understood that such rotation schedules are always randomly assigned to S. Similarly, if two experimental treatments and a control treatment are employed, one might wish to counterbalance treatments A, B, and C. Again, however, S should be randomly assigned to orders ABC, BCA, and CAB. Other designs such as Latin squares are discussed in Edwards (1960).

One must never assume that counterbalancing eliminates all possible contaminants. It is recommended that experimental data be examined for order effects even when counterbalanced designs are employed. For example, Evans (1968) has reported that hypnotic investigations in which *Ss* are tested in the order of waking followed by hypnosis seldom reveal differences between the two conditions, whereas hypnotic performance is superior to waking performance when the reverse order is employed.

5. *The Halo Effect*

The halo effect refers to the tendency of an investigator to ascribe certain tendencies to the *S* based on his knowledge of the *S*'s role in the experiment. The implication is that the *E* should not be aware of the treatment the *S* has received. This can be achieved in a number of ways, and the simplest procedure is to have one member of the research team administer the treatment and another collect the data in a "blind" setting. It is generally unacceptable for an experimenter to administer a treatment and then measure the *S*'s response. Not only is he capable of committing "unintentional" errors in the hypothesized direction, but he is also likely to communicate such expectations to the *S*. Therefore, assessment of ergogenic aids should be conducted in at least a single-blind setting. The necessity of more rigorous blinds will be discussed later.

6. *Experimenter Expectations*

A great deal of research has been conducted in recent years which indicates that experimenter expectancy effects can influence the outcome of various types of behavioral investigations. This effect has come to be known as the Rosenthal effect. The typical experimental paradigm is something like the following. The senior investigator assigns "naïve" experimenters to various groups of *Ss* for the purpose of evaluating certain responses. The senior investigator presents the various experimenters with different working hypotheses, and the result is that different experimental results (i.e., expectancies) are anticipated by the experimenters.

This approach has been employed in a wide variety of psychological experiments (Rosenthal and Rosnow, 1969), and the findings have frequently supported the expectancy hypothesis. However, Barber and Silver (1968) have suggested that the influences may not be as significant as proposed here. Also, Wessler (1968) reported that psychomotor performance is not influenced by experimenter expectancy effects. Furthermore, Martens (1970) has suggested that psychomotor performance would probably be less susceptible to this effect than cognitive and affective factors. On the other hand, Hicks (1970) has recently demonstrated that the S's physiological responsivity is influenced by the experimenter's expectation.

While the actual influence of experimenter expectancy effects (Rosenthal effect) on muscular performance has not been demonstrated, implications derived from numerous psychological investigations suggest that data collection should be performed in a double-blind setting in order to minimize the influence of experimenter expectancy effects and demand characteristics.

7. *Demand Characteristics*

Not only do investigations dealing with experimenter effects demonstrate the possibility that experimenters communicate (intentionally or unintentionally) expectancies to the S, but such studies also reveal that the S is not a passive receiver of stimuli. Orne (1962) has likened the S's performance in an experiment to problem-solving behavior, in which the S views his task as being one of determining the experiment's true purpose and then responding in accordance with the perceived hypothesis. Orne (1962) has proposed that the totality of cues responsible for communicating the experimental hypothesis to the S be referred to as "demand characteristics."

Intiuitively, one would think that a postexperimental interview with the S would clarify the extent to which demand characteristics were operating. Unfortunately, the problem seems to be far more complex. For example, in a study by Levy (1967) in which Ss were actually given the experimental hypothesis, 75% would not admit to prior knowledge during the debriefing. Furthermore, Evans (1968) has argued that postexperimental interviews suffer from the "pact of ignorance" situation which ". . . implicitly exists between *S* and *E*, particularly when deception is an integral part of the procedure" (p. 478). Evans (1968) suggests that *S* often deduces more information about the actual hypothesis than he should, and the experimenter just as often prefers not to realize this.

Unfortunately, it seems as though the problem has gone far beyond the matter of subtle cues in experimentation dealing with ergogenic aids. Investigators in this area have typically employed before–after designs in which the working hypothesis has been openly conveyed. For example, the usual procedure for investigating the efficacy of oxygen breathing in facilitating treadmill performance has consisted of testing Ss while they breathe room air and then retesting them while they breathe high concentrations of oxygen. Enhanced performance under such circumstances might result from the oxygen mixture, but equally tenable would be the possibilities that (a) the S suppressed his base-line performance (pretest) in order to permit an increase on the posttest; (b) the S endured the pain necessary for maximal performance; (c) a learning effect occurred; (d) *E* intentionally or unintentionally urged the S to perform better under the oxygen condition; or (e) *E* intentionally or unintentionally recorded the data to favor the oxygen conditions. In order to minimize such methodological problems neither S nor *E* should be aware of the contents of the gas mixture (double-blind). Also, the administration of the gases should be counterbalanced (AB, BA) and the order randomly assigned to the S.

8. *The Hawthorne Effect*

The halo effect relates to the tendency of raters to ascribe certain traits to given ratees on the basis of other qualities possessed by the same individual (Thorndike, 1920). This effect is experimenter oriented, whereas phenomena such as the Rosenthal effect and demand characteristics represent reciprocal situations; that is, the S becomes an active receiver of stimuli (intended or unintended and subtle or overt) from the experimenter. In contrast to these response mechanisms is the Hawthorne effect, which tends to be more S oriented. The Hawthorne effect suggests that the S's performance may increase during an experiment, not because of manipulation of the independent variable, but simply because the S received a treatment. Any treatment versus no treatment might be another way of stating the matter.

Most experimental designs intended for use with human Ss do not control for influences from the Hawthorne effect. For example, the manipulation of the independent variable is typically regarded as effective when the experimental group or treatment surpasses the control group or treatment on the dependent variable. The tacit assumption under such conditions is that the experimental variable evokes the increment. Unfortunately, one can never be confident under such circumstances that the observed increment simply was not a result of any treatment versus no treatment.

The experimental contaminant known as the Hawthorne effect derives its name from the famous experiment conducted at the Hawthorne Plant of the Western Electric Company in Chicago. This investigation is perhaps the best-known example of the inherent dangers associated with a single-group before–after experiment. Not only did this investigation demonstrate the necessity of control groups in human experimentation, but the primary implication was that a third group should receive a sham or placebo treatment in order to control for the problem of effects due to any treatment versus no treatment.

The Hawthorne study was conducted by the Western Electric Company in connection with the National Research Council, and the initial concern related to studying the influence of the quality and quantity of illumination on work efficiency in industrial settings (Roethlisberger and Dickson, 1939). These experiments lasted for a period of 2½ years, and the results prompted further experimentation dealing with rest pauses, shorter working days and weeks, fatigue and monotony, interpersonal relations, and supervision.

The initial experiment consisted of four illumination studies. In the first study, variations of 3, 6, 14, and 23 fc were evaluated, and in this particular shop the output was up and down. Also, variations of 5, 12, 25, and 44 fc in another shop were characterized by a continuous increase in output. While variations of 10, 16, 27, and 46 fc increased output in a stepwise fashion, production did not decrease when the illumination was decreased. In other words, it seems that production increased because the workers were in an experiment and not because of enhanced illumination.

The above before–after design did not include a control group and, therefore, it would be difficult to ascribe the increases to illumination. However, a second study was conducted in which an experimental group worked under intensities of 24, 46, and 70 fc, while a control group worked under a fairly constant* intensity. Both groups improved appreciably, but there was no significant difference between the two groups. Therefore, it appears that simply involving Ss in an experiment enhances performance.

In the third study, involving artificial light alone, a control group worked at 10 fc illumination and an experimental group worked at intensities varying from 10 to 3 fc. In the latter case the intensity was decreased 1 fc at a time. The production rate of the experimental group did not begin to decrease until the illumination reached 3 fc, at which time the workers protested that they could hardly see what they were doing. It should be emphasized, however, that the workers maintained

* The intensities for the controls varied from 16 to 28 fc because of the increased daylight that accompanied the advancing season.

their efficiency up to this point in spite of the visual handicap. It seems reasonable to assume that they were able to function efficiently at these low levels of illumination simply because they were part of an experiment.

In the fourth investigation two female Ss worked in a room in which the illumination was eventually reduced to 0.06 fc. This intensity represents the amount of light approximately equal to that of a moonlit night. Not only did the Ss maintain their efficiency at this intensity, but they also reported that they became less tired under these conditions as compared with working under "bright lights." Furthermore, they did not experience eye strain. These self-reports, as well as the efficiency of work, probably reflect demand characteristics. At any rate, Roethlisberger and Dickson (1939) interpreted this performance as reflecting "psychological factors." Further tests were conducted in another shop where light was increased daily. The workers reported that they liked the brighter lights and, again, it seems reasonable to interpret such responses as reflecting demand characteristics. Furthermore, while the electrician actually increased the light daily at the outset, he then began to replace the lights with the same size bulbs. The Ss presumably thought the lights had been "stepped up," and they commented favorably. This, too, seems to reflect demand characteristics. In the same experiment the workers were informed that the lighting would be decreased, and initially it was, but the electrician then began replacing the bulbs with those of the same size. While the workers continued to remark that the weaker light was not as pleasant, their production did not change appreciably at any point.

The most interesting finding from the Western Electric study is what has come to be known in the behavioral sciences as the Hawthorne effect. The implication is that placing an experimental group, and perhaps even a control group, in a special position alerts Ss to the fact that they are involved in a scientific investigation. Furthermore, it is conceivable that Ss in such situations frequently respond in a manner consonant with the experimenter's overt or covert expectations.

Such an experimental contaminant could easily operate in most experimental paradigms involving the assessment of ergogenic aids. For example, to administer a substance such as amphetamine sulfate to Ss and then test the influence of the drug on strength of grip may evoke changes due to the Hawthorne effect rather than the substance under investigation. Also, the employment of a control group does not provide adequate insurance since the superiority of the experimental treatment may simply reflect a comparison of any treatment with no treatment. In order to adequately test for the Hawthorne effect, a third group or treatment is desired. This third group or treatment should consist of a sham; that is, an innocuous treatment should be employed in addition to the experimental and control treatments. Innocuous treatments of the type proposed are commonly referred to as sham or placebo treatments, and this design is illustrated below.

PLACEBO PARADIGM

$O_1 \cdots X \cdots O_2$
$O_1 \cdots C \cdots O_2$
$O_1 \cdots P \cdots O_2$

In the above example Ss in the experimental group (X) could be tested on strength of grip, administered amphetamine sulfate, and retested; Ss in the control (C) could be tested and then retested following a comparable time period in which no treatment was involved; and the placebo group (P) could receive an inert substance such as sodium bicarbonate prior to being retested. The efficacy of amphetamine sulfate would be acknowledged only if Group X exceeded Groups C and P on the task. In other words, if Group X surpassed Group C but not Group P, it would be concluded that any substance was superior to no treatment. Of course, if a traditional before–after paradigm employing an experimental and a control group were used, such a conclusion would never be arrived at. It should also be emphasized that the administration of presumably potent substances and inert placebos should always be conducted under double-blind conditions. This point will be pursued further in the next section.

In the example just cited Ss could have been randomly assigned to experimental, control, and placebo groups and then tested on strength of grip following the respective treatments. Of course, this would be appropriate only if the requirement of minimum sample size were met. Also, a repeated measures design in which the order of treatments were counterbalanced (XCP, CPX, PXC) and randomly assigned to Ss would be another possibility. The important point is not whether an after-only, before–after, or repeated measures design is used, but rather that a placebo treatment is employed in a double-blind setting.

9. *Placebo Plots*

The previous section outlines the efficacy of employing a placebo plot in research dealing with ergogenic aids. While there are situations in which placebo plots are not possible, this limitation is usually governed by the investigator's imagination. Unfortunately, placebo treatments themselves are not free of experimental problems. Indeed, such treatments occasionally introduce experimental contamination rather than eliminate it. The present section is a review of selected placebo studies and certain methodological contaminants thought to be associated with the use of placebo treatments.

The term placebo is taken from Latin and means "I will please." The term usually is reserved for describing an inert substance, but soothing or ingratiating remarks or acts are also used as placebos. An example of the first instance would be that of a physician or experimenter giving the patient or *S* an inert substance such as sodium bicarbonate but informing the recipient that the placebo is an amphetamine that reduces fatigue. A placebo treatment involving an act was illustrated in the light-bulb experiment discussed earlier. That is, the workers in the Hawthorne study were made to believe that the electrician was increasing or decreasing the lighting when, in fact, the replacement bulbs were of the same size. This "act," it will be recalled, evoked responses consonant with expectations for actual changes in illumination. In other words, a placebo can be either an inert substance or an act used in controlled experimentation to tease out the influence of the Hawthorne effect.

Drug experimentation offers a fruitful model for the investigator concerned with the efficacy of selected ergogenic aids. For example, the assessment of a new drug is usually carried out in a double-blind setting in which the experimental *S*s are administered the drug, and a second group of *S*s receives a placebo; sometimes a control group is used and it receives nothing. This is carried out in a double-blind setting in which neither *E* nor *S* realizes which substance has been used; that is, the coded treatments are not broken until the study is completed.

There are numerous reasons why a double-blind paradigm must be employed. Boshes (1960) cites the example of a patient who suffered from chronic asthma for 27 years. Finally, the patient responded to a new experimental drug, and when it was removed the asthma returned. The patient's asthma was not relieved when the psysician substituted a placebo. Also, shifts from the placebo to the agent and from the agent to the placebo were carried out several times. The results were consistent and always favored the new agent. The pharmaceutical firm was contacted for a new supply of the agent, and they replied that the physician had actually been given a placebo! In other words, the firm's placebo (presumed agent) was effective in relieving the patient's asthma, but the physician's placebo was not! The physician's placebo apparently carried with it an unintended message (Rosenthal effect) concerning its inert composition.

The necessity of double-blind paradigms has even been demonstrated for surgical procedures. For example, Cobb *et al.* (1959) evaluated the effect of ligating the internal mammary arteries on patients with angina pectoris. The investigation was performed in a double-blind setting in which the internal mammary arteries were ligated in eight patients, and nine "placebo" patients received only skin incisions. All 17 patients were then followed for 3–15 months. Over half of the patients in both groups experienced significant subjective improvement, and striking improvement of the exercise tolerance of two placebo Ss was observed. Also, one of these Ss did not demonstrate the abnormal exercise ECG which occurred preoperatively (actual sham). These investigators concluded that ". . . subjective benefit from this operation is more likely to be on a psychological basis" (Cobb *et al.*, 1959, p. 1118).

Glick and Margolis (1962) have evaluated the research designs of 34 studies involving a specific drug (chlorpromazine). The studies involving single-blind designs were associated with clinical improvement in 59.7% of the cases, whereas the double-blind studies involving placebo controls had improvement in only 37.5% of the cases. In other words, a significant ($P < 0.01$) difference in treatment effectiveness was observed which was design dependent. While these findings clearly substantiate the necessity of double-blind designs, alternative approaches have been suggested (Plutchik *et al.*, 1969).

Placebos have been demonstrated to be capable of reducing pain induced by a wide variety of sources. This has special meaning for the assessment of muscular performance since pain is frequently associated with muscular effort. Indeed, Ikai and Steinhaus (1961) have suggested that the perception of pain may be the limiting factor in the expression of muscular strength. Boshes (1960) has reported that morphine is effective in reducing intense pain in about 75% of the cases and a placebo is about 35% effective under the same circumstances. In other words, a placebo is just as effective as a powerful drug in 50% of the cases. He also reported that morphine and placebos, respectively, are about 52 and 40% effective in treating moderate pain. In addition, any drug is about 60–70% effective if the patient is anxious, and the placebo is about as effective. Pain, of course, is highly personal, subjective, and complex. A thorough discussion of pain and placebo response can be found in Sternbach (1968).

Several articles indicate that factors other than a substance's actual potency may influence a drug's effectiveness. For example, Schapira *et al.* (1970) reported that tablet color plays a role in drug response. In their investigation, patients were administered oxazepam in red, yellow, and green tablets. Color was randomly assigned in a double-blind crossover study. While not statistically significant, trends indicated that anxiety improved most when green tablets were administered and depression was most improved with yellow tablets. In addition, Hussain and Ahad (1970) have reported that the form in which a drug is administered may be the important factor. They reported that capsules were preferred over tablets by patients with anxiety states. Also, capsules were found to be taken more regularly than tablets, and psychological dependency was higher for capsules.

Unfortunately, placebo plots are not always successful because investigators fail to consider additional factors in the experimental milieu that produce interactive effects. For example, Luoto (1964) has reported that neurotic introverts are positive placebo reactors, and neurotic extroverts are negative placebo reactors. These findings have been corroborated by Morgan (1970), who reported that the muscular performance of extroverts decreased following ingestion of a placebo, whereas that of introverts increased under the same condition. In other words, placebo response seems to be related to personality type, and the implication is that psychometric data will facilitate the interpretation of results in experimentation involving muscular performance.

V. Summary

Ergogenic (work-producing) aids are substances and phenomena that enhance muscular performance above levels anticipated under normal conditions. The present volume represents a synthesis of the research that has been conducted on selected ergogenic aids. The emphasis is on substances such as drugs, oxygen, and foods, as well as phenomena such as mental practice, warm-up, hypnosis, music, social facilitation, information feedback, and anxiety states.

Various substances and phenomena purported to possess ergogenic attributes have been shown to be potent at an acute but not chronic level. Also, such aids interact with the task per se and, therefore, task specificity represents an important consideration. It has also been demonstrated that certain aids evoke paradoxical distance effects; that is, they are ergogenic up to a point, at which time further increases impair performance. Another important variable is the consumer of the substance or phenomenon in that certain "types" of individuals respond negatively and others positively to the same ergogenic aids.

The present chapter has dealt with numerous methodological factors that should be considered in the design of experiments involving ergogenic aids. Throughout the following chapters the various authors frequently comment about the methodological adequacy of certain investigations. Indeed, it seems reasonable to argue that many of the investigations dealing with ergogenic aids have been characterized by inadequate designs. The present chapter emphasizes the necessity of controlling the many artifacts associated with behavioral research. Emphasis is placed on guidelines associated with ethical and legal considerations, as well as the inherent methodological problems produced by such considerations. For example, the matter of informed consent is reviewed along with its concomitant interaction with sensitization of the Ss to hypothesized outcomes. Special reference is made to the phenomenon of volunteerism and the associated problems of external and ecological validity. A plea is made for double-blind placebo investigations and several designs are suggested in order to minimize contamination due to demand characteristics, experimenter expectancies, and the halo and Hawthorne effects. Such matters must be considered in designing experiments involving ergogenic aids, as well as interpreting the outcomes of published research in this area.

References

Asnes, D. P. (1970). *N. Engl. J. Med.* **282,** 634.

Ayres, L. P. (1911). *Amer. Phys. Educ. Rev.* **16,** 321.

Barber, T. X., and Silver, M. J. (1968). *Psychol. Bull.* **70,** 1.

Bartley, S. H. (1965). "Fatigue: Mechanism and Management." Thomas, Springfield, Illinois.

Beecher, H. K. (1958). "Experimentation in Man." Thomas, Springfield, Illinois.

Beecher, H. K. (1969). *Science* **164,** 1256.

Blix, G., Ed. (1967). "Symposium on Nutrition and Physical Activity." Almquist & Wiksell, Uppsala.

Boshes, B. (1960). *Ann. Intern. Med.* **52,** 182.

Bourne, G. H. (1968). *In* "Exercise Physiology" (H. B. Falls, ed.), pp. 155–171. Academic Press, New York.

Brown, J. S. (1961). "The Motivation of Behavior." McGraw-Hill, New York.

Campbell, D. T., and Stanley, J. C. (1963). "Experimental and Quasi-Experimental Designs for Research." Rand McNally, Chicago, Illinois.

Carron, A. V. (1968). *Res. Quart.* **39,** 463.

Chapanis, A. (1967). *Ergonomics* **10,** 557.

Cobb, L. A., Thomas, G. I., Dillard, D. H., Merendino, K. A., and Bruce, R. A. (1959). *N. Engl. J. Med.* **260,** 1115.

Cochran, W. C. (1963). "Sampling Techniques." Wiley, New York.

Cohen, J. (1969). "Statistical Power Analysis for the Behavioral Sciences." Academic Press, New York.

Corbin, C. B. (1967). *J. Gen. Psychol.* **76,** 143.

Curran, W. J., and Beecher, H. K. (1969). *J. Amer. Med. Ass.* **10,** 77.

Dempster, W. J. (1970). *Lancet* **1970,** May 16, 1050.

de Vries, H. A. (1966). "Physiology of Exercise for Physical Education and Athletics." W. C. Brown, Dubuque, Iowa.

Edwards, A. L. (1960). "Experimental Design in Psychological Research." Holt, New York.
Evans, F. J. (1968). *Behav. Sci.* **13**, 477.
Eysenck, H. J. (1958). "Sense and Nonsense in Psychology." Penguin, Baltimore, Maryland.
Falls, H. B. (1969). *Res. Quart.* **40**, 45.
Fowler, W. M., Jr. (1969). *J. Health Phys. Educ. Rec.* **40**, 37.
Ganslen, R. V. (1968). *In* "Exercise Physiology" (H. B. Falls, ed.), pp. 197–218. Academic Press, New York.
Glick, B. S., and Margolis, R. (1962). *Amer. J. Psychiat.* **118**, 1087.
Graubard, S. R., ed. (1969). *Daedalus* **98**, 219.
Havighurst, C. C. (1970). *Science* **169**, 153.
Hicks, R. G. (1970). *Psychophysiol.* **7**, 10.
Hussain, M. Z., and Ahad, A. (1970). *Brit. Med. J.* **2**, 466.
Ikai, M., and Steinhaus, A. H. (1961). *J. Appl. Physiol.* **16**, 157.
Johnson, L. C., and O'Shea, J. P. (1969). *Science* **164**, 957.
Johnson, W. R. (1961). *J. Sports Med. Phys. Fitness* **1**, 71.
Karpovich, P. V. (1965). "Physiology of Muscular Activity," 6th ed. Saunders, Philadelphia, Pennsylvania.
Konz, S., and McDougal, D. (1968). *Hum. Factors* **10**, 233.
Levy, L. H. (1967). *J. Pers. Soc. Psychol.* **6**, 365.
Londeree, B. R., Updyke, W. F., and Burt, J. J. (1969). *Res. Quart.* **40**, 725.
Luoto, K. (1964). *J. Abnorm. Soc. Psychol.* **68**, 54.
Malina, R. M. (1969). *Res. Quart.* **40**, 134.
Martens, R. (1969). *Res. Quart.* **40**, 317.
Martens, R. (1970). *J. Mot. Behav.* **2**, 52.
Massey, B. H., Johnson, W. R., and Kramer, G. F. (1961). *Res. Quart.* **32**, 63.
Mathews, D. K., Stacy, R. W., and Hoover, G. N. (1964). "Physiology of Muscular Activity." Ronald Press, New York.
Melmon, K. L., Grossman, M., and Morris, R. C., Jr. (1970). *N. Engl. J. Med.* **282**, 427.
Morgan, W. P. (1970). *In* "Psychology of Sport and Physical Activity" (M. A. Mordy and L. F. Locke, eds.), Monograph XIII, pp. 5–11. *Quest* Board, Columbus, Ohio.
Morgan, W. P. (1972). *In* "Psychomotor Domain: Movement Behaviors" (R. N. Singer, ed.). Lea & Febiger, Philadelphia, Pennsylvania.
Namboodiri, N. K. (1970). *Amer. J. Sociol.* **76**, 83.
Nelson, R. C., and Lambert, W. (1965). *Res. Quart.* **36**, 296.
News and Comment section. (1970). *Science* **169**, 161.
Orne, M. T. (1962). *Amer. Psychol.* **17**, 776.
Pierson, W. R., and Rasch, P. J. (1964). *Res. Quart.* **35**, 313.
Plutchik, R., Platman, S. R., and Fieve, R. R. (1969). *Arch. Gen. Psychiat.* **20**, 428.
Ricci, B. (1967). "Physiological Basis of Human Performance." Lea & Febiger, Philadelphia, Pennsylvania.
Richardson, A. (1967). *Res. Quart.* **38**, 263.
Rimoin, D. L. (1970). *N. Engl. J. Med.* **282**, 634.
Rimoin, D. L., Merimee, T. J., Rabinowitz, D., Cavalli-Sforza, L. L., and McKusick, V. A. (1969). *N. Engl. J. Med.* **281**, 1383.
Roethlisberger, F. J., and Dickson, W. J. (1939). "Management and the Worker." Harvard Univ. Press, Cambridge, Massachusetts.

Rohles, F. H., Nevins, R. G., and Springer, W. E. (1967). *Aerosp. Med.* **38**, 286.
Rosenthal, R. (1966). "Experimenter Effects in Behavioral Research." Appleton, New York.
Rosenthal, R., and Rosnow, R. L., eds. (1969). "Artifact in Behavioral Research." Academic Press, New York.
Rosnow, R. L., Rosenthal, R., McConochie, R. M., and Arms, R. L. (1969). *Educ. Psychol. Meas.* **29**, 825.
Schapira, K., McClelland, H. A., Griffiths, N. R., and Newell, D. J. (1970). *Brit. Med. J.* **2**, 446.
Shor, R. E. (1964). *Int. J. Clin. Exp. Hypn.* **12**, 258.
Simonson, E., ed. (1971). "Physiology of Work Capacity and Fatigue." Thomas, Springfield, Illinois.
Singer, R. N. (1965). *Res. Quart.* **36**, 473.
Steinhaus, A. H., and Wendhut, G. (1953). *J. Appl. Physiol.* **5**, 677.
Sternbach, R. A. (1968). "Pain, a Psychophysiological Analysis." Academic Press, New York.
Thorndike, E. L. (1920). *J. Appl. Psychol.* **4**, 25.
Uhrbrock, R. S. (1961). *Personnel Psychol.* **14**, 9.
Van Itallie, T. B., Sinisterra, L., and Stare, F. J. (1960). *In* "Science and Medicine of Exercise and Sports" (W. R. Johnson, ed.), pp. 285–300. Harper, New York.
Wessler, R. L. (1968). *Percept. Mot. Skills* **26**, 911.
Williams, J. M., Hoepner, B. J., Moody, D. L., and Ogilvie, B. C. (1970). *Res. Quart.* **41**, 446.
Winer, B. J. (1962). "Statistical Principles in Experimental Design." McGraw-Hill, New York.
Wrightsman, L. S. (1966). *Amer. Psychol.* **21**, 812.

Part II

PHENOMENA

Chapter 2

Trait and State Anxiety

*Rainer Martens**

I. Introduction

None of us is a stranger to anxiety. We have all had moments when we fought hard to control our anxiety. Most of us can recall those anxious moments before an important final examination, or seeing a red light blinking in the rear-view mirror, or just before an important competitive sporting event. Several behavioral manifestations may have be-

* The present chapter was written while the author was supported in part by a research grant to the Motor Performance and Play Research Laboratory via the Adler Zone Center by the Department of Mental Health of the State of Illinois and by U.S. Public Health Research Grant MH-07346 from the National Institute of Mental Health.

come obvious in those moments, e.g., increased heart rate, increased palmar perspiration, and noticeable dryness of the mouth. Strangely enough, while we suspect that anxiety has existed for some time, only recently have we begun to realize its enormous impact on human life. Anxiety has been called the official emotion of our society. It has been likened to an ever-reproducing fungus that manages to creep into every corner of human endeavor. There is no doubt that anxiety is a pervasive psychological phenomenon.

Anxiety, for most people, manifests definite negative connotations. These negative connotations are reinforced by our observations of the bizarre behavior of severely anxious people, the attribution of mental illness to the inability to cope with anxiety, and the disruption of our own behavior when confronted with stressful situations. It must then seem somewhat paradoxical to the reader that anxiety is a topic in a book on ergogenic aids and muscular performance. An ergogenic aid refers to the facilitation of human performance; i.e., it has a definite positive connotation. Although anxiety is usually regarded as negative affect, does it in fact facilitate the quality or quantity of human muscular performance? The answer to that question is the subject of this chapter. To begin it is necessary to obtain some definitional agreement in an area replete with ambiguous terms.

A. Anxiety: What Is It?

Prolific research in the area of anxiety has not resulted, as one might have hoped, in a clear understanding of this pervasive phenomenon. One of the major deterrents to more rapid progress has been the failure to clearly define anxiety and related terms as empirical and theoretical constructs. Too often different terminology is used for defining the same construct, and, then too, identical constructs are referred to by different nomenclature. The end result is considerable confusion on the part of the student.

Before the relationship between anxiety and muscular performance can be seriously considered, it is essential that answers to the following questions be obtained. What is anxiety and how is it measured? Are there different kinds of anxiety? How does anxiety differ from stress? Does stress produce anxiety? How does anxiety differ from fear? Are anxiety and arousal the same thing? While we all share general notions of what anxiety is, precision in definition is needed to make anxiety a useful experimental construct.

Early experimental work with anxiety failed to distinguish between anxiety as a transitory state that fluctuates over time (state anxiety) and as a personality trait that remains stable (trait anxiety). Spielberger (1966) believes that the conceptual status of anxiety has been muddled by a failure to distinguish between state and trait anxiety. According to Spielberger, "Anxiety states are characterized by subjective, consciously perceived feelings of apprehension and tension, accompanied by or associated with activation or arousal of the autonomic nervous system" (p. 17). Trait anxiety, on the other hand, is "a motive or acquired behavioral disposition that predisposes an individual to perceive a wide range of objectively nondangerous circumstances as threatening, and to respond to these with state anxiety reactions disproportionate in intensity to the magnitude of the objective danger" (p. 17). He notes that the relation between state and trait anxiety is analogous to the relation between kinetic and potential energy. State anxiety is like kinetic energy; i.e., it is a reaction taking place now at some level of intensity. Trait anxiety is like potential energy; i.e., it is a latent disposition for a reaction to occur if triggered by appropriate stimuli.

We may further clarify what is meant by anxiety by discovering how it differs from such concepts as arousal, stress, and fear. Anxiety as a state influences behavior along two dimensions, intensity and direction. Usually two alternatives in direction are available. The individual can avoid or approach, although he may choose to "freeze," which may be inferred as avoidance behavior. Arousal, activation, energy mobilization, and other similar terms have been used to define the intensity dimension of behavior. This intensity dimension has come to imply a condition of the organism varying on a continuum from deep sleep to intense excitement. (The term "arousal" will be used hereafter.) It should be noted that the level of arousal is not synonymous with the degree of overt muscular activity. Vigorous muscular activity requires high levels of arousal, but high arousal does not require overt muscular activity.

The distinction between arousal and anxiety then is that arousal is the intensity dimension of behavior elicited by anxiety states. Arousal also differs from anxiety in that arousal is built into the organism as the reaction to any form of intense stimulation, while anxiety is learned. This of course does not imply that arousal is not mediated by learning, for it certainly is. Anxiety also differs from arousal in that anxiety is limited to arousal produced by the perception of danger.

Many writers in the area of anxiety have felt it useful to distinguish between anxiety and fear. Epstein (1967) has elaborated on the distinction, stating that fear is a reaction to things or specific situations, whereas anxiety is a general state of apprehension or uneasiness that occurs in many different situations. Epstein defines fear as an avoidance motive.

The threat to the organism is clearly perceived and the direction for avoidance or withdrawal is known. Avoidance or withdrawal is normally attempted but not always successfully completed. Anxiety, on the other hand, is a state of arousal following perception of danger and the desire to withdraw or avoid the source of anxiety is high, but the source is unknown and the direction to withdraw is unclear. Basowitz *et al.* (1955) have made a similar distinction, observing that anxiety excludes any realistic assessment of its source, i.e., the sources are either denied or misperceived in such a way that anxiety is diffuse in its occurrence and not objective in its referents. Fear, however, is defined as specific in its occurrence and pertinent in its referents.

The usefulness of distinguishing between anxiety and fear, however, must be questioned. Situations eliciting state anxiety are often considered to be the result of specific fears which through learning have become generalized. As we shall see in discussing stress, identifying the objective source of the anxiety or threat seems to be somewhat less important than the perception of the situation. The perception of threat is the critical feature. Whether the threat is objective or subjective makes a useful semantic distinction, but not a useful empirical one. Furthermore, to the organism undergoing the state anxiety, whether the source is objective is irrelevant. He perceives it as a real threat and that is why he responds to it.

It is also necessary to distinguish anxiety from stress. The term stress is in vogue these days and what often was previously termed competition, conflict, or something else is now included under the rubric of stress research. Many workers in the area of stress research so view anxiety research, suggesting that stress is a broader concept encompassing anxiety.

The term stress should probably be acknowledged as one of the most ambiguous terms in the behavioral sciences. In different investigations, it has been defined as a stimulus variable, a response variable, and an intervening variable. Attempting to obtain some synthesis in the meaning of the term, Cofer and Appley (1964) outlined what the literature indicates the critical features of stress to be.

1. Stress is a state of the organism.
2. It involves an interaction between the individual and the environment.
3. It is more extreme than an ordinarily motivated state.
4. A perceived threat must be present.
5. The integrity of the organism is somehow involved.
6. A normal adjustive (coping) response cannot be found.

On the basis of these identifiable features of stress, Cofer and Appley define psychological stress as "the state of an organism where he perceives that his well-being (or integrity) is endangered and that he must devote all of his energies to its protection" (p. 453).

To further clarify the nomenclature used to describe the concepts employed in anxiety and particularly in stress research, a model developed by McGrath (1970) appears quite useful. According to McGrath four factors or classes of events occur in stress research. First, the individual is in some physical–social system which we may summarily call his environment. McGrath refers to this class of events as the "objective situational demand"; i.e., the environment places some demand on the organism. This has been also referred to as load, input, or stressor. Next, the subject must perceive the objective demand and make some decision about it, resulting in "subjective demand." The individual then makes a "response(s)" to the subjective demand. The response(s) can be at the physiological, psychological, or behavioral level. Finally, there are the "consequences" to the response(s).

Properties of the individual may influence this four-stage model of stress. Within our concern here, trait anxiety is an important predisposition influencing subjective demand. McGrath states that stress (or state anxiety) occurs when there is an imbalance between the demand and the response capability of the individual. For stress to occur, however, the demand is perceived in some way (subjective demand) and the response capability must be perceived as inadequate. Furthermore, the consequences must be perceived as important and there must be anticipation of adverse consequences arising from failure to meet the demands. Therefore McGrath modified his definition of stress to say "Stress has to do with a (perceived) substantial imbalance between demand and response capability, under conditions where failure to meet demand has important (perceived) consequences" (p. 20).

McGrath points out that, while we normally think of stress in terms of too great a demand, it is equally probable that too little demand places stress on the organism. A large body of experimental evidence concerned with sensory deprivation or isolation has shown that this lack of demands may also be stressful. An underload then, just as an overload, can lead to stress or heightened anxiety states.

Contrasting Cofer and Appley's as well as McGrath's conception of stress with Spielberger's definition of state anxiety, it is readily apparent that the two concepts are substantively synonymous. Both stress and state anxiety refer to a similar state of the organism resulting from the perception of threat. The conclusion that stress and state anxiety are homomorphisms was initially suggested by Aiken (1961). In the literature the term stress has been used more frequently than state anxiety to refer to this state of the organism, while the general term anxiety has been frequently used to refer only to trait anxiety. In this chapter the distinction between trait anxiety and state anxiety will be maintained. The term stress, however, will be used synonymously with state anxiety. When the term anxiety is used it will refer in a general way to both trait and state anxiety.

B. State Anxiety: Is It an Ergogenic Aid?

The answer to this question is quite clear. Anxiety states can never act as ergogenic aids. A "state" describes an existing condition, while an aid implies a change in those conditions which results in improved responses. While state anxiety cannot be considered an ergogenic aid, substances and phenomena that change anxiety states can be. In considering the influence of changing anxiety states on muscular performance, two factors must be considered: (a) the influence that changes in anxiety states have on both the direction and intensity of behavior and (b) the state of the organism at any particular moment.

State anxiety motivates behavior, as do other emotions. Motivated behavior as noted earlier has two dimensions, direction and intensity. Because the direction of behavior motivated by high anxiety levels is to avoid or withdraw, anxiety is considered negative affect and therefore may be considered negative motivation. Disregarding other factors, intense state anxiety results in the individual not performing at all. Other factors, however, cannot be disregarded and operate on the individual to remain in the situation. This may of course lead to an approach–avoidance conflict, which may lead to increased anxiety states (but that is part of the situational demand). For example, in a competitive sport situation the anxiety state or level of stress elicited by fear of failure or fear of physical harm may be accompanied by a strong desire for success, recognition, and positive reinforcement. The situational demand engenders some desire to avoid the situation, but the anticipated positive outcome motivates the individual to approach the situation. Usually only when stress becomes very intense or when the positive attributes associated with the situation are perceived as highly unattainable or undesirable, will the individual withdraw. This rarely occurs and within the experimental research has not been given serious attention. Although the desired direction for behavior resulting from high anxiety states is quite clear, actual movement in that direction seldom occurs. Therefore, in the present discussion the concern will be primarily with the intensity dimension of behavior that accompanies changes in anxiety states.

This intensity dimension of behavior, or arousal, accompanying changes in anxiety states and its relationship to the quality and quantity of muscular performance has been the focus of considerable research. The remainder of this chapter reviews the experimental evidence concerning this relationship and the question as to whether certain substances and phenomena may act as ergogenic aids to muscular performance.

II. Influence of Anxiety on Muscular Performance

This section will focus on the influence of trait and state anxiety, and the interaction between the two, on muscular performance. A review by the author (Martens, 1971) provides the framework for much of the following discussion. It is beyond the scope of this chapter to consider the influence of state and/or trait anxiety on the physical or emotional health of the individual. The interested reader will find no difficulty in locating abundant literature in this area.

The review of literature is organized around the two most popular theoretical positions in this area: the drive theory hypothesis and the inverted U hypothesis.

A. The Drive Theory Hypothesis

Almost all studies investigating the relationship between trait anxiety and motor behavior in the absence of a stressor have used the Taylor (1953) Manifest Anxiety Scale (MAS) as the measure of trait anxiety. These studies have been undertaken for one of two reasons: (a) to test hypothesized relationships predictable from drive theory and therefore to test drive theory and (b) to determine the applicability of drive theory for predicting motor behavior. The former purpose also serves the latter but not vice versa. Before reviewing the efficacy of drive theory notions for predicting the motor behavior of individuals varying in trait anxiety as measured by the MAS, it may be useful to briefly review the basic tenets of drive theory.

The essential components of drive theory for our purposes are based on the assumption that the excitatory potential (E) which determines the strength of a given response (R) is a multiplicative function of total effective drive state (D) and habit strength (H). Symbolically this is represented as $R = f(E) = f(D \times H)$. The theory also assumes that the level of D is a function of the magnitude of r_e, a persistent emotional response aroused by aversive stimuli. The MAS was devised for the purpose of selecting individuals differing in r_e or trait anxiety and hence drive level.

Spence and Spence (1966) have outlined the basic predictions of drive theory when concerned with the acquisition of complex skills. The basic premises of these theorists are that during the early stages of learning the responses are mostly wrong. For example, when acquiring a complex motor skill it is primarily the wrong responses that are dominant and strong. Therefore, these incorrect responses have the highest probability of being emitted. But as learning of the correct responses increases with practice, the habit strength of these responses would be expected to equal and then exceed that of competing responses. As a result, once the task has been learned the correct responses are more likely to be emitted. Spence and Spence then predict that the increased drive associated with high anxiety increases the likelihood of the dominant response being emitted. Thus, the following hypothesis, which is illustrated in Fig. 1, is put forth.

> While the performance of a high anxiety group would be expected to be inferior to that of a low anxiety group in the early stages of learning, it should become superior in later stages.

1. *Trait Anxiety*

This section consists of a review of the literature concerning whether individuals varying in trait anxiety as assessed by the MAS differ in

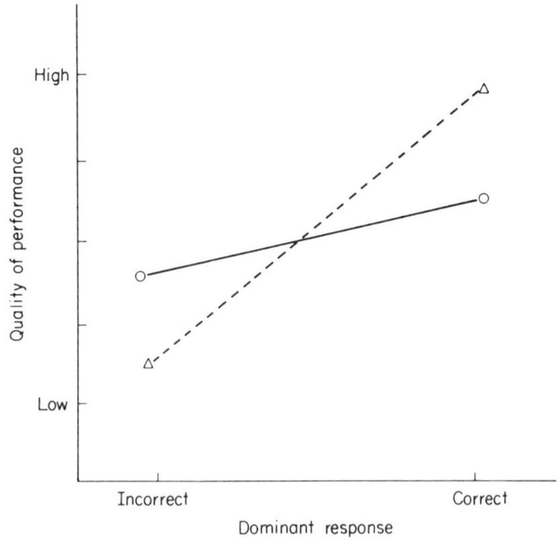

Fig. 1. The drive theory hypothesis (△, high anxiety; ○, low anxiety).

performance on motor tasks. Since 1953 at least 28 studies have used the drive theory hypothesis to examine this question. Because several studies have had more than one finding applicable to the hypothesis, a total of 35 findings are extant. The experimental procedure most frequently used to test this hypothesis has been to administer the MAS to a large number of individuals from which the individuals scoring at both extremes of the scale are selected as subjects. Both the low- and high-anxious subjects then perform a motor task under identical conditions. Some measure of the speed or accuracy of muscular performance is the dependent variable.

The 28 studies investigating the relationship between trait anxiety and motor performance in the absence of experimentally induced changes in state anxiety are summarized in Table I. Inspection of this table reveals that the predominant samples were college students. The tasks varied widely; tracking tasks and response time, however, were the most prevalent. In the result column, an equals sign represents no difference between the anxiety groups, and a "greater than" sign may be translated as "better than." An attempt was made to interpret the results of these studies as being consistent with drive theory (positive), as opposite to drive theory predictions (negative), as nonsignificant (none), or as uninterpretable. Thirteen different findings were determined to be consistent with the theory, none was in opposition to the theory, 15 found no differences, and seven were uninterpretable. In general, these findings parallel the enigmatic general anxiety literature.

Drive theory, with its many criticisms, has never been criticized for its lack of theoretical precision. Therefore, it would seem that the interpretation of experimental tests of the drive theory hypothesis should be relatively easy. Unfortunately, that is far from true when the theoretical notions are extended to complex behavior. The major difficulty in interpreting the results in Table I was determining the habit hierarchies for the motor responses on the various motor tasks. (Habit hierarchy refers to the dominancy of the correct and incorrect responses.) An individual's habit hierarchy is based on his past experience in a given task and related tasks; for each motor task then and within each group of people the hierarchy was a variable. For an interpretation to be made, it was necessary to make a subjective decision as to the habit strength of the correct and incorrect responses in determining if the study supported or refuted the theory. For those findings in which an interpretation was made, it was necessary to categorize habit hierarchies into such vague classifications as learning versus performance. The assumption was that, while the skill was being acquired and the learning curves had not reached an asymptote, the incorrect response was dominant. After the

TABLE I

Summary of Research on the MAS and Motor Behavior Relationship in the Absence of a Stressor[a]

Sample	Task	Result[b]	Interpretation	Investigator
College males and females	Stylus maze	LA = HA	None	Axelrod *et al.* (1956)
College males	Matching foot patterns while walking	HA > LA	Uninterpretable	Baker (1961)
College football players	Football ability	LA = HA	None	Carder (1965)
College males	Stabilometer	Early, LA = HA	None	Carron (1968)
		Late, LA > HA	Uninterpretable	
Fifth grade boys and girls	Perceptual–motor discrimination	Easy task HA > LA	Positive	Castaneda *et al.* (1956)
		Difficult task, LA > HA	Positive	
College males and females	Response time	LA = HA	None	Desiderato (1964)
High school girls	Agility, balance, and coordination	LA = HA	None	Diehl (1965)
College males	Time estimation	Learning phase, LA > HA	Positive	Duthie and Roberts (1968)
		Performance phase, LA = HA	None	
College males and females	Stylus maze	LA > HA	Positive	Farber and Spence (1953)
College males and females	Response time	LA = HA	None	Farber and Spence (1956)
College males	Response time	LA > HA	Uninterpretable	Grice (1955)
College males	Sport achievement	LA = HA	Uninterpretable	Hammer (1967)
High school and college males	Sport achievement	LA = HA	Uninterpretable	Hammer (1968)
College males and females	Tracking	LA > HA	Positive	Hammes and Wiggins (1962)
Military men	Response time	LA > HA	Negative	Kamin and Clark (1957)

College males	Coincident timing	Learning phase, LA = HA	None	Martens (1969)
		Performance phase, HA > LA	Positive	
College males	Coincident timing	Learning phase, LA > HA	Positive	Martens and Landers (1969)
		Performance phase, LA = HA	None	
Male VA patients	Pursuit rotor	LA = HA	None	Matarazzo and Matarazzo (1956)
College females	Stylus maze	LA = HA	None	McGuigan *et al.* (1959)
College males and females	Stylus maze	Easy		Meisels *et al.* (1967)
		Error, HA > LA	Positive	
		Time, LA > HA	Negative	
		Difficult		
		Error, LA > HA	Positive	
		Time, LA > HA	Positive	
College females	Stylus maze	LA = HA	None	Nash *et al.* (1966)
Fourth grade boys and girls	Perceptual–motor discrimination	LA > HA	Positive	Palermo *et al.* (1956)
College males	Ring peg	LA = HA	None	Ryan and Lakie (1965)
High school males	Tracking	LA = HA	None	Singh (1968)
College males	Steadiness	LA = HA	None	Vaught and Newman (1966)
College males	Response time	HA > LA	Positive	Wenar (1954)
Male VA patients and college males	Tracking	LA > HA	Positive	Wiggins *et al.* (1962)
College males	Writing letters inverted	Easy, LA > HA	Uninterpretable	Wright *et al.* (1963)
		Difficult, HA > LA	Uninterpretable	

[a] From Martens (1971). Permission to reproduce obtained from the *Journal of Motor Behavior*.
[b] LA, low anxiety; HA, high anxiety.

TABLE II

SUMMARY OF RESEARCH ON THE INTERACTION EFFECTS OF THE MAS AND STRESS[a]

Sample	Task	Stressor	Result[b]	Interpretation	Investigator
College males	Matching foot patterns while walking	Shock	LA > HA	Uninterpretable	Baker (1961)
College males	Stabilometer	Shock	Stress early, LA > HA	Positive	Carron (1968)
			Stress late, LA and HA inferior	Uninterpretable	
			Delta score, LA = HA	Uninterpretable	
College males	Stabilometer	Shock	LA = HA	Uninterpretable	Carron and Morford (1968)
High school boys and girls	Response time	Auditory stimulus	HA > LA	Positive	Castaneda (1956)
High school girls	Ability, balance, and coordination	Performance filmed for evaluation	LA = HA	None	Diehl (1965)

College males and females	Response time	Shock	LA = HA	None	Farber and Spence (1956)
College males and females	Tracking	Illumination intensity	LA = HA	None	Hammes and Wiggins (1962)
Military men	Response time	Shock	LA > HA	Negative	Kamin and Clark (1957)
College males	Coincident timing	Audience	Error, LA = HA	None	Martens (1969)
			Trials to criterion, HA > LA	Uninterpretable	
College males	Coincident timing	Competition and failure	LA = HA	None	Martens and Landers (1969)
College females	Response time	Shock	LA = HA	None	Nash *et al.* (1966)
College females	Pursuit rotor	Failure	LA = HA	None	Price (1951)
College males	Ring peg	Competition	LA > HA	Positive	Ryan and Lakie (1965)
College males	Steadiness	Competition	LA > HA	Uninterpretable	Vaught and Newman (1966)
College males	Response time	Stimulus intensity	LA = HA	None	Wenar (1954)

[a] From Martens (1971). Permission to reproduce obtained from the *Journal of Motor Behavior*.

[b] LA, low anxiety; HA, high anxiety.

learning curve had become asymptotic, and acquisition was indicated, the correct response was assumed to be dominant.

While only seven findings were labeled uninterpretable, the inability to accurately determine the habit hierarchy for motor responses renders all interpretation tenuous. Even in experiments where a skill was clearly being acquired, the prediction of habit hierarchy remained subjective, especially when repeated trials were part of the procedure.

While the results are clearly equivocal if one attempts to interpret them in terms of drive theory, perhaps some consistencies in the findings are manifested around other variables. Such variables as the acquisition phase versus the performance phase were considered, as were task difficulty and the nature of the task—particularly tasks emphasizing the speed or rate of performance versus those emphasizing the quality or accuracy of performance. Inspection of the studies in Table I, however, does not reveal any such trends.

2. *Trait–State Anxiety Interaction*

This section reviews the relationship between the MAS and motor behavior when changes in state anxiety are experimentally manipulated. The equivocal findings of the previous section do not preclude the possibility that, in situations where a stressor is deliberately introduced, differences in motor performance among groups varying in trait anxiety may support the drive theory hypothesis. In fact, Spence and Spence (1966) have suggested that it would be wise to deliberately include stressful stimulation in order to increase the probability that anxiety groups will differ. Drive theorists are unclear as to whether differences in performance should be expected in the absence of a stressor. However, they do concur that differences should be found when state anxiety is manipulated for groups characterized by low and high trait anxiety.

Summarized in Table II are the studies that have investigated the trait–state anxiety interaction. These findings are also inconsistent. When these studies were interpreted in terms of the drive theory hypothesis, within the limitations discussed previously, three findings supported the theory predictions, one was opposite of the theory, eight findings showed no differences, and six were uninterpretable. Upon further inspection of these studies, no consistencies were apparent when distinguishing between learning and performance, speed and accuracy, or task difficulty.

Many writers have conjectured that the type of stressor imposed may elicit specific kinds of responses, which may differentially affect performance. Saltz (1970), for example, cited evidence that, for studies investigating verbal behavior, the results were more interpretable when distinguishing between the forms of induced stress used in the experimental situation. He noted that high-anxious individuals showed disrupted behavior under failure-induced stress but not under pain-induced stress. Low-anxious individuals, however, were disrupted by pain-induced stress but not by failure-induced stress. No consistencies are revealed in the findings in Table II when one distinguishes between pain- and failure-induced stress for motor behavior.

The major methodological weakness of the studies investigating the trait–state anxiety interaction is that most studies have assumed the induced stressor to be effective in changing anxiety states. Much greater confidence could be placed in the findings of these studies if corroborative evidence were available indicating that the stressors actually produced changes. When negative findings are obtained and corroborative evidence as to the effectiveness of the stressor is not available, it is impossible to determine whether the interaction between trait and state anxiety had no influence on motor behavior, or whether anxiety states were not changed. Of the studies in Table II, only those by Diehl (1965) and Martens (1969) reported corroborative physiological data as to the effectiveness of the induced stressors.

3. *Conclusions*

For two reasons the continued use of drive theory to predict motor behavior does not seem warranted. First, the results using the MAS have failed to reveal any consistent findings in either the absence or presence of an external stressor, and, second, it is not possible to adequately test the theory until the habit hierarchies of responses to various motor tasks can be independently determined. At present, no method for establishing habit hierarchies for motor responses is known. It is remarkable that Taylor spelled that out quite clearly in 1956, but because the MAS and the drive theory hypothesis continue to be used, it is apparent that her advice was not understood, unheeded, or unknown.

B. The Inverted U Hypothesis

The second theoretical viewpoint to be considered has been as popular, if not more so, than the drive theory hypothesis but has received less direct experimental attention. Instead, the inverted U hypothesis has been commonly proposed as a *post hoc* explanation for results not fitting the drive theory hypothesis. While drive theory predicts a linear relationship between drive level or arousal and performance, the inverted U hypothesis proposes that the relationship between arousal and the quality of performance is curvilinear. The inverted U hypothesis is illustrated in Fig. 2, which indicates that the quality of performance increases up to a certain point, after which additional increases in arousal result in increasingly inferior performance.

Many studies have indirectly supported the inverted U hypothesis for motor behavior by comparing the performance of low- and high-anxiety groups under only two levels of stress, assuming that a continuum with at least three points legitimately could be constructed. When the low-anxiety–low-stress group and the high-anxiety–high-stress group were inferior to the other groups, the inverted U hypothesis was considered to be supported. While studies obtaining these results indirectly support the inverted U hypothesis, it is only one of several possible explanations to account for the results. A direct test of the inverted U hypothesis must have at least three widely separated points on the arousal continuum.

Wide variation in experimental manipulation of arousal, drive, or state anxiety has resulted in a diversified body of literature in this area. Arousal has been commonly manipulated by the selection of low-, moderate-, and high-drive subjects using the MAS, by squeezing a dynamometer to induce muscular tension, and by psychological stressors such as ego-involving instructions, failure, or noxious stimuli. For the more general literature on this relationship, the reader is directed to reviews by Courts (1942b), Lazarus *et al.* (1952), and Duffy (1962). Malmo (1957,

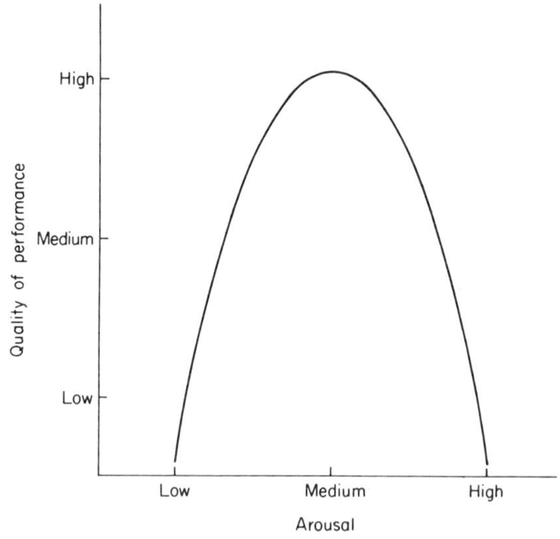

Fig. 2. The inverted U hypothesis.

1959) has discussed the inverted U hypothesis within a neuropsychological framework. Finally, this relationship has been discussed in terms of an extension of drive theory by Broen and Storms (1961), Hebb (1955), and Spence and Spence (1966). In this section the evidence that has directly tested the inverted U hypothesis and motor behavior will be reviewed.

Five studies have investigated the inverted U hypothesis by varying trait anxiety. Matarazzo *et al.* (1955) administered the MAS to a large number of male college sophomores. These students were divided into seven anxiety groups, ranging from low to high, and each performed a motor maze task. A comparison of the seven anxiety groups' performance scores supported the inverted U hypothesis. Similarly, using three anxiety groups, Singh (1968) found that the performance of the moderate-anxiety group on a mirror tracing task was superior to that of the low- and high-anxiety groups. Studies by Matarazzo and Matarazzo (1956) and Harrington (1965), however, revealed no differences in motor performance among groups with increasing trait anxiety levels. Although the evidence for the inverted U relationship is equivocal when trait anxiety is used to vary arousal, it may be that, similar to the drive theory hypothesis, the relationship is expected to hold only when individuals varying in trait anxiety are subjected to changing anxiety states.

Only one study has directly tested the inverted U hypothesis by examining the interaction between trait and changing anxiety states on motor behavior. Martens and Landers (1970) selected low-, moderate-, and high-trait-anxiety junior high school boys and subjected them to a low, moderate, or high stressor (fear of physical pain). Palmar sweat prints, heart rates, and subjective stress reports were obtained from each subject to determine the effectiveness of the experimental manipulation of state anxiety. Although the heart rate results failed to clearly show that three levels of state anxiety were effectively created, the palmar sweat prints and subjective stress reports did.

The performance results supported the inverted U hypothesis separately for trait anxiety and state anxiety. That is, the moderate-trait-anxiety group performed significantly better on a tracking task than the low- and high-trait-anxiety groups, regardless of the stress condition. Similarly, the moderate-stress group performed significantly better than the low- or high-stress groups, regardless of the trait anxiety level. The inverted U relationship for the three stress groups is understandable and is supported by the sweat print and subjective stress reports. However, the separate inverted U for the trait anxiety scores is perplexing, particularly when the physiological data did not reveal any differences among the three trait anxiety groups. It was expected that individuals with high predispositions to respond to stressful stimuli would have been more affected by the high levels of stress than individuals with low predispositions. The results, however, failed to show any interaction between trait anxiety and changing anxiety states.

While no clear support for the inverted U is found when trait anxiety is used to vary arousal level, an examination of the studies using induced muscular tension to vary arousal may be more enlightening. Freeman (1933), in one of the very early studies testing this relationship for motor responses, found some experimental support for the inverted U hypothesis. Subsequently, Courts (1942a), using six levels of increasing induced muscular tension, found a double inverted U or "M" relationship. No plausible explanations for this unusual relationship were offered by Courts and the finding has never been replicated. The only other support for the inverted U hypothesis came from Marteniuk (1968), who reported that moderate levels of induced muscular tension produced the best reaction times. In the same study, however, the relationship between movement time and increasing arousal was negative linear.

Additional nonsupport for the inverted U hypothesis came from studies by Eason and White (1960), Adams (1954), and Bell (1959). Eason and White (1960) found that performance on a rotary pursuit was negatively correlated with increased muscular tension. The studies by Adams (1954) and Bell (1959) failed to reveal any differences between motor performance and induced muscular tension. Finally, studies by Parker (1970), Warm *et al.* (1967), and Weybrew (1963) have not supported the inverted U hypothesis on time-estimation tasks. In the latter two studies, the results showed that, as muscular tension increased, the time estimated decreased.

One final study that has investigated the inverted U relationship in a field setting warrants some attention. This study was done by Lowe (1971) under the direction of J. McGrath on little league baseball players. In this intriguing field study, arousal was operationally defined by the criticalness of the game in relationship to the other games of the season and by the criticalness of the situation within any one game. For example, the criticalness of the game increased when the two teams playing one another were closer in the league standings and nearer first place and the number of games remaining was small. The later the inning, the closer the score, the more outs, the more men on base, all made the situation more critical. Physiological and observational data also were obtained to corroborate the operational definition of arousal.

Lowe's results showed that both heart rate and breathing rate increased as the criticalness of the situation increased. The initial analysis of the hitting performance of these little leaguers was found to support the inverted U notion. Lowe and McGrath, however, reckoned that the best pitchers were used in the toughest games and that the pitcher threw harder in the more critical situations, resulting in the task being more difficult under these more stressful situations. The investigators then completed a questionable statistical adjustment for this difference and found that when the task difficulty was held constant, the relationship between performance and arousal was positive linear. They concluded, on the basis of this finding, that in this situation the inverted U relation between arousal and performance is an artifact that is obtained only when task difficulty and arousal are varied simultaneously. They suggested that the true relation between arousal and performance is positive linear.

While only further study in other field settings can determine the viability of Lowe and McGrath's conclusion, their methodology for investigating the arousal–performance relationship is worth noting. Certainly the need for more field studies in which the demand situations increasing arousal are natural rather than artificial is apparent. One of the real weaknesses of the research in this area has been the relatively weak manipulation of the arousal variable.

Associated with this weak manipulation of arousal level is the critical need in each investigation to provide corroborative physiological and/or other data to verify that changes in arousal have occurred. Unfortunately, only a few recent studies have provided such evidence. As noted earlier, without corroborative data, when the inverted U hypothesis is not supported, one does not know if it is because the hypothesized relationship is untrue or if the arousal level was not manipulated. For example, in the study by Parker (1970) using the induced muscular tension paradigm, no significant changes in heart rate or skin resistance due to the induced tension were found. With this information her failure to find an inverted U relation between time estimation and increasing levels of induced tension became more understandable. One must question just how many studies that have not supported the inverted U have failed to effectively manipulate the arousal variable. Closely related to this problem is the impossibility of knowing for sure that arousal level was manipulated on both sides of the inflection point, even when significant differences between corroborative data were reported.

Are there other reasons, besides the failure to assess the effectiveness of manipulating the independent variable when testing the inverted U relation, that may account for these inconsistent findings? Some experimental work by Eason and Branks (1963) and Pinneo (1961) points to the importance of remembering that behavior varies on two continua, direction and intensity. Eason and Branks found that the relationship between performance and arousal cannot be successfully predicted by considering arousal level alone but that the direction of attention is also important. Pinneo discussed the possibility that subjects have to divide their attention between attempting to perform the experimental task and maintaining the required degree of muscular tension. The implication from these studies is that the nature of the task and the method of manipulating arousal need greater attention.

In a similar formulation, Easterbrook (1959) and Wachtel (1967) proposed that as individuals concentrate more intently on cues relevant to the task their level of arousal increases and performance improves. Additional increases in arousal, such as lifting moderate weights, without appreciably distracting the subject's attention from the relevant task cues may lead to further improvement in performance. If, however, additional increases in arousal, such as lifting heavy weights, becomes distracting or draws the subject's attention to the lifting of the weights rather than the performance of the task, his performance may deteriorate. The performance decrement associated with high levels of arousal may be due to the subject's attention to stimuli irrelevant to the task.

As this review of the inverted U hypothesis concludes, it is necessary to interject that the findings are incongruent with what most textbooks indicate. Levitt (1967) states in reference to the general literature that "one of the closest approximations to a true scientific principle is the so-called Yerkes–Dodson Law" (p. 117). Cratty (1967) and Singer (1968) both indicate that this relationship for motor behavior is unequivocal, an unrefutable law. From the present review only two things seem readily apparent. First is the lack of clear support for the inverted U hypothesis, and second is that much additional and improved research is needed. Particular emphasis needs to be given to the nature of the task and the form of arousal manipulation. Oxendine (1970), Latane and Arrowood (1963), and Schnore (1959) have indicated the potential importance of considering the type of motor activity when considering the relationship between arousal and performance. Other factors that may need to be considered are the stage of practice, the relationship of the stressor to the task, the reinforcements in the situation, and certain personality variables.

C. The IPAT Anxiety Scales

While a large number of trait and state anxiety scales have been developed, research studies investigating the relationship between anxiety and muscular performance have used only a few. Of course, the MAS has been the most frequently used trait anxiety scale, but the anxiety scales of the Institute for Personality and Ability Testing (IPAT) have also received some use. The two scales, the Anxiety Scale (Cattell, 1957) and the 8-Parallel-Form Anxiety Battery (Scheier and Cattell, 1960), have been used primarily in studies with a definite applied purpose. For example, most investigations have used the IPAT scales to determine changes in anxiety as a result of participation in some physical activity such as wrestling (Morgan, 1970a,b; Newman, 1967), swimming (Karbe, 1966; Lampman, 1967), football (Langer, 1966), and horseback riding (Hutson, 1965). The anxiety scales were given at various times before and after competition or to measure other expected changes in state anxiety associated with the physical activity.

Using the IPAT in this experimental procedure, Morgan (1970a) reported that the perceived difficulty of a college wrestling match did not influence anxiety level, but a significant decrease in anxiety level did occur from preseason level to prematch level. Among high school wrestlers, however, Newman (1967) failed to find any changes in anxiety as a function of time to competition. And in contrast to Morgan's finding, Lampman (1967) found that anxiety level increased as the time to compete neared for college swimmers, as did Langer (1966) for college football players. In another study, Morgan (1970b) reported changes in anxiety level among college wrestlers undergoing a 4% weight loss.

Because the experimental paradigms of these investigations indicate that they are concerned with assessing changing anxiety states as a function of competition or participation in physical activity, it is appropriate to question whether the IPAT scales are assessing state anxiety. According to Cattell, these scales measure "free-floating, manifest" anxiety. Exactly what is meant by "free-floating, manifest" anxiety is not clear, but examining both scales one can see that the questions are definitely structured to assess anxiety proneness or trait anxiety and not immediate anxiety states (content validity). Furthermore, Spielberger *et al.* (1970) have reported evidence that the IPAT scales have concurrent validity in assessing trait anxiety. The IPAT scales are significantly correlated with the MAS (0.85 for college females and 0.73 for college males) and with Spielberger's Trait Anxiety Scale (0.75 for college females and 0.76 for college males), both of which are well-established trait anxiety scales.

Based then on the content and concurrent validity of the IPAT scales, it appears that neither scale is an appropriate instrument for the measurement of state anxiety. If the instrument is to be used for measuring trait anxiety, the significant changes in anxiety level reported in the above studies reflects poorly on its reliability. Trait anxiety is a relatively constant condition of the individual and should not fluctuate significantly in response to particular situations.

The question can then be asked, how does one account for the frequently reported changes in state anxiety when using the IPAT scales? While the scales have some validity for measuring trait anxiety, they seem also to be responsive to changes in state anxiety. It would appear that these scales are measuring in some way both trait and state anxiety and not distinguishing between the two. Therefore, it seems reasonable to conclude that because of the ambiguity in the type of anxiety measured, and because of the importance in maintaining a distinction between trait and state anxiety, the IPAT anxiety scales are not the best instruments to use. If one wishes to assess state anxiety, he should consider scales specifically designed for that purpose, for example, Zuckerman's (1960) Affect Adjective Check List, Kern and Bialek's Subjective Stress Scale (Berkun *et al.*, 1962), and the State Anxiety Scale of Spielberger (Spielberger *et al.*, 1970). To measure general trait anxiety the scale with the most impressive credentials would seem to be Spielberger's Trait Anxiety Scale.

III. Modulation of Anxiety States

The present section deals primarily with means of reducing excessively high state and trait anxiety. Because of the pervasiveness of anxiety and the general attitude that anxiety is negative affect, experimental attention has focused not on increasing anxiety, but rather on decreasing both trait and state anxiety. Therefore, the induction of moderate or high anxiety levels from low anxiety levels will not receive attention here.

Following the dichotomization used in this text, various modulators of anxiety may be categorized into substances and phenomena. The only substances receiving substantial experimental attention are the psychotropic drugs. While many phenomena could be considered, due to space limitation only two behavior therapies and the role of physical activity in the reduction of anxiety will be discussed.

A. Psychotropic Drugs

The pharmacotherapeutic control of anxiety when extreme anxiety states are the primary symptoms has been the center of much research. For an in-depth consideration of the use of psychotropic drugs to reduce anxiety states see Wittenborn (1966). A number of psychotropic substances such as barbiturates, several phenothiazines, meprobamate, chlordiazepoxide, and particularly diazepam and oxazepam have been used successfully to reduce anxiety states. The question of drug choice seems to be based on which side effects the patient can best tolerate, since all of the drugs have some predictable side effects.

Current thinking among psychopharmacologists is that there is no such thing as "the anxiety state," but that there are many anxiety states. It is not surprising then that no one drug has been shown to be generally efficacious in the treatment of anxiety states, but instead that various drugs have been successful for different individuals. In conjunction with this, the medical profession is quick to point out that drug therapy is only a temporary solution to extreme anxiety problems. The psychotropic drugs buy time to seek out the underlying causes of anxiety.

B. Behavior Therapies

To go beyond temporary alleviation of abnormal anxiety states, several behavior therapies that attempt to break the stimulus–response chain have been used. Two therapies, implosion and systematic desensitization, have received recent acclaim. Both techniques will be discussed briefly.

1. *Implosive Therapy*

Implosive therapy is one of the newer techniques based on the principle of extinction. Extinction occurs when a conditioned stimulus is presented in the absence of the unconditioned stimulus, resulting in a diminishing conditioned response. The emphasis in implosive therapy is on the extinction of anxiety-evoking conditioned stimuli (cues) that perpetuate anxious behavior. According to Wenrich (1970) the basic principle of implosion is the following. "If a conditioned stimulus is presented without an accompanying unconditioned stimulus, an intense emotional reaction will be generated; and with repeated presentation of these anxiety-eliciting stimuli, the reaction will subside and cease altogether" (Wenrich, 1970, p. 17).

One of the primary advantages of implosive therapy is that it is not essential that the specific cues eliciting anxiety be identified, but that only a reasonable approximation is sufficient since it makes use of the principle of generalization of extinction. Implosive therapy consists of the therapist interviewing the patient in order that reasonable hypotheses of the cues eliciting anxiety can be obtained. From the interview, the therapist determines a cue hierarchy. The patient is then presented with a cue low on the hierarchy and asked to imagine and verbalize it. This is repeated until the anxious behavior elicited by this cue is extinguished. The next higher cue on the hierarchy is then presented and worked through until extinction has occurred. This procedure is followed until all cues have been extinguished.

To determine the initial success of the therapist in selecting the appropriate cues physiological and behavioral observations are made of the patient. If the cues elicit anxiety, the assumption is that the individual has been conditioned to them previously. Of course, the more accurate the hypothesized cues initially and the more realistically they are presented, the greater the extinction effect.

2. *Systematic Desensitization*

Systematic desensitization is a behavior therapy based on the principle of reciprocal inhibition, which is based on the principle of counterconditioning. Counterconditioning is a process whereby a new conditioned response, which is incompatible with the conditioned response to be eliminated, is conditioned to the conditioned stimulus. If counterconditioning has been effected, the presentation of the conditioned stimulus elicits the new conditioned response rather than the original conditioned response. According to Wolpe and Lazarus (1966) the principle of reciprocal inhibition is as follows. "If a response inhibitory of anxiety can be made to occur in the presence of anxiety-evoking stimuli, it will weaken the bond between these stimuli and the anxiety" (p. 12).

In systematic desensitization the response inhibition of anxiety is complete relaxation. The process involves three steps: (a) training in deep muscle relaxation, (b) construction of anxiety hierarchies, and (c) counterposing relaxation and anxiety-evoking stimuli from the hierarchies. The construction of anxiety hierarchies is similar to the procedures followed in implosive therapy, although greater precision is needed. The third phase of the technique involves the integration of the relaxation procedure and the anxiety-evoking stimuli from the hierarchy. With the patient relaxing, a very low anxiety-evoking cue is presented and the patient is told to visualize it. He is then told to stop visualizing it and relax. A series of increasing anxiety-evoking stimuli are presented to the patient, juxtaposed with relaxation. Eventually the previously noxious stimulus can be imagined without any anxiety whatever. This occurrence is then transferred to a real-life situation.

How viable are the behavior therapies of implosion and systematic desensitization? At present, there is not sufficient evidence available to reach any sound conclusions. Only a few studies have used implosive therapy. The evidence available is largely positive, but it consists primarily of a limited number of case studies. While more evidence has accrued supporting the use of systematic desensitization, it is of a similar form. However, considerable experimental attention is being focused on these techniques and their viability will be determined soon.

C. Physical Activity

Although this chapter's primary concern has been with the influence of state and trait anxiety on muscular performance, some consideration needs to be given to the influence of physical activity on state and trait anxiety.

In their zeal for their profession, many physical educators have written in rather grandiose terms about the numerous positive psychological attributes associated with participation in physical activity. Although these attributes may exist, many question the generality of these positive psychological outcomes attributed to physical activity. Therefore, some experimental attention has focused on this question in order to determine if positive psychological attributes do arise from participation in physical activities, and more importantly if so how the positive attributes can be maximized and the negative attributes minimized.

With respect to anxiety many early references have stated that physical exercise and increased physical fitness lower anxiety. Lacking direct experimental evidence, studies that show a relationship between lower anxiety levels and increased physical fitness or physical competence have been cited. For example, Jacobson (1936) compared the ability of athletes to relax with that of nonathletes. The results showed that the athletes could relax more quickly and completely. Of course, relaxation is certainly not synonymous with anxiety, but it is one common behavioral manifestation of low anxiety states.

Two better-controlled studies by de Vries (1966) provide evidence that neuromuscular tension is lower after exercise than after a simple relaxation period. Through electromyographic observation he found a significant decrease in neuromuscular tension in the elbow flexors after exercising by bench stepping. From the data obtained, de Vries suggested that exercise may be more effective in reducing tension among individuals who have high initial tension levels.

Although much more work needs to be done in this area, these studies suggest that physical activity reduces state anxiety by lowering tension. What about the influence of physical activity on trait anxiety? Some indirect evidence can be found in the personality literature in physical education. Several studies have shown that highly skilled performers, or athletes compared to nonathletes, are lower in trait anxiety. More thorough reviews, however, have shown that this finding is not consistent (Husman, 1968). Ryan (1968) notes that inconsistent findings should be expected when such a diversity of instruments to assess anxiety and different samples have been used.

More directly related to the question, Cattell (1960), Cureton (1960), and Tillman (1965) have reported correlational evidence that better overall fitness is related positively to lower trait anxiety scores. Jetté (1969) also reported evidence that middle-aged men who trained regularly were less anxious than those who did not. Popejoy (1967), however, investigating the effects of a 20-week training program for middle-aged women on trait anxiety, found no significant differences, although when the high-anxious subjects were looked at separately a decrease in anxiety was observed. Although these studies generally suggest that physical activity is related to decreasing levels of trait anxiety, none of them provides insight as to the etiology of trait anxiety reduction by physical activity.

A series of investigations on the relationship between physical fitness and trait anxiety have been completed in the Physical Fitness Research Laboratory, University of Illinois (Franks and Jetté, 1970). In general these studies have shown low correlations between all fitness measures and trait anxiety. However, when a mental or physical stressor was introduced before the fitness measures were obtained, higher multiple correlations were obtained. These authors suggested that this supports the relationship between low anxiety and tolerance for stress.

From their review, Franks and Jetté concluded that, for physical activity to influence trait anxiety, individuals need to have a relatively high level initially. Furthermore, their findings led to the conclusion that training must occur over a long period of time and be vigorous enough to produce fitness changes. Finally, they observed that training should not be of such severe intensity that the subjects cannot adjust to it.

Although some evidence appears to support the notion that physical activity, particularly physical exercise, can reduce high trait anxiety, considerable experimental work needs to be done to determine the specific parameters of this problem. For example, what constitutes a vigorous enough fitness program for various populations, but which is not too intense? Does participation in activities other than fitness programs, such as individual and team sports, also reduce trait anxiety? Or is it possible that this is dependent on many other factors such as winning or losing, other personality dispositions, and interpersonal relations? Too little is known about the reduction of trait or state anxiety for physical activity to be considered an effective modulator.

IV. Conclusion

This literature review may appear to have revealed little. In the sense that no clear relationships between either trait or state anxiety and muscular performance were elucidated, that conclusion is true. In the sense, however, that this diffuse literature has been reviewed in terms of the two most common theoretical positions with an indication of what really is known rather than what is conjectured, this review may be useful.

It is apparent that drive theory has not adequately predicted between inferior and superior motor performance. The construct validity of the MAS with respect to motor behavior is nil. Furthermore, drive theory was shown not to be a viable theory for predicting complex motor behavior because of the inability to *a priori* determine habit hierarchies for motor responses. It is clear that drive theory and the MAS have failed to contribute to the understanding of muscular performance.

With respect to the inverted U hypothesis, many, if not most, believe that this relationship is firmly established. The evidence reviewed for varying levels of trait anxiety, induced muscular tension, and psychological stress showed no clear support for this relationship for motor responses. Some evidence indicated that a number of other variables mediate the relationship between arousal and performance. Such factors as the nature of the task, the stressor changing anxiety states, and other personality factors must be considered.

What are the implications of the failure to find any clear and simple relations between muscular performance and arousal? What directions should future research take in this area? Has anything been gained from the accrued evidence? Let us consider the answers to these questions.

It is doubtful if any overly simple relations such as those predicted by the drive theory hypothesis or the inverted U hypothesis will ever be supported when other variables are left uncontrolled. The relationship between muscular performance and arousal changes is obviously more complex than initially thought. Therefore, the continued investigation of simple relations by the use of univariate designs in which only one or at most two independent variables are manipulated does not appear to be fruitful. Instead, the use of multivariate designs in which the interactions between several relevant independent and several dependent variables are observed appears to be the next step in experimental research in this area.

Several other points that were mentioned earlier need reiteration. For example, the work by Eason and Branks (1963) indicates that the directional aspect of behavior cannot be ignored in the investigation of the relationship between changing anxiety states and muscular performance. Also it should be apparent that each investigation testing changes in anxiety states needs to provide evidence that such changes occurred. And once again the importance of maintaining the distinction between trait and state anxiety when using anxiety inventories is underlined.

What directions should future research in this area take? Work by Sarason *et al.* (1960) indicates that a situational anxiety approach may be a more viable strategy. Sarason's situational approach is based on the observation that anxieties are manifested by a wide range of situations. What may be anxiety provoking to one person may not necessarily be anxiety provoking to another. Sarason believes that it is rather pretentious to think that at this time we can measure such a pervasive construct as general anxiety. Instead, Sarason has approached the study of anxiety by investigating the relationship between a specific trait anxiety and behavior in that specific situation. His attention has been centered on the anxieties elicited in academic testing situations. This approach has been much more successful than the general anxiety approach when studying verbal behavior.

Endler and Hunt (1966), following a somewhat similar approach, have shown that a larger proportion of behavioral variance can be explained when individual differences, the situation, and the mode of response are jointly considered. Most psychologists today recognize that to explain any behavior the individual and the situation within which the behavior occurs must not be viewed separately.

Because of the success of these investigators, the situational anxiety approach warrants consideration when investigating the relationship between anxiety and muscular performance. For example, much of our performance efforts occur in competitive situations. What is the effect of these competitive situations on individuals varying in "competitive trait anxiety"? Perhaps before discovering a general relationship between anxiety and muscular performance, we need to determine the relationship between specific anxieties and specific motor responses. By developing a competitive trait anxiety scale, by varying the competitiveness of the situation, by considering such variables as task complexity, etc., and by improving methodology, a better understanding of the relationship between competitive anxiety and muscular performance may be obtained.

Initially it was stated that anxiety as a state cannot be an ergogenic aid. Those substances, such as psychotropic drugs, and phenomena, such as behavior therapies and physical activity, which change anxiety states may act as ergogenic aids. To determine if they do, the relationship between anxiety and muscular performance must be understood. This review has clearly shown that at the present time that relationship is not known and that it is much more complex than initially thought. Current interest in the manipulation of trait and state anxiety has centered on changing abnormally high anxiety levels. The manipulation of anxiety states as an ergogenic aid probably will not be concerned with these abnormal states. Rather, ergogenic aids will be used to increase or decrease the arousal level of "normals," without pushing the subject to withdraw, to a point similar to the inflection point of the inverted U. We are a long way from knowing how to effectively use substances and phenomena for this purpose.

References

Adams, J. A. (1954). *J. Exp. Psychol.* **48,** 127–130.

Aiken, L. R. (1961). *Psychol. Rec.* **11,** 365–372.

Axelrod, H. S., Cowen, E. L., and Heilizer, F. (1956). *J. Exp. Psychol.* **51,** 131–138.

Baker, R. F. (1961). Unpublished doctoral dissertation, Univ. of California, Los Angeles.

Basowitz, H., Persky, H., Korchin, S. J., and Grinker, R. R. (1955). "Anxiety and Stress, an Interdisciplinary Study of a Life Situation." McGraw-Hill, New York.

Bell, A. H. (1959). *Percept. Mot. Skills* **9,** 111–115.

Berkun, M., Bialek, H., Kern, R., and Yagi, K. (1962). *Psych. Mon. Gen. Appl.* **76,** 1–39.

Broen, W. E., Jr., and Storms, L. H. (1961). *Psychol. Rev.* **68,** 405–415.

Carder, B. (1965). Unpublished master's thesis, Univ. of California, Santa Barbara.

Carron, A. V. (1968). *Res. Quart.* **39,** 463–469.

Carron, A. V., and Morford, W. R. (1968). *Percept. Mot. Skills* **27,** 507–511.

Castaneda, A. (1956). *J. Abnorm. Soc. Psychol.* **53,** 225–228.

Castaneda, A., Palermo, D. S., and McCandless, B. R. (1956). *Child Develop.* **27,** 327–332.

Cattell, R. B. (1957). Institute for Personality and Ability Testing. IPAT Anxiety Scale Questionnaire, Champaign, Illinois.

Cattell, R. B. (1960). *In* "Exercise and Fitness," pp. 138–151. Athletic Institute, Chicago, Illinois.

Cofer, C. N., and Appley, M. H. (1964). "Motivation, Theory and Research." Wiley, New York.

Courts, F. A. (1942a). *J. Exp. Psychol.* **40,** 504–511.

Courts, F. A. (1942b). *Psychol. Bull.* **39**, 347–367.
Cratty, B. J. (1967). "Social Dimensions of Physical Activity." Prentice-Hall, Englewood Cliffs, New Jersey.
Cureton, T. K. (1960). *In* "Exercise and Fitness," pp. 152–182. Athletic Institute, Chicago, Illinois.
Desiderato, O. (1964). *Psychol. Rep.* **14**, 51–58.
de Vries, H. A. (1966). "Physiology of Exercise for Physical Education and Athletes." W. C. Brown, Dubuque, Iowa.
Diehl, B. (1965). Unpublished master's thesis. Univ. of California, Santa Barbara.
Duffy, E. (1962). "Activation and Behavior." Wiley, New York.
Duthie, J. H., and Roberts, G. C. (1968). *In* "Contemporary Psychology of Sport" (G. Kenyon, ed.), pp. 583–589. Athletic Institute, Chicago, Illinois.
Eason, R. G., and Branks, J. (1963). *Percept. Mot. Skills* **16**, 525–543.
Eason, R. G., and White, C. T. (1960). *Percept. Mot. Skills* **10**, 199–210.
Easterbrook, J. A. (1959). *Psychol. Rev.* **66**, 183–201.
Endler, N. S., and Hunt, J. McV. (1966). *Psychol. Bull.* **65**, 336–346.
Epstein, S. (1967). *In* "Progress in Experimental Personality Research" (B. A. Maher, ed.), Vol. 4, pp. 1–89. Academic Press, New York.
Farber, I. E., and Spence, K. W. (1953). *J. Exp. Psychol.* **45**, 120–125.
Farber, I. E., and Spence, K. W. (1956). *J. Pers.* **25**, 1–18.
Franks, B. D., and Jetté, M. (1970). *Proc. Nat. Coll. Phys. Educ. Ass. Men.* 48–57.
Freeman, G. L. (1933). *Amer. J. Psychol.* **45**, 17–52.
Grice, G. R. (1955). *J. Abnorm. Soc. Psychol.* **50**, 71–74.
Hammer, W. H. (1967). *J. Sports Med. Phys. Fitness* **7**, 31–34.
Hammer, W. H. (1968). *In* "Contemporary Psychology of Sport" (G. Kenyon, ed.), pp. 61–71. Athletic Institute, Chicago, Illinois.
Hammes, J. A., and Wiggins, S. L. (1962). *Percept. Mot. Skills* **14**, 59–61.
Harrington, E. F. (1965). Unpublished master's thesis, Univ. of California, Berkeley.
Hebb, D. O. (1955). *Psychol. Rev.* **62**, 243–254.
Husman, B. F. (1968). *In* "Contemporary Psychology of Sport" (G. Kenyon, ed.), pp. 56–70. Athletic Institute, Chicago, Illinois.
Hutson, M. F. (1965). Unpublished master's thesis, Univ. of North Carolina, Greensboro.
Jacobson, E. (1936). *Amer. J. Psychol.* **48**, 98–108.
Jetté, M. (1969). Unpublished doctoral dissertation, Univ. of Illinois, Urbana.
Kamin, L. J., and Clark, K. W. (1957). *J. Abnorm. Soc. Psychol.* **54**, 262–263.
Karbe, W. W. (1966). Unpublished doctoral dissertation, New York University.
Lampman, J. J. (1967). Unpublished master's thesis, Univ. of Florida, Gainesville.
Langer, P. (1966). *Percept. Mot. Skills* **23**, 1191–1199.
Latane, B., and Arrowood, A. J. (1963). *J. Appl. Psychol.* **47**, 324–327.
Lazarus, R. S., Deese, J., and Osler, S. J. (1952). *Psychol. Bull.* **49**, 293–317.
Levitt, E. E. (1967). "The Psychology of Anxiety." Bobbs-Merrill, New York.
Lowe, R. (1971). Unpublished doctoral dissertation, Univ. of Illinois, Urbana.
McGrath, J. E., ed. (1970). *In* "Social and Psychological Factors in Stress," pp. 10–21. Holt, New York.
McGuigan, F. J., Calvin, A. D., and Richardson, E. C. (1959). *Amer. J. Psychol.* **72**, 434–438.
Malmo, R. B. (1957). *Psychol. Rev.* **64**, 276–287.
Malmo, R. B. (1959). *Psychol. Rev.* **66**, 367–386.
Marteniuk, R. G. (1968). *Res. Quart.* **39**, 1025–1031.

Martens, R. (1969). *J. Pers. Soc. Psychol.* **12**, 252–260.
Martens, R. (1971). *J. Mot. Behav.* **3**, 151–180.
Martens, R., and Landers, D. M. (1969). *J. Mot. Behav.* **1**, 1–10.
Martens, R., and Landers, D. M. (1970). *J. Pers. Soc. Psychol.* **16**, 29–37.
Matarazzo, R., and Matarazzo, J. D. (1956). *J. Consult. Psychol.* **20**, 70.
Matarazzo, J. D., Ulett, G. A., and Saslow, G. (1955). *J. Gen. Psychol.* **53**, 79–95.
Meisels, M., Youssef, Z. I., and Doran, M. J. (1967). *Psychonom. Sci.* **9**, 193–194.
Morgan, W. P. (1970a). *Int. J. Sport Psychol.* **1**, 7–13.
Morgan, W. P. (1970b). *Med. Sci. Sports* **2**, 24–27.
Nash, E. L., Phelan, J. G., Demas, G., and Bittner, A. (1966). *Percept. Mot. Skills* **22**, 483–487.
Newman, R. E. (1967). Unpublished master's thesis, South Dakota State Univ., Brookings.
Oxendine, J. B. (1970). *Quest* **13**, 23–32.
Palermo, D. S., Castaneda, A., and McCandless, B. R. (1956). *Child Develop.* **27**, 333–337.
Parker, N. K. (1970). Unpublished doctoral dissertation, Univ. of Illinois, Urbana.
Pinneo, L. R. (1961). *J. Exp. Psychol.* **62**, 523–531.
Popejoy, D. I. (1967). Unpublished doctoral dissertation, Univ. of Illinois, Urbana.
Price, H. G. (1951). Unpublished doctoral dissertation, State Univ. of Iowa, Iowa City.
Ryan, E. D. (1968). *Proc. Nat. Coll. Phys. Educ. Ass. Men*, pp. 70–75.
Ryan, E. D., and Lakie, W. L. (1965). *J. Pers. Soc. Psychol.* **1**, 342–345.
Saltz, E. (1970). *Psychol. Rev.* **77**, 568–573.
Sarason, S. B., Davidson, K. S., Lighthall, F. F., Wait, R. R., and Ruebush, B. K. (1960). "Anxiety in Elementary School Children." Wiley, New York.
Scheier, I. H., and Cattell, R. B. (1960). "Handbook and Test Kit for the IPAT 8-Parallel-Form Anxiety Battery." Institute for Personality and Ability Testing, Champaign, Illinois.
Schnore, M. M. (1959). *J. Exp. Psychol.* **58**, 117–128.
Singer, R. N. (1968). "Motor Learning and Human Performance." Macmillan, New York.
Singh, N. P. (1968). *Psychol. Stud.* **13**, 111–114.
Spence, J. T., and Spence, K. W. (1966). *In* "Anxiety and Behavior" (C. D. Spielberger, ed.), pp. 291–326. Academic Press, New York.
Spielberger, C. D., ed. (1966). *In* "Anxiety and Behavior," pp. 3–22. Academic Press, New York.
Spielberger, C. D., Gorsuch, R. L., and Lushene, R. E. (1970). "The State–Trait Anxiety Inventory." Consulting Psychologists Press, Palo Alto, California.
Taylor, J. A. (1953). *J. Abnorm. Soc. Psychol.* **48**, 285–290.
Taylor, J. A. (1956). *Psychol. Bull.* **53**, 303–320.
Tillman, K. (1965). *Res. Quart.* **36**, 483–489.
Vaught, G. M., and Newman, R. E. (1966). *Psychonom. Sci.* **6**, 519–520.
Wachtel, P. L. (1967). *Psych. Bull.* **68**, 412–429.
Warm, J. S., Smith, R. P., and Caldwell, L. S. (1967). *Percept. Mot. Skills* **25**, 153–160.
Wenar, C. (1954). *J. Abnorm. Soc. Psychol.* **49**, 335–340.
Wenrich, W. W. (1970). "A Primer of Behavior Modification." Brooks-Cole, Belmont, California.
Weybrew, B. B. (1963). *Percept. Mot. Skills* **17**, 118.

Wiggins, S. L., Brokaw, J. R., Heckel, R. V., and Salzberg, H. C. (1962). *Percept. Mot. Skills* **15**, 759–762.
Wittenborn, J. R. (1966). "The Clinical Psychopharmacology of Anxiety." Thomas, Springfield, Illinois.
Wolpe, J., and Lazarus, A. A. (1966). "Behavior Therapy Techniques." Pergamon, Oxford.
Wright, J. H., Gescheider, G. A., and Battig, W. F. (1963). *Percept. Mot. Skills* **16**, 368.
Zuckerman, M. (1960). *J. Consult. Psychol.* **24**, 457–462.

Chapter 3

Information Feedback

Robert M. Malina

I. Introduction

A. Overview

Man's inherent capacity to learn is perhaps his most significant native endowment and is a prime determinant of his ability to cope successfully with his environments—natural, man-made, and human. Although learning is manifested in a variety of forms, the learning of motor skills is of major concern in any attempt at understanding the adaptive process in man. The product of properly oriented motor learning is skill. Physical skill represents an adaptation in movement responses resulting in an approach to perfection of performance. Such motor learning is seen in a variety of activities ranging from simple muscular responses to complex movement sequences. Nevertheless, desirable motor learning involves the development of neuromuscular patterns of coordination and the adaptation to perceptual stimuli, resulting in precision, speed, and efficiency of performance. As such, any consideration of ergogenic aids should include an examination of the factors that might facilitate and enhance the learning of motor skills.

Studies of motor learning have unequivocally stressed the importance of providing the learner with as specific and as immediate knowledge of his performance as possible. This knowledge generally provides information on the accuracy, adequacy, or correctness of the performance. The central role of knowledge of results in studies on the acquisition of skill is clearly indicated in the following comment from Irion's (1966, p. 34) historical survey of psychomotor skills research:

> Whatever the confusions and misinterpretations may be in the data or in the theory, there can be small doubt that knowledge of results is the single most important variable governing the acquisition of skillful habits.

B. Terminology

A variety of terms has been employed in the literature concerning the choice of names and the meaning of knowledge of results in motor learning and performance. As one would expect, taxonomic difficulties have ensued and prevailed. As yet, there is not complete agreement on an appropriate term to precisely describe this rather complex concept. For example, Bilodeau and Bilodeau (1961, p. 250) write:

> . . . there is no agreement on the definition, never mind the function. Indeed, there is not even widespread agreement as to name; knowledge and feedback represent the core words, modified by other such words as results, performance, psychological, achievement, intrinsic, extrinsic, extra, supplementary, augmented, degraded, proprioceptive, incentive, social, etc. Feedback appears to be the more descriptive and harmless appellation.

In a more recent review, Bilodeau (1966) echoed much the same situation, a variety of terms used to define, describe, or otherwise identify the same experimental procedures. Bilodeau (1966) prefers the term information feedback (IF): "Perhaps IF is the least noxious of the available expressions, if only because information has a more contemporary ring than knowledge" (p. 256). In light of the semantic (as well as theoretical) difficulties, the term information feedback will be used throughout this review. It refers to the experimentally controllable information or stimuli made available to the performer either during the course of his response or after the completion of the response. This operational definition of information feedback is essentially identical with that of Bilodeau (1966, p. 256): ". . . IF refers to stimuli under the experimenter's control, and related to response (R), presented during the course or at the end of a response." This definition excludes the internal or intrinsic information associated with the performance of the response task itself.

Information feedback thus includes information concerning the technique of performing a particular task and the actual outcome of the task either during the course of its performance or at the completion of its performance. This information may be direct or indirect, and it may vary as a function of factors such as precision and completeness. Through various types of experimental designs, such information of performance has been made readily available, withheld, altered, delayed, and/or confounded. In some cases, information feedback has been augmented and supplemented by auditory or visual cues such as buzzers or lights. Thus, in view of the wide range of variability in the approaches to the role of information feedback in skill acquisition and performance, the inherent complexity of the problem is apparent. A number of reviews have appeared over the past 10–15 years relevant to the functions and properties of knowledge of results or information feedback in motor skill learning and performance (Ammons, 1956; Annett, 1961; Annett and Kay, 1957; Bilodeau and Bilodeau, 1961; Bilodeau, 1966). Information feedback is also generally considered in reviews of psychomotor skill learning (for example, see Fitts, 1964; Noble, 1968). As one would expect, the general conclusion from such reviews is that information feedback is a critical variable affecting learning and controlling performance in a wide variety of motor tasks.

C. Task Scope

Much of the research on the nature of information feedback in skill learning, however, has been limited to psychomotor tasks, relatively fine motor tasks limited in extent, for example, lever positioning, knob turning, etc. In most cases, such tasks are discrete rather than continuous. Bilodeau (1966), for example, limits her extensive review to an emphasis on information feedback and positioning responses in discrete-trial presentation, commenting that "the topic of IF, or the stimulus consequences of behavior, is so broad that it puts no limits to one's coverage" (p. 259). Gross motor skills, on the other hand, have been noticeably omitted from information feedback analyses to a large extent. Although gross skills are the result of the coordination of perceptual and motor factors, the "grossness" of such skills perhaps renders them unsuitable for analysis in terms of the rigid controls required in studies of information feedback as the critical variable. Nevertheless, as will be indicated later in the chapter, several attempts have been made at examining the role of information feedback in the learning and performance of gross motor tasks.

Since the performance requirements of skills tasks vary considerably and since the area of information feedback as the critical variable in learning tasks is so broad in scope, the present review will concern the effects of information feedback in the learning and performance of motor tasks in which speed, accuracy, or speed and accuracy are primary. Speed and accuracy are generally considered factors essential to skillful performance in a variety of psychomotor and gross motor tasks. Although contrasting approaches have been used to describe neuromuscular performance, speed and accuracy are invariably stressed as being prime requisites of highly skilled performance. Johnson (1961), for example, recognized four dimensions of skill: speed, accuracy, form, and adaptability. Klausmeier (1961) related skillful performance to speed, efficiency, accuracy, consistency, and flexibility, and McCormick (1957) has indicated that performance of any kind of motor task can be analyzed in terms of the speed, accuracy, and strength required for adequate execution of the skill. The foregoing descriptions of skillful performance are generalized statements and need to be verified by appropriate techniques of analysis and identification.

II. Speed and Accuracy as Identifiable Factors in Motor Performance

A. Factor Analyses

The factor analysis method has been used by a variety of investigators in an attempt to understand the basic causal variables underlying skilled performance in motor tasks. As a result a number of so-called primary or unitary abilities termed factors, including speed and accuracy in most analyses, have been isolated (for a general discussion of the forms and functions of factor analysis, see Liba and Safrit, 1969).

Larson and Yocom (1951), with the aid of factor analysis techniques, have included speed and accuracy as two separate components of physical fitness. Both, however, were regarded as isolated factors, with speed referring to the number of successive movements per unit time and accuracy referring to the individual's ability to direct willful movements toward an object that may be distant (as in the throw for accuracy). McCloy and Young (1954) have included accuracy of direction as a basic factor in the effective learning of motor skills: "This factor is involved in the ability of a performer to project implements rapidly . . ." (p. 9). McCraw (1949) has identified an accuracy factor in an analysis of motor learning. The factor was termed "aiming control in static body position in sport-type motor learning" (p. 333). No mention of speed, however, was evident in this analysis. In a comprehensive analysis of physical fitness performance items, Fleishman (1964) identified nine comprehensive factors with no factors for speed or accuracy as such (see below for further discussion).

Factor analyses of psychomotor skills have also produced speed and accuracy factors. In perhaps the most comprehensive study of psychomotor tasks, Fleishman and his co-workers (Fleishman, 1953, 1954, 1964; Fleishman and Ellison, 1962; Hempel and Fleishman, 1955) have isolated 11 factors important in psychomotor skill learning and performance. Two of these relate to the accuracy and speed components of skill. The first was an aiming factor described as the ability to execute a precise, quick series of accurately directed movements demanding visual adjustment and motor control (eye–hand coordination). This factor, however, has been identified by paper and pencil tests only. These tests required the subject to mark dots or lines with a pencil in a specified small area. The second factor was called manual dexterity, which involved the ability to execute controlled arm or hand movements at a rapid rate. This factor appeared to combine the eye–hand coordination aspect of the aiming factor with speed.

Bourassa and Guion (1959), in a factorial study of dexterity tests, have identified a manual dexterity factor similar to Fleishman's and a factor tentatively called visual feedback, which they defined as ". . . the ability to use fine visual cues in the manipulation and placing of small objects" (p. 202). The authors have further indicated that the visual feedback factor may be similar to Fleishman's aiming factor derived from the paper and pencil tests. The evidence, however, did not justify the designation of this factor in accord with Fleishman's.

Guilford (1958) has also presented a theoretical scheme of classifying physical fitness and psychomotor factors. Included in this system was a dynamic precision factor, which was grossly designated as dynamic balance but which was regionally characterized by arm and hand aiming. This factor, like Fleishman's aiming factor, was heavily loaded on the paper and pencil type of tests. Two pertinent regional speed factors were also included in Guilford's scheme, arm speed and finger speed.

The foregoing factor analyses would seem to suggest a lack of relationship between gross motor tasks and fine or psychomotor tasks, and perhaps independence of speed and accuracy factors involved in both categories of tasks. Hempel and Fleishman (1955), for example, reported that ". . . the abilities contributing to performance on gross physical tasks are quite independent of those contributing to fine manipulative skill" (p. 15). Fleishman (1964, p. 26) has more recently reiterated this observation: ". . . the present evidence indicates that abilities in physical proficiency are somewhat independent of the kinds of psychomotor abilities . . . and *are usually considered separately*" (italics mine). The evidence for the above conclusions was derived from factor analyses of gross physical performance and fine manipulative tasks separately. The factors identified in the gross performances were devoid of any accuracy, speed, or speed and accuracy factor. This was probably due to the omission of accuracy and speed items in the gross physical proficiency tests employed. This is a critical feature since the results of any factor analysis are limited by the test variables employed, and if a factor that may be present in the tests is absent in the test battery employed, it will fail to appear in the final list of comprehensive factors.

B. Summary

If physical proficiency and psychomotor abilities should be considered separately, one may legitimately inquire as to the applicability of principles derived from studies of psychomotor tasks to studies of gross motor tasks. Or, are such different classes of motor abilities a function of observing skilled performance at different levels of complexity? In agreement with the findings of Fleishman (1964) and Hempel and Fleishman (1955), Seashore (1942) did not observe an interrelation between fine and gross motor abilities in a factor analysis of such skills. However, one of Seashore's factors, restricted essentially to the fine motor skills analyzed, had a good loading on the baseball throw for distance, a skill requiring careful direction of the ball by the hands. This observation prompted Seashore (1942, p. 273) to conclude

> Some activities which upon superficial analysis are called large muscle activities do involve finer motor coordinations. The problem for research, then, is not one of looking for dependency of fine and gross coordinations,

but rather is one of determining the respective roles of all the ability variables which are contributory to the whole activity.

III. Role of Information Feedback in Learning and Performance

A. Introduction

As was evident in the discussion of the proper appellation of the knowledge of results or information feedback concept, there are divergent views as to the precise role of information feedback in motor learning and performance. In one of the first theoretical discussions of the properties and functions of feedback, Brown (1949) indicated three functions of feedback (which Brown termed knowledge of results) in psychomotor tasks: as a reward, as a form of information, and as motivation. It should be noted that Brown's discussion was actually a proposal for a program of research to determine how information feedback operates in the performance of psychomotor tasks. Irion's (1966) historical survey of skill acquisition research indicates that Brown's (1949) report ". . . exerted its influence principally through the researches of the Bilodeaus . . ." (p. 30). This point will become increasingly clear later in this discussion.

B. Feedback Models

Annett and Kay (1957) presented views similar to those of Brown (1949), but they differentiated between information feedback as a directional indicator and as augmented feedback. The authors, however, in taking a perceptual approach to the problem, emphasized the performer's perception of the feedback as the critical factor. Smode (1958), on the other hand, discussed achievement information feedback, which ". . . tells S how the results of his responses conform to some objective reference" (p. 297). On the basis of his review, Smode reported three generalizations attributed to achievement information feedback. First, it improves the level of performance in overlearned tasks; second, it augments the rate of improvement early in the practice of a new skill; and, third, it augments interest in and decreases fatigue during the performance of a particular task. Annett (1961) surveyed some of the literature on information feedback and performance and reported that the information value of feedback is a function of both the new information and the preexisting information. In addition, Annett (1961) noted that

". . . the information rather than motivation content of KR (knowledge of results) is important to learning whilst motivation is an important variable in performance" (p. 12).

In a comprehensive review, Bilodeau (1966) indicated three empirical and three theoretical properties of information feedback. The empirical properties of information feedback are as follows: it is response strengthening; it is performance sustaining; and it eliminates previously established responses. Information feedback's theoretical basis stems from its directive, motivating, and reinforcing properties. Not all investigators agree, however, on the theoretical properties assigned to information feedback in terms of how it specifically operates in facilitating and enhancing skills performance.

Various forms of information feedback are evident in discussions of its operation. Miller (1953), for example, distinguished between action feedback and learning feedback. The former is defined as the information available during the performance of a task which tells the subject what to do next and thus allows him to alter his present response. Learning feedback, on the other hand, is defined as the information available after the termination of the response which indicates to the performer what he should have done. Bilodeau (1966) agrees with Miller's twofold distinction but prefers to label learning feedback as terminal feedback. Annett and Kay (1957) also distinguished among different types of information feedback in terms of intrinsic and extrinsic feedback. Intrinsic feedback refers to information arising from the internal environment, that is, the subject's proprioceptive stimulation from his own neuromuscular system. Conversely, extrinsic feedback refers to the information arising from the external environment, that is, that provided by the display or by the investigator. Thus,

> . . . the receiving of signals from internal and external sources is intrinsic in most skilled performances. Knowledge of results is not then something which a scientist has ingeniously introduced into a training situation—it is something which will be inherent in that situation from the moment when the trainee is given any rudimentary idea as to what he is to try to do. (Annett and Kay, 1957, p. 72)

Bilodeau (1966), however, is of the opinion that the kinesthetic stimulation accompanying the performance of a motor act is not information feedback unless some standard of comparison is provided.

C. Summary

It is evident in the preceding discussion that there is a variety of types of feedback and that not everyone agrees as to what is or is not information feedback. Nevertheless, it is apparent that feedback can take a variety of forms in motor tasks. It is equally apparent that whenever an individual performs a motor act, there is always some information of his performance available to him, be it externally controllable in the form of information feedback, or be it internal in the form of kinesthetic stimulation.

IV. Effects of Information Feedback on Performance

A. Introduction

Although speed and accuracy were indicated as the variables of concern at the outset of this discussion, most available studies of information feedback have dealt exclusively with some form of discrete accuracy task as the critical variable. Nevertheless, such observations provide relevant background for the understanding of speed and accuracy as important variables in human performance.

The typical sequence of events in information feedback experiments is one in which a response is made (i.e., a task is performed), followed by a clear-cut break in the activity before a subsequent response is made. Information feedback is generally provided in the break between the responses (Bilodeau, 1966).

B. Selected Investigations

Many of the significant features of information feedback research are illustrated in Fig. 1 from the work of Bilodeau *et al.* (1959). Four groups of subjects were used in the study of lever-displacing accuracy. Group 0 had no information feedback, Group 2 had information feedback withdrawn after two trials with feedback, Group 6 had information feedback withdrawn after six trials with feedback, and Group 19 (controls) received information feedback throughout the study. The data illustrated in Fig. 1 clearly indicate a gradual improvement in lever-displacing accuracy when information feedback in the form of the amount and direction of error was provided (the control comparison—a decrease in the mean absolute error). No improvement without information feedback (Group 0) was likewise evident. There was also a marked reduction in lever-displacing accuracy when information feedback was removed during the course of the experiment (Groups 2 and 6). The right-hand part of Fig. 1 compares trials 20–24 for Group 0 (note that these trials represent the first trials with information feedback after 19 trials without feedback) with trials 1–5 for the control group (i.e., the first five trials with information feedback). This comparison shows no difference between the groups and thus demonstrates the absence of a latent learning effect; that is, there was no detrimental effect on the accuracy of performance and the rate of learning when information feedback was introduced immediately or late in practice.

In an investigation of the effects of achievement information feedback on learning a tracking task, Smode (1958) found that the groups receiving a high level of achievement information feedback during the performance of the task reached and maintained a superior level of tracking accuracy throughout the training period. Smode concluded, therefore, that ". . . the high-level information feedback clearly facilitated performance" (p. 303), and the observed gains were attributed to an increased motivational level. Stockbridge and Chambers (1958) assessed the role of additional or supplementary information feedback in learning an aiming task. The subjects were required to aim at moving targets. The evidence indicated that the additional information feedback significantly improved aiming accuracy. This advantage, however, was reduced to an insignificant level when the supplementary information feedback was removed.

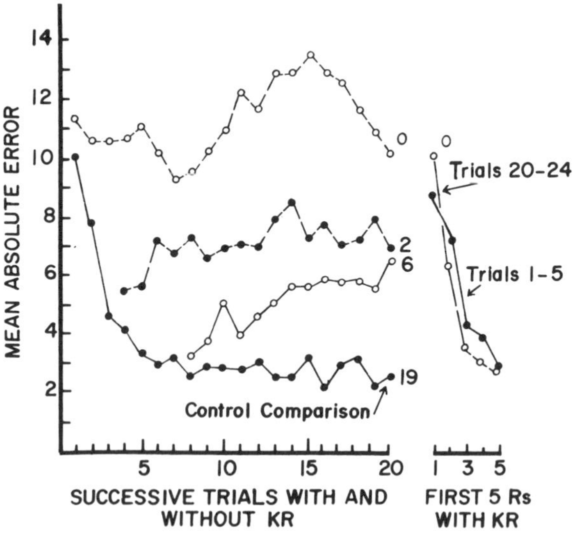

Fig. 1. Mean absolute error in positioning a manual lever to 33° on successive trials with and without KR. Number to the right of each curve represents experimental group number. (Reprinted from Bilodeau *et al.*, 1959. Copyright by the American Psychological Association, and reproduced here with permission of Professor I. McD. Bilodeau and the American Psychological Association.)

Williams and Briggs (1962) examined the effects of augmented feedback on tracking accuracy. During a training program experimental groups were given augmented feedback (in the form of auditory clicks) when tracking accuracy was within or outside fixed tolerance limits. Performance in the groups receiving augmented information feedback was superior to that of a control group which did not receive augmented feedback. Interestingly, within the experimental groups, the augmented information feedback condition which provided such feedback when the subject was outside the fixed tolerance limits (i.e., an off-target criterion as opposed to an on-target criterion) proved to be the most effective training condition.

The problem of augmented feedback is confounded by the effects of utilizing different forms of information feedback either singly or in various combinations. Battig (1954), for example, examined the effects of various information feedback cues on performance in a complex coordination task of manipulating a joy stick. Six groups were used: standard practice, no practice, verbal stimulus, verbal response, kinesthetic response, and verbal stimulus–kinesthetic response. After eight training sessions with the respective information cues, the standard practice group performed at a level superior to that of all other groups. Since the role of visual information was maximized in the standard practice setting for the positioning task under study, Battig (1954) concluded that ". . . the results point to the importance of visual cues for this particular skill" (p. 379). Karlin and Mortimer (1961) reported the results of two experiments in which verbal, visual, and auditory cues were used as augmented information feedback singly or in combination. The first experiment considered the effects of visual, verbal, and combined visual–verbal information feedback on the learning and retention of a crank-turning task that required the performer to turn the crank at a constant rate of speed. Using several measurement parameters, Karlin and Mortimer (1961) found that verbal information was inferior in learning but superior during retention tests when time within scoring tolerance and magnitude of constant error were used as performance measures. In terms of variability of performance, verbal information proved to be inferior to both the visual information and the combined visual–verbal information feedback conditions during both learning and retention. The second experiment reported by Karlin and Mortimer (1961) considered the effects of visual, verbal, and auditory augmented information feedback as well as their withdrawal on a compensatory tracking task. As expected, the augmented information feedback improved performance during the learning trials. The verbal feedback group performed significantly better than the auditory feedback and control groups, but not significantly better than the visual feedback group. However, it should be noted that all three forms of augmented information feedback were effective in learning and retention of the tracking task, with the verbal being the most effective and the auditory the least effective. Upon the withdrawal of the augmented information feedback, the four groups maintained their relative positions to each other, i.e., the verbal feedback group had the best performance followed by the visual, auditory, and control groups. It should be noted that the verbal group differed significantly only from the control group, while the visual and auditory groups did not differ significantly from the controls.

Robb (1968) assessed a variety of information feedback conditions on the learning of an arm movement pattern. The feedback conditions involved the following: concurrent* visual feedback, concurrent proprioceptive feedback and terminal knowledge of graphs, a combination of the first two feedback conditions, concurrent visual feedback interspersed with passive watching, and concurrent visual feedback at slow and standard speeds. Concurrent visual feedback proved to be the most effective variable in the learning of the arm movement pattern. Interestingly, performing the movement pattern at a slower rate than the standard proved to be a detriment to performance on the criterion test. The last-mentioned observation, as will be discussed later, might be of particular importance in assessing the role of information feedback in tasks requiring both speed and accuracy.

The foregoing discussion indicates a significant role for augmented information feedback in motor skills. It functions in general to improve motor performance. However, the effectiveness of augmented feedback is related to the type of feedback used, the kind of performance measured, and the measures of performance used.

The preceding discussion also indicates that visual information, although important, is not always the critical factor in the performance of positioning and tracking tasks. Nevertheless, the importance of visual information is generally stressed in tasks requiring a great deal of precision. Using a two-hand positioning task, Elwell and Grindley (1938) found a marked deterioration in accuracy of positioning without visual feedback. The authors concluded that visual cues were essential to the direction and regulation of skillful performance in this task. In a study of the role of incomplete visual information feedback in the performance of a coordination task requiring the subject to manipulate accurately an airplane type of control stick, Abbey and Cowan (1960) found a marked

* Concurrent feedback as defined by Robb (1968) appears to be similar in most respects to the action feedback described by Miller (1953).

superiority in the performance of a group receiving complete visual information feedback as compared to a group receiving incomplete visual feedback. Baker and Young (1960) examined the line-inscribing accuracy of blindfolded subjects with varying amounts of training with error information feedback. The results indicated a direct relationship between the amount of gain in accuracy of performance and the amount of training with feedback. They also noted a marked decline in performance when error information feedback was denied, the deterioration in performance being independent of the amount of training with feedback. Baker and Young (1960) thus concluded that ". . . when feedback is withheld the finer discriminations cannot be made and performance immediately falls to that level achieved early in training" (p. 264).

Garvey and Knowles (1954), working with a joy stick positioning task, reported generally similar observations emphasizing the role of visual information feedback in performance. The accuracy with which a joy stick could be pointed at a target without visual feedback as to the stick's position was somewhat reduced, but it was still adequate for most applied joy stick situations. The latter observation illustrates an important point in the assessment of feedback effects on motor performance. What might be adequate in one situation might not be so in another. The performance requirements of particular tasks and skills do in fact vary and need to be emphasized. Smith and Smith (1961), as a further example, investigated the accuracy of tossing balls at targets photographically portrayed at varying distances. The results showed quite clearly that visual direction alone was not an adequate basis for accurate ball-tossing behavior. Rather, the authors emphasized the importance of the performer's perceptions of his own activity and performance, for instance, the perceived location of the point of impact relative to the target, which might result in adjustments to correct for "under" or "over" errors.

The time interval between the completion of a response and the provision of information feedback has received considerable attention. Using a skill in which the subjects tossed a ball over the shoulders at a target without seeing the target, Lorge and Thorndike (1935) investigated the role of delayed information of results. Without information feedback, the subjects showed no improvement in accuracy but, with information of ball–target contact, the subjects gained in accuracy decisively. Longer delays, however, tended to decrease the increment in accuracy as compared to delays of shorter duration. In a more recent study similar in design to that of Lorge and Thorndike (1935), Lavery (1964) examined the effects of delayed information feedback on the accuracy of tossing magnetized pellets at a target. There were two groups of subjects, one receiving immediate information feedback (zero delay) and the other receiving information feedback only after the following throw had been made (one-trial delay). Both groups improved in the accuracy of tossing performance, but the group receiving information feedback with a one-trial delay attained a higher level of accuracy. Better accuracy performance was also attained when information feedback was more specific (accuracy scores plus information of the direction and distance of each toss from the target center as compared to accuracy scores only). In a similar study, Alexander (1950) assessed the role of information feedback delay in the accuracy of dart throwing. The subjects were required to toss darts over a barrier in a darkened enclosure and were informed of their accuracy at varying delay intervals. The results showed statistically insignificant differences among the various feedback intervals, but Alexander noted two somewhat significant observations. First, the groups that received shorter feedback delays were better able to guess the position of target contact; and, second, the visual observation of the flight of the dart over the barrier or the kinesthetic feeling as the darts were thrown provided immediate information to the subjects.

In a study of the effects of information feedback delay on the accuracy of lever positioning using a trial-delay technique, Bilodeau (1956) reported an improved level of accuracy for all groups, including those for which information feedback was delayed. However, the experimental groups with no delay and shorter delays of information feedback performed at higher accuracy levels. In fact, as the number of trials over which feedback was delayed was increased, the errors in lever positioning increased progressively. Comparing the various delay conditions, Bilodeau suggested that, with no delay, the information feedback served a "directive function," which indicated to the performer the degree to which his response differed from the goal and thus provided him with an indication of the changes in response necessary to improve the next response. In the trial-delay cases, however, the delayed information feedback functioned as an "incomplete error-signal," which lacked information about the changes in response made between the last response and the one to which the information feedback applied. The information feedback, therefore, did not indicate to the performer the changes necessary to improve his last response.

Archer and Namikas (1958) delayed additional information feedback in the learning of a rotary pursuit tracking skill task while permitting vision of the target. The delay of the additional information feedback was not an effective factor in the attainment of this skill. Archer and Namikas suggested that the additional information feedback exerted negligible effects, whereas the visual feedback provided an adequate basis for tracking performance. Thus, the foregoing results indicate no obvious benefit for the provision of additional information feedback. Bilodeau and Rosenquist (1964) reported observations similar to those of Archer and Namikas (1958). Using a 1-second buzzer or a continuous buzzer signal as the supplementary information feedback, these authors did not observe differential training effects in a rotary pursuit task, leading them to conclude that rotary pursuit performance is "not sensitive" to additional feedback.

The specific operation of information feedback in the acquisition and retention of motor tasks thus requires further examination. Lavery (1962) examined the effects of qualitative (direction of error) and quantitative (extent as well as direction of error) information feedback on the acquisition of three ball-manipulating tasks under a variety of conditions. Improvement in performance with the various combinations of information feedback took place from day to day. However, the training conditions involving immediate information feedback produced higher performance scores than training conditions involving information feedback only after 20 trials were completed. In the retention trials, on the other hand, those subjects receiving information feedback only after the completion of 20 trials performed better, leading Lavery (1962) to comment that, with information feedback provided immediately after the response, ". . . the subjects pay more attention to it than to any other cues which seem superfluous (inefficient) but which could be useful in retention" (p. 306). Lavery tested this suggestion in a subsequent experiment in which the subjects were instructed to concentrate on cues inherent in the performance task that would aid them when information feedback was not available. When tested for retention after acquisition under these conditions, there was no difference between subjects receiving immediate information feedback and subjects receiving information feedback after the completion of 20 trials. Hence, Lavery (1962) concluded that ". . . any training method that encourages the subject to perceive and interpret the cues inherent in the task, will favour retention" (p. 309). In a subsequent study, Lavery and Suddon (1962) noted significantly better retention on three tasks following a five-trial delay compared to a zero-trial delay training program. The authors interpreted their observations as being in accord with that presented above; that is, information feedback which enhances the cues inherent in the performance task results in better retention.

Although kinesthetic cues are usually relegated to the realm of intrinsic feedback and are not information feedback as defined at the outset, the observations of Lavery (1962) emphasize the significance of concentrating on cues inherent in the performance task, which of course include kinesthetic cues. The role of kinesthetic information in facilitating or enhancing skill acquisition and retention is not clear. Some limited evidence, however, indicates a greater or lesser role for kinesthetic awareness in motor skill acquisition at various stages of learning. Phillips and Summers (1954), using bowling as the learning skill, found kinesthetic awareness to be of greater importance in the initial rather than final stages of learning the skill. Taylor and Smith (1956), investigating the learning curves for an industrial skill, obtained opposite results. They noted that, early in learning the operation of a power sewing machine, spatial, verbal, and perceptual factors were more important than speed and kinesthetic factors, which had only a slight effect on the acquisition of the skill. Later in performance, however, the perceptual or visual factors became less important, while the role of kinesthetic factors increased and became dominant. Similarly, in an analysis of patterns of skilled and unskilled psychomotor performances, Fleishman (1957) speculated that kinesthetic abilities played a progressively more important role at higher levels of proficiency.

Relevant to the preceding discussion in general, and more specifically relevant to Lavery's (1962) suggestion of emphasis on the cues inherent in the performance task, are the observations of Bell (1968). Bell examined the effects of augmented information feedback on the badminton long serve, a skill that entails considerable accuracy in striking the shuttlecock and placing it in a specific part of the playing area. Although Bell's groups improved in performance during the training sessions, the augmented information feedback apparently had little effect on a posttest and retention test. On the basis of these observations, Bell (1968, p. 29) offered the following conclusion:

> Where sufficient knowledge of results is inherent in the task, the direction of practice through the use of additional knowledge of results does not further affect the acquisition or retention of gross motor skill at beginning levels of performance.

Thus, perhaps information feedback varies in its effectiveness depending on the subject's level of proficiency in a motor task. Undoubtedly a part of the learning process in such experimental tasks is learning the information value of the information feedback per se and then incorporating it into the performance of the subsequent response. Proficient performers probably make better use of the information available to them. Whether the relationship between proficiency of performance and the enhancing effects of information feedback is linear, however, needs further study, especially in the domain of gross motor tasks.

Much of the discussion presented in this chapter has been limited to relatively simple tasks, although several complex coordination tasks have been studied. These, by and large, have incorporated accuracy of performance as the primary response variable. Although speed of performance is involved in these tasks, it is seldom considered in information feedback studies. With regard to the effects of various information feedback conditions on tasks requiring both speed and accuracy to a high degree, data are generally lacking. This is unfortunate, for speed and accuracy are frequently desirable in many skills, especially gross motor skills such as throwing with great speed and accuracy, lunging or fencing with speed and accuracy, stroking a tennis ball with maximum velocity and accuracy of placement, and so on. The skills indicated above are primarily ballistic, and it is difficult to modify a ballistic movement during its execution. Hence, information feedback effects would function in the form of the learning feedback described by Miller (1953).

In an attempt to apply information feedback concepts derived from essentially psychomotor tasks, Malina (1963, 1969; see also Malina and Rarick, 1968) studied the effects of different information feedback practice conditions on the speed and accuracy of overhand throwing performance. Five groups of high school boys were used, a control group (Group 1), which received no practice, and four experimental groups, each of which received the same number of practice sessions under different information feedback conditions as follows: (a) Group 2, speed information feedback only; (b) Group 3, accuracy information feedback only; (c) Group 4, speed and accuracy information feedback; and (d) Group 5, no information feedback. Results for speed and accuracy performance over the testing and practice sessions are indicated in Figs. 2 and 3. Accuracy appeared to be affected by withholding accuracy information feedback to a greater extent than speed was affected by withholding speed information feedback. On the other hand, both speed and accuracy improved under the training conditions in which the respective type of information feedback was provided. Improvement in accuracy, however, was more variable than improvement in speed. For example, it was not until the second half of the practice program that the groups receiving accuracy information feedback showed definite indications of improvement.

The general findings of Malina's (1963, 1969) information feedback study agree in principle with the results of Fulton (1942, 1945) and Solley (1951, 1953) in studies of speed and accuracy in lunging skills, and of Woods (1967) in a study of velocity and accuracy in the forehand tennis stroke. In these studies, practice conditions emphasized speed, accuracy, or speed and accuracy. Greater proficiency was generally evident in the emphasized factor or factors, while proficiency in the unemphasized

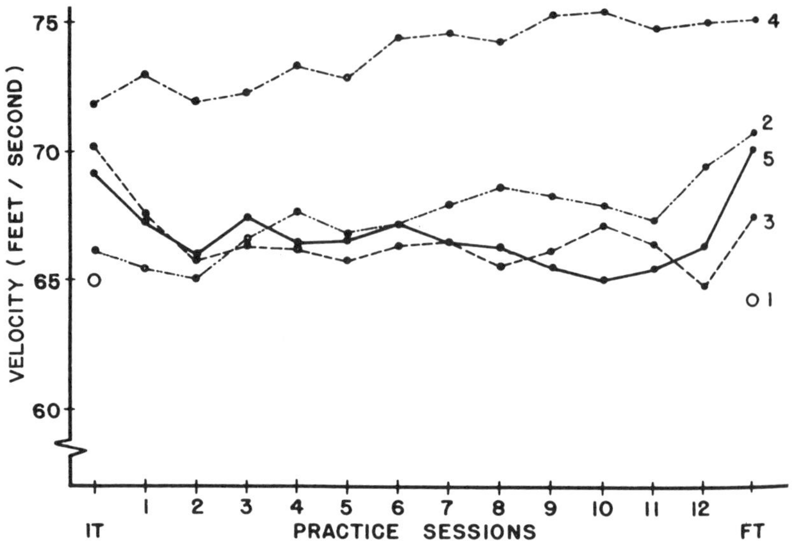

Fig. 2. Mean group performance in throwing velocity during training under different conditions of information feedback. Number to the right of each curve represents test-group number; IT, initial test; FT, final test. (Reprinted from Malina, 1969, with permission of the author and the American Association for Health, Physical Education, and Recreation.)

factor or factors was reduced and more variable. Although the directive used throughout Malina's (1963, 1969) study was to strive for maximum accuracy (i.e., a bull's eye) and maximum speed, the speed information feedback group (Group 2) improved in speed and regressed in accuracy, while the exact opposite was true for the accuracy information feedback group (Group 3) during the practice program. The subjects apparently directed their attention toward the factor for which information feedback was readily available to the neglect of the factor for which it was withheld. On the other hand, the speed–accuracy feedback group (Group 4) improved in both speed and accuracy during the practice program, suggesting that when the premium was on both variables and information feedback was provided for both, the subjects directed their attention to both speed and accuracy. The degree to which a subject is able to utilize the information value of the information feedback is of course dependent on his ability to effectively combine the speed and accuracy information in subsequent trials. The performance curves of the speed–accuracy information feedback group suggest that the subjects experienced difficulty in combining speed and accuracy effectively early

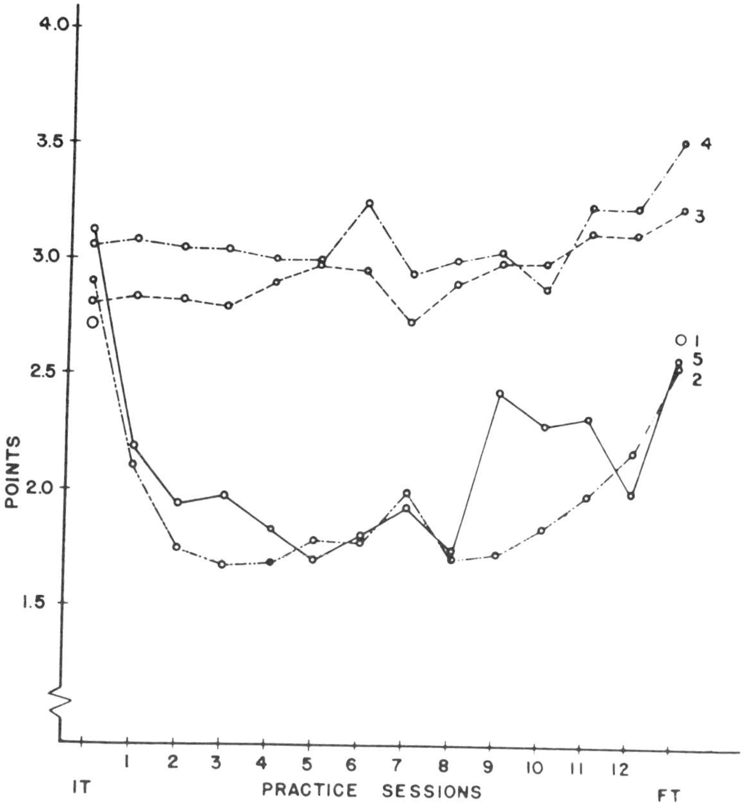

Fig. 3. Mean group performances in throwing accuracy during training under different conditions of information feedback. Number to the right of each curve represents test-group number; IT, initial test; FT, final test. (Reprinted from Malina, 1969, with permission of the author and the American Association for Health, Physical Education and Recreation.)

in the training program when speed improved and accuracy was relatively stable. As practice continued the subjects learned to effectively incorporate both speed and accuracy into the throw, showing an improvement in accuracy with a moderately stable speed. This interpretation seems to be in agreement with Ammons' (1956, p. 287) discussion of the specificity of knowledge of performance:

> The point of optimum specificity of knowledge of performance is related to some extent to the stage of learning. At the start of learning a new task, the subject can use little information. As learning proceeds, he is able to use more and more. Learning is, in fact, dependent upon the subject's acquisition of techniques for utilizing a greater range of information.

The performance curves of the speed–accuracy information feedback group also suggest that speed and accuracy information feedback functioned differently at different points in the training program. Speed information seemed to dominate early in practice, while accuracy information appeared to dominate later.

The accuracy performance curves of the speed information feedback (Group 2) and no information feedback (Group 5) groups suggest that the subjects were adapting to the lack of accuracy information feedback during the later training sessions. This was more evident in Group 2 (Fig. 3), which received speed information feedback only, and suggests that vision of the bull's eye prior to and during the throwing act (up to ball release), was sufficient to guide the subject's accuracy performance. By doing so (i.e., by concentrating on the target), the subjects perhaps disregarded their subjective impressions of the accuracy or inaccuracy of the preceding throw and concentrated only on the speed information feedback and the bull's eye in directing the subsequent throw. Further exploration of this suggestion is necessary, for it is entirely possible that the subjects might eventually have surpassed their initial accuracy levels had the practice program been continued.

Improvement or reduction in performance on the final test situation, in which information feedback was identical for all groups, was specific to the type and completeness of information feedback provided or withheld during the practice program. There was, however, one significant exception. Group 5, which practiced without information feedback, showed no appreciable change in throwing speed on the final test relative to the initial test (Fig. 2). Malina (1969) speculates that the subjects could not effectively combine the speed and accuracy information feedback made available to them during the final test since they had just completed a practice program during which neither speed nor accuracy information feedback was provided to them. Since the contributory components of throwing speed are rather gross, i.e., speed in throwing is generally produced by an all-out effort during which momentum is imparted to the ball by a sequence of gross bodily movements, the adjustments essential for improved speed were perhaps easier to make than the finer adjustments necessary to improve throwing accuracy, i.e., visual localization, direction, timing, and so on. Hence, the subjects improved in throwing speed at the expense of accuracy.

At the expense of belaboring my own observations (Malina, 1963, 1969), I shall consider the role of information feedback in effecting speed and accuracy changes. The available information feedback served a "directive function" (Bilodeau, 1956) or a "directive effect" (Elwell and Grindley, 1938). According to Ammons (1956, p. 287)

> Other things being equal, the more exactly a subject knows how he has performed, the more likely he is to be able to make appropriate corrections. The effect, then, is primarily a directive one.

As such, the information feedback indicated the degree to which the throw differed from the goal (i.e., maximum accuracy and maximum speed) and thus provided an indication of the adjustments in performance necessary to improve the next throw. This directive function of information feedback is obvious in the performances of Groups 2 and 3, the speed and accuracy information feedback groups, respectively. In the case of Group 4, which received both speed and accuracy information feedback during the training program, the directive function of the available feedback is more complex. The subjects had to interpret the directive content of both forms of information feedback in terms of the corrections necessary to improve the subsequent throw. As such, the subjects had to combine both directives in the next throw in order to improve in speed and accuracy of performance. However, there remains the possibility that one form of information feedback might have prevailed over the other. According to the "law of prior entry" (Young, 1961, p. 277), that is, "If two stimulations are physically simultaneous, the impression for which the subject is attentively predisposed is the first to make its conscious effect," either speed or accuracy may have taken preference. This would nevertheless be dependent on the subject's attention set to either variable or both, although prior to each throw the subjects were directed to strive for both accuracy and speed.

The directive function of information feedback is perhaps also related to the favorable motivational state produced by the available feedback. As indicated earlier, one of the properties of information feedback is its motivating effect on subsequent performance. Accordingly, the more an individual knows about his performance, the more highly motivated he is likely to be. As such, providing complete speed and accuracy information feedback probably created a favorable attitude in the subjects of Group 4. This heightened motivational level perhaps contributed to a greater effort, which resulted in improved speed and accuracy performance.

The precise role of withholding information feedback in effecting speed and accuracy changes during the course of the training program is not clear. On the one hand, withholding or denying information feedback removed the directive function. Without information feedback, there was no information available concerning the changes in response necessary to improve the subsequent throw. The subjects, therefore, had difficulty making the adjustments necessary to correct the preceding response. On the other hand, withholding or denying information feedback may have created "frustration states." Since information feedback affects the motivational level of the individual, it is entirely possible that withholding such feedback may have effected adverse motivational states. According to Annett and Kay (1957, p. 79)

> In so far as it is normal to receive feedback when making a response we might expect a situation in which the operator is denied knowledge to be frustrating. There need be nothing intrinsically motivating about knowledge of results but in so far as its removal militates against goal attainment its removal will be frustrating.

The deterioration in performances experienced by the subjects of Groups 2, 3, and 5 in the variable or variables for which information feedback was not provided may have been affected by both the absence of a directive function and the presence of adverse motivational states. However, it should be noted that Groups 2 and 3 trained with speed and accuracy information feedback, respectively. Thus, a third factor may have functioned to facilitate or inhibit performance in the variable for which information feedback was not provided, i.e., the law of prior entry discussed earlier. The observed performance changes during the training program suggested that the predisposed attention states of Groups 2 and 3 to the speed and accuracy information feedback, respectively, may have exerted a somewhat facilitatory effect on performance in the variable for which information feedback was not available. For example, the accuracy of Group 2 showed fewer fluctuations than the accuracy of Group 5, which received no information feedback. Similarly, the speed curve of Group 3 showed less variability than the speed curve of Group 5. As such, it appeared that the speed and accuracy performance of Group 5 during the training program was marked by greater variability and fluctuation than the performance of the two groups that received partial information feedback. This was perhaps due to the absence of a directive effect, since no information feedback was available to Group 5, as well as to adverse motivational states created by the lack of information feedback.

V. Summary

The complexities surrounding the role and effects of information feedback in facilitating and enhancing human motor performance are many. The material discussed here represents only a minor segment of the vast area encompassed by information feedback in motor learning and performance research. As such, a precise understanding of the changes that occur in human performance as a result of specific information feedback conditions or alterations is essential and merits further research.

Evident throughout this discussion is the definition of information feedback as experimentally controllable information. However, in many of the reports cited, operational definitions of information feedback do in fact vary. This represents a considerable limitation, especially when trying to compare studies that have employed different experimental designs, tasks, and types of subjects. By and large, most of the studies reviewed have incorporated some task that uses movements of the hand and arm, which are relatively easy to correct under the generally rigid experimental conditions imposed. A large class of motor activities of concern to those interested in human movement characteristic of the well-trained athlete or of the novice has gone largely unexplored in information feedback studies, perhaps only for the lack of imagination in devising appropriate training or performance conditions.

A variety of studies has shown that information feedback is a significant factor in the development of proficiency in tasks requiring a high degree of accuracy, speed, or both accuracy and speed. Providing information feedback generally improves performance, while withholding, restricting, and perhaps delaying feedback has the effect of impeding the acquisition of proficiency in motor performance. As indicated earlier, the situation is complex and, to say the least, more research is needed to further elucidate the ergogenic effects of information feedback on human performance.

References

Abbey, D. S., and Cowan, P. A. (1960). *Percept. Mot. Skills* **11**, 43.

Alexander, L. T. (1950). Dissertation, Ohio State Univ., Columbus, as cited by Ammons (1956).

Ammons, R. B. (1956). *J. Gen. Psychol.* **54**, 279.

Annett, J. (1961). "The Role of Knowledge of Results in Learning: A Survey." U. S. Naval Training Device Center Technical Report 342–3, 53. pp.

Annett, J., and Kay, H. (1957). *Occup. Psychol.* **31**, 69.

Archer, E. J., and Namikas, G. A. (1958). *J. Exp. Psychol.* **56**, 325.

Baker, G. H., and Young, P. (1960). *Can. J. Psychol.* **14**, 257.

Battig, W. F. (1954). *J. Exp. Psychol.* **47**, 371.

Bell, V. L. (1968). *Res. Quart.* **39**, 25.

Bilodeau, E. A., and Bilodeau, I. McD. (1961). *Annu. Rev. Psychol.* **12**, 243.

Bilodeau, E. A., Bilodeau, I. McD., and Schumsky, D. A. (1959). *J. Exp. Psychol.* **58**, 142.
Bilodeau, I. McD. (1956). *Amer. J. Psychol.* **69**, 434.
Bilodeau, I. McD. (1966). *In* "Acquisition of Skill" (E. A. Bilodeau, ed.), pp. 255–296. Academic Press, New York.
Bilodeau, I. McD., and Rosenquist, H. S. (1964). *J. Exp. Psychol.* **68**, 53.
Bourassa, G. L., and Guion, R. M. (1959). *J. Appl. Psychol.* **43**, 199.
Brown, J. S. (1949). *In* "Research Planning Conference on Perceptual and Motor Skills." USAF Human Resources Research Center Conference Report 49-2, pp. 81–87.
Elwell, J. L., and Grindley, G. C. (1938). *Brit. J. Psychol.* **29**, 39.
Fitts, P. M. (1964). *In* "Categories of Human Learning" (A. R. Melton, ed.), pp. 243–285. Academic Press, New York.
Fleishman, E. A. (1953). *Psychol. Bull.* **50**, 241.
Fleishman, E. A. (1954). *J. Exp. Psychol.* **48**, 437.
Fleishman, E. A. (1957). *J. Appl. Psychol.* **41**, 263.
Fleishman, E. A. (1964). "The Structure and Measurement of Physical Fitness." Prentice-Hall, Englewood Cliffs, New Jersey.
Fleishman, E. A., and Ellison, G. D. (1962). *J. Appl. Psychol.* **46**, 96.
Fulton, R. E. (1942). *Res. Quart.* **13**, 30.
Fulton, R. E. (1945). *Arch. Psychol.* **5**(300), 1–53.
Garvey, W. D., and Knowles, W. B. (1954). *J. Appl. Psychol.* **38**, 191.
Guilford, J. P. (1958). *Amer. J. Psychol.* **71**, 164.
Hempel, W. E., Jr., and Fleishman, E. A. (1955). *J. Appl. Psychol.* **39**, 12.
Irion, A. L. (1966). *In* "Acquisition of Skill" (E. A. Bilodeau, ed.), pp. 1–46. Academic Press, New York.
Johnson, H. W. (1961). *Percept. Mot. Skills* **13**, 163.
Karlin, L., and Mortimer, R. G. (1961). "Psychological Study of Motor Skills: Phase II." U. S. Naval Training Device Center Technical Report 558-2.
Klausmeier, H. J. (1961). "Learning and Human Abilities." Harper, New York.
Larson, L. A., and Yocom, R. D. (1951). "Measurement and Evaluation in Physical, Health, and Recreation Education." Mosby, St. Louis, Missouri.
Lavery, J. J. (1962). *Can. J. Psychol.* **16**, 300.
Lavery, J. J. (1964). *Amer. J. Psychol.* **77**, 437.
Lavery, J. J., and Suddon, F. H. (1962). *Percept. Mot. Skills* **15**, 231.
Liba, M. R., and Safrit, M. J. (1969). *In* "New Perspectives of Man in Action" (R. C. Brown, Jr., and B. J. Cratty, eds.), pp. 130–146. Prentice-Hall, Englewood Cliffs, New Jersey.
Lorge, I., and Thorndike, E. L. (1935). *J. Exp. Psychol.* **18**, 186.
McCloy, C. H., and Young, N. D. (1954). "Tests and Measurements in Health and Physical Education." Appleton, New York.
McCormick, E. J. (1957). "Human Engineering." McGraw-Hill, New York.
McCraw, L. W. (1949). *Res. Quart.* **20**, 316.
Malina, R. M. (1963). Dissertation, Univ. of Wisconsin, Madison.
Malina, R. M. (1969). *Res. Quart.* **40**, 134.
Malina, R. M., and Rarick, G. L. (1968). *Res. Quart.* **39**, 220.
Miller, R. B. (1953). "Handbook on Training and Training Equipment Design." USAF Wright Air Development Center Technical Report 53–136.
Noble, C. E. (1968). *Annu. Rev. Psychol.* **19**, 203.
Phillips, M., and Summers, D. (1954). *Res. Quart.* **25**, 456.

Poulton, E. C. (1970). "Environment and Human Efficiency." Thomas, Springfield, Illinois.

Robb, M. (1968). *Res. Quart.* **39,** 175.

Seashore, H. G. (1942). *Res. Quart.* **13,** 259.

Smith, P. C., and Smith, O. W. (1961). *J. Exp. Psychol.* **62,** 223.

Smode, A. F. (1958). *J. Exp. Psychol.* **56,** 297.

Solley, W. H. (1951). *Mot. Skills Res. Exch.* **3,** 76.

Solley, W. H. (1953). *Res. Quart.* **23,** 231.

Stockbridge, H. C., and Chambers, B. (1958). *J. Appl. Psychol.* **42,** 148.

Taylor, J. G., and Smith, P. C. (1956). *J. Appl. Psychol.* **40,** 142.

Williams, A. C., and Briggs, G. E. (1962). *J. Exp. Psychol.* **64,** 519.

Woods, J. B. (1967). *Res. Quart.* **38,** 132.

Young, P. T. (1961). "Motivation and Emotion." Wiley, New York.

Chapter 4

Mental Practice

Charles B. Corbin

I. Introduction

Practice is one method of effecting a change in behavior and promoting learning. One specific practice technique is mental practice (MP), also referred to as imaginary practice (Perry, 1939), covert rehearsal (Corbin, 1967a,b), symbolic rehearsal (Sackett, 1935), implicit practice (Morrisett, 1956), and conceptualization (Egstrom, 1964). Mental practice is repetition of a task, without observable movement, with the specific intent of learning.

Practicing mentally has been advocated by golfers, bowlers, and sportsmen of all types. Indeed, each of us at one time or another has thought about his mistakes or his "best shots" in performing a motor skill. The bowler "thinks" of the curve ball hitting squarely in the pocket. Children imagine hitting a ball squarely, knocking it over the fence. Each of us can cite similar instances in which MP seems to aid in the development of skilled motor behavior. Even the cartoonist Charles Schultz recognized the MP phenomenon in one of his cartoons (Fig. 1).

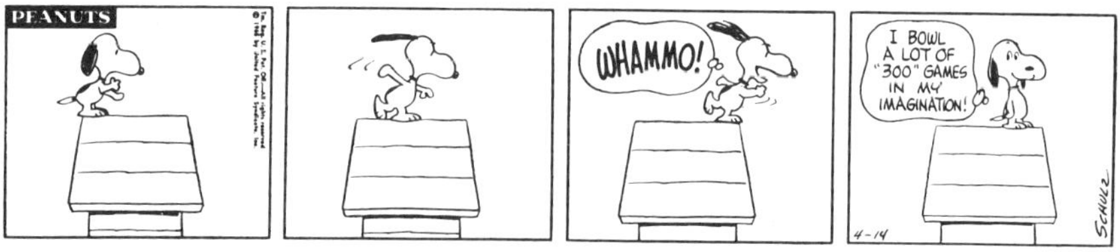

Fig. 1.

Courtesy of United Feature Syndicate, Inc., © 1965.

Others have contributed to the popularization of MP as a practical technique for learning skills. Morrison (1932, 1940) has written two books suggesting the value of MP in improving golf skills. Shaw (1939) in *Newsweek* and Phillips (1955) in the *Reader's Digest* told of the value of MP for golf and chess. These and other articles have focused attention on the MP phenomenon to the extent that more than 50 research studies, articles, and books have appeared in recent years.

So that the reader might better understand the nature of MP research, it seems appropriate to describe a "typical" study investigating the MP variable. The following paradigm is an example of a research design frequently employed to investigate the effects of MP as compared with the overt performance of a skill task.

In this typical study eighty subjects are randomly assigned to each of four different groups. In this case twenty are assigned as controls, twenty as MP subjects, twenty as physical practice (PP) subjects, and twenty as combined MP–PP subjects. Characteristically the study lasts 7–21 days. During this time all subjects except the controls practice daily. Experimental conditions might be as follows: (a) control group, no practice; (b) MP group, practice the basketball free shot mentally while reading a description of the skill, thirty trials; (c) PP group, overtly practice the basketball free shot, thirty trials; and (d) MP–PP group, practice overtly fifteen trials and mentally fifteen trials. This design is illustrated in the following tabulation.

Control group	Mental practice group	Physical practice group	Combined mental–physical practice group	Total
20 subjects	20 subjects	20 subjects	20 subjects	80 subjects

At the end of the 7- to 21-day period all subjects are tested in basketball free shooting. Means of groups are statistically compared to see if groups differ in performance as a result of the practice condition administered. If the MP group mean exceeds that of the control group, MP is said to be effective in facilitating skill performance. Many studies have reported a similar design, noting that the MP group scores significantly better than the control group but not as well as the PP and combined MP–PP groups.

The design of most MP research is similar to that of the above study. The following is a synthesis of the literature relating to MP as an ergogenic aid.

II. Early Research in Mental Practice

In the early 1900's, Washburn (1916) wrote a book dealing with the phenomenon of imagining in movement. Although many of the ideas expressed in this book were pure speculation rather than scientific fact, Washburn did make some observations that provide a basis for current study of the effects of MP on the development of skilled motor behavior. She suggested that "tentative movements" or movements of slight magnitude actually occur during imagining. She speculated that ". . . centrally excited sensations are much less steady and enduring than peripherally excited sensations" (Washburn, 1916, p. 37). Implicit in Washburn's work is the notion that real or peripheral experience is superior to imagined or central experience in effecting changes in performance. Her work also implied that imagined or central experience is of some value in effecting changes in skilled motor behavior.

Washburn also suggested the existence of varying degrees of nervous sensation. This indicated that imaginary and real sensations are basically of the same variety except that imaginary sensations are of less magnitude; however, all sensations were alleged to involve overt muscle responses. These early ideas presented by Washburn suggested many of the ideas currently being investigated.

Freeman (1931) investigated neuromuscular spread during muscular exercise, including the actual implicit muscular activity accruing during mental activity. He suggested the possibility that coordination could be improved as a result of muscular activity. Freeman's study tended to verify Washburn's earlier notion of the occurrence of actual "slight" muscular contractions during mental activity. However, no evidence was presented supporting the notion that this implicit muscular activity would increase the skill involved in the performance of a motor task.

Jacobson's (1932) work was the first to scientifically resolve the question as to whether actual muscular activity does occur during imagining. In his thorough study of muscular phenomena during imagining, Jacobson showed that electromyographic (EMG) responses occur during imagining. Although his results upheld Washburn's idea that muscular activity occurs during imagining, his research further suggested that greater muscular activity develops during imagining by subjects with movement experience. The fact that Jacobson trained subjects to relax, thus eliminating extraneous muscular activity, added to the validity of his work. Although Jacobson's classic work did not directly resolve the question as to whether imagining can improve skilled motor behavior, it did add significantly to our understanding of muscular activity during imagining.

III. Mental Practice and Task Specificity

A. Mental Practice and "Ideational" Tasks

The first research that actually studied the relative value of actual practice versus MP was conducted using what Sackett (1934, 1935) referred to as "ideational or symbolic activities." Although these "ideational" activities did involve skilled behavior, they included tasks such as mirror drawing, maze tracing, and card sorting which emphasized the symbolic rather than the motor aspects of skilled performance.

Siipola (1935) found that previous observation of a mirror drawing task without actual motor practice facilitated later execution of the task. Although this study did not actually involve imaginary practice, it did suggest that having a "mental picture" of a specific motor task would facilitate the learning of such a task.

Mental rehearsal as a practice condition was first isolated by Sackett (1934, 1935). Subjects rehearsed a maze tracing task either verbally, by imagining, or by overt action of recalling the maze. All methods facilitated the learning of the maze task, but the imaginary method appeared to be the best. The work of Sackett, like that of Siipola, suggested that imaginary practice has some effects on the improvement of performance of perceptual motor tasks, although Sackett was less than enthusiastic about the use of MP for motor skill learning.

Eggleston (1936) conducted a study of the relative value of actual practice versus imaginary practice in the learning of simple tasks. The Whipple Digit Symbol Test was employed as a task of ideational learning and card sorting as a task of sensory motor learning. After a practice period, a final test was given. The results showed MP and physical practice (PP) to be beneficial in facilitating performance of both tasks. Eggleston (1936) concluded that, in both ideational and sensory motor learning, PP is slightly superior to MP (imaginary practice) in many or all respects but that MP is an effective method of learning.

One study was conducted to investigate the relative efficiency of actual practice and imaginary practice in five selected tasks (Perry, 1939). The five skills primarily involved "ideational or symbolic activities." Tasks included card sorting and mirror tracing. Perry employed 52 subjects of elementary school age to test the effects of MP on the improvement of these ideational tasks. The conclusion was that MP may have been as effective or even more effective than PP, depending on the task. However, the investigation suggested that MP was most effective when objective facts rather than subjective facts were involved. Perry also suggested that imaginary practice may allow more time for practice than does overt practice. However, the type of task selected precluded any conclusions about tasks that are primarily perceptual–motor in nature, as opposed to ideational.

On the basis of his review of MP investigations, Buxton (1942, p. 193) suggested that the reported findings "illustrate the possibility that skill acquisition is a suitable type of learning task in which to study this phenomenon (MP). Although the studies reviewed were not studies of motor skill but of "ideational" tasks, they indicate that MP, imagining, and reminiscing might be studied in regard to their effect on perceptual–motor skills.

Morrisett (1956) attempted to sort out the effect of MP on different dimensions of skill performance. He suggested that all tasks require each of three basic skill dimensions but that skills are predominately either symbolic (stimulus–response association), perceptual (stimulus discrimination), or motor (high in skeletal muscular activity). Morrisett (1956) hypothesized that tasks requiring perceptual and/or symbolic factors would be facilitated by MP, while tasks that are predominately motor in nature would show little or no effect from implicit practice. His investigations used tasks emphasizing each of the three factors (symbolic, perceptual, and motor). He concluded that MP improved the performance of symbolic or ideational tasks the most, and had little influence on the performance of motor skills. Morrisett's results do not seem to negate the suggestion of Buxton and others that MP may be of value in facilitating skill acquisition but, nevertheless, he indicated that successful task performance is determined by the relative amounts of motor and symbolic learning involved in the practice conditions.

B. Mental Practice and Motor Skill Tasks

Probably the first study using a motor skill task was reported by Vandell *et al.* (1943). This classic study has served as the basis for much of the current MP research. These investigators evaluated the effects of MP on the acquisition of a motor skill. Three groups of 12 boys served as subjects in this experiment. The groups consisted of (a) a group of 12 college freshmen, (b) a group of 12 junior high school boys, and (c) a group of 12 high school boys. The motor skill was not the same for all of the groups studied. Each group was divided into three conditions: one group of four receiving no practice, one group of four practicing overtly and physically for 20 days, and one group of four practicing mentally for 20 days. The college students performed a dart-throwing task, the high school students a basketball-throwing task, and the junior high school boys a dart-throwing task. The groups were equated on motor ability, I.Q., educational age, chronological age, and physique, and the experimenters had a personal conference with each subject to encourage maximum performance. Impressive improvements were made by both PP and MP groups. This led to the conclusion by the investigators that MP was about as effective as PP in developing motor skill. This study was of great importance because it was the earliest of its type. The validity of the results might be questioned because of the lack of statistical analysis and the small number of subjects employed. Nevertheless, the study did provide impetus to continued investigation of the facilitatory effects of MP on skilled motor behavior.

In 1949, Twining conducted a study using the ring toss as the criterion. One important difference between this study and previous studies was that Twining used statistical procedures in interpreting his data. The study showed the MP group to perform better than the no-practice group. In addition, Twining suggested a limit to the length of time for which subjects could concentrate on MP.

Hoban and Van Ormer (1950) conducted a study of MP in which they suggested a concept of "kinesthetic imagery" and speculated that the type of instruction given previous to the MP might be of great importance in its effectiveness. They reported that instructions may affect a subject's ability to "verbally manipulate" the steps of the task. The implication was that MP, in itself, is a skill that can be learned and developed. For this reason, it might be wise to offer different types of approaches to MP in order to gain the greatest benefits from such types of practice.

Harby (1952) studied MP in a manner different from most of the work done previously. In this study, he attempted to determine whether watching moving pictures would aid in the development of a physical skill. Although only one of the experimental groups showed significant gains in skill, Harby concluded that MP was effective in improving basketball free-throwing ability. He also concluded that a combination of mental–physical practice was the best type of practice. While it was not the intent of Harby's study to investigate the reasons why MP produced learning, he did indicate that movies might be more effective than other types of MP because they lengthen the attention span of subjects.

Steel (1952, 1962) using the baseball throw and Trussell (1952) using juggling as criterion tasks found no significant improvement in skilled motor performance after MP. However, both investigators concluded that MP and PP combined was an effective practice technique.

The results of a later study by Clark (1960) indicated that MP facilitated the development of skill in basketball shooting. Like previous investigators Clark suggested that combined MP and PP was superior to either type of practice used separately. Another contribution of Clark's study was the notion that some degree of physical skill must be present for an individual to gain maximal effects from MP.

A study by Corbin (1967a) investigating acquisition and retention of a wand-juggling task among subjects of varying skill levels revealed no MP benefits for acquiring and retention of skill and no differences among performers of different skill levels in ability to use MP. He suggested that MP must be based on experience in order for the practice to be effective. A follow-up study (Corbin, 1967b), which required all subjects to "experience" or actually practice the juggling task under controlled conditions prior to MP, found MP to be effective in producing learning in the task. It appears that the previous "experience" interacted with MP and facilitated performance of this relatively complex motor skill.

Phipps (1968) investigated the effects of MP on the acquisition of skills classified as simple, of intermediate difficulty, and of complex difficulty. Of significance was the finding that MP was not effective in improving performance of a complex skill in the absence of actual experience or without physical practice, while performance of a simple task was improved through MP without prior experience of the skill. Apparently, the level of skill complexity is related to the need for "experience" prior to MP.

C. Mental Practice and Physical Fitness Development

Shaw (1940) conducted a study to determine whether more vivid imaginary experiences would be accompanied by more muscular activity than the less vivid experiences. The EMG responses during actual and "mental" weight lifting were compared. Shaw concluded from the results of his study that MP did produce actual muscular activity and that the more vivid imaginary experiences produced greater muscular contractions. This evidence tended to support Washburn's (1916) earlier theory pertaining to "tentative movements."

The fact that EMG responses were evoked by imagining prompted Kelsey (1961) to study the effects of MP on muscular endurance. He studied the effects of MP on the endurance capacity of the abdominal and thigh flexor muscles. Kelsey concluded that muscle responses during MP were sufficient to improve muscular endurance. A similar study by Steel (1962) supported Kelsey's contention that MP is effective in promoting gains in muscular endurance. Results of studies such as those by Kelsey (1961) and Steel (1962) led Richardson (1964) to suggest that MP may have implications in the practice of physiotherapy. However, more recent studies by Cronk (1967) and Rodriguez (1967), who studied the effects of MP on arm and abdominal strength, did not support the contention that MP facilitates physical fitness gains.

IV. Theories of Mental Practice

More than 50 different research studies have been conducted investigating the MP phenomenon. Various explanations for the MP "effect" have been advanced. Some of the most tenable explanations follow.

A. A "Gross Framework" Theory of Mental Practice

The "gross framework" idea has been advocated by Lawther (1968) as a condition necessary for optimal motor learning, especially for the beginner. The learner must be able to conceptualize the entirety of the task or the "gestalt" if he is to improve in skill performance. Specifically, the learner's attention must be directed to the general impression or the gross outline of the skill rather than to the details of the movement. It is certainly possible that MP could be of value in helping the learner establish the "gross framework." The work of Corbin (1967a,b) and others suggesting experience to be necessary for effective use of MP would seem to fit well in this conceptualizing explanation of MP. The previous experience, either actual or vicarious (demonstration, movies, etc.), would be necessary for the initial conceptualizing of the "gross framework" of the skill to be learned. This explanation could account for MP "effects" being somewhat less than those of overt practice or PP. This MP theory would imply that once the "gross framework" or concept of the skill had been firmly set through previous experience and MP, additional MP would not evoke additional benefits. Other explanations would be necessary to account for any further improvement in skill once the gross concept of the skill had been established.

B. Selective Attention and Mental Practice

One important concern in learning a skilled motor task is that of selective attention. If the learner is to gain in skill proficiency, attention must be directed toward the important aspects of the skill to be learned. The learner must be selective in attending to various acts involved in performing the skill. These "key" skill components are incorporated in the "practiced" skill, while the nonnecessary movements are "selected out" or eliminated. Bruner (1960), in his classic work "The Process of Education," points to the need for attention to the fundamentals of understanding. He notes that details are rapidly forgotten unless placed in a structured pattern. It is possible that repeated MP of the skill to be learned could benefit the learner by calling attention to important details of the desired movement. Further, the mental repetition would serve to reinforce the specific details of the movement, which would prevent forgetting of these important details.

C. A Feedback Theory of Mental Practice

The early work of Washburn (1916) suggested that "tentative movements" of slight magnitude actually occur during imagining. The work of Shaw (1940) and Jacobson (1944) clearly established a factual basis for Washburn's contention. Further, Bowdlear (1927) long ago noted that trial and error is necessary for effective skill learning. He suggested rational analysis to be only partly effective in skill learning. Rather, as one tries a skill and fails he "gets the hang of things" even though he never clearly determines the necessary conditions required for success.

The fact that errors produce adjustment prior to additional trials can be explained in terms of a simplified feedback theory. Sensory or perceptual interpretations are made and the reason for the error is surmised before additional trials are attempted. The information gained from the interpretation is fed back to facilitate adjustment in future skill performance trials. The value of feedback in skill learning for overt practice or PP is obvious. It is possible, however, that feedback theory may apply to MP as well.

For one to use MP effectively he must construct a real and controlled image of the skill to be learned. This image, although overtly unseen, produces a slight but real muscular contraction. The innervation of the muscles involved in the skill being imagined may well be capable of providing kinesthetic feedback necessary to make adjustments in future trials, thus improving skilled motor performances.

D. Insight through Mental Practice

The idea that the "gross framework" is necessary for effective performance is consistent with Gestalt theory, which suggests the need for an understanding of the "whole" or "total" in learning. In addition, Gestalt theorists point to the need for insight in successful problem solving. Improvements in performance, they suggest, do not necessarily come in proportion to the length of time spent in practice. Rather, learning occurs with periodic changes in behavior resulting from insight.

Most individuals have experienced "insightful" behavior after periods of practice. Regardless of the skill to be learned, some mental imagining is necessary prior to and during the improvement of performance through insight. It is possible that MP provides the opportunity for behavioral changes resulting from insight. Involvement in MP would not insure improved performance or learning but would provide for a new perceptual organization through insight.

The suggestion that experience is necessary for MP relates to insight theory, in that prior experience of at least a gross mental image must be present in order for MP to provide an opportunity for learning through insight.

E. Motivation and Mental Practice

It is possible that performance differences between groups (MP versus control groups) might reflect differing levels of motivation between such groups. There are at least two different theories that relate to such possible motivational differences.

First, attention to verbal instructions, demonstrations, or whatever creates an interest or a level of motivation in the performer; that is, the performer practices mentally for some time and as a result has a desire to try out the specific skills practiced. The MP group would surpass the control group because of the motivation to actually try the skill that was practiced mentally.

A second, and related, theoretical view suggests that MP groups may perform better than control groups as a result of the "Hawthorne effect." Control groups frequently are given no treatment, while MP groups attend practice sessions. The fact that one group gets "something" and the other "nothing" justifies the concern that the "Hawthorne effect" may be operating. In such experiments the MP group's superiority cannot be attributed solely to motivation resulting from experimental involvement. It is interesting to note that an investigation by Williams (1970) showed no difference between MP and control groups when compared on arousal as measured by EMG responses. Mental practice apparently can be interpreted in favor of a learning hypothesis not attributable to different arousal (motivational) variables induced by "experimenter bias."

F. A Connectionist Theory of Mental Practice

Just as Washburn's theory of "tentative movements" (1916) is of importance to the feedback theory of MP, it also plays an important role in connectionist theory. Since mental practice produces specific muscle responses of slight magnitude, it can be argued that these "tentative movement" responses form a "connection" with the MP stimulus. Repetition of the stimulus (MP) with the desired response (EMG potential) results in a strong connection between the stimulus and the response. Thus, repeated MP results in an improved overt performance of the task that was practiced mentally.

V. Acquisition and Retention of Skilled Motor Behavior

Most frequently the research designed to determine the effect of MP has been confined to acquisition of skill. In these studies a skill is mentally practiced for a period of time ranging from 1 day to several weeks. In all but a few cases skilled performance has been tested at the completion of the prescribed practice period. Only a few investigations have studied retention of skilled motor behavior resulting from MP.

The typical experiment in this area of inquiry involves three groups of randomly assigned subjects consisting of control and PP groups. Experimental groups are typically administered a treatment of MP or PP and then tested for skill acquisition. A summary of the types of MP investigations completed to date is presented in Table I. Most of these investigations have been limited to the study of skill acquisition.

Several investigators have followed subjects after initial acquisition of a skill to determine the extent to which MP is effective in facilitating retention of skilled motor behavior. For example, Sackett (1934), Johnson (1967), and Corbin (1967a,b) have studied retention of skilled performance after MP. The results of these studies are inconclusive.

The wide variety of experimental conditions used in the studies reported in Table I indicates that different MP conditions produce different MP results. The following section will consider some of the conditions that may affect skill learning resulting from MP.

VI. Conditions Affecting Mental Practice

A. Length of Practice Sessions and Duration of the Learning Experience

While educators and psychologists have long acknowledged the phenomenon of reactive inhibition (i.e., the tendency of task repetition to

TABLE I

SUMMARY OF MP RESEARCH

Criterion task studied	Length of practice session	Duration of experiment	Subjects	Type of MP
Mirror tracing	1 minute	1 day	Elementary school boys	Undirected
Pursuit rotor	3 minutes	2–6 days	Elementary school girls	Read instructions
Maze task	5 minutes	1 week	Junior high school boys	View movies
Card sorting	10 minutes	2 weeks	Junior high school girls	Listen to directions
Dot symbol test	15 minutes	9 days	High school boys	Observe live performer
Tapping speed	20+ minutes	10 days	High school girls	Overt vocalization
Finger dexterity		20 days	College men	Subvocalization
Dart throwing		3 weeks	College women	Write instructions
Basket shooting	1 trial	5 weeks	Coed groups	Combined audiovisual
Ring toss	10 trials	6–12 weeks	Varsity athletes	Other combinations
Baseball throw	15 trials		Adult men and women	
Ball juggling	20 trials			
Wand juggling	25 trials			
Volleyball serve	30 trials			
Triple jump	30+ trials			
Tennis stroke				
Shot put				
Handball serve				
Gymnastics stunts				
Soccer kicks				
Badminton serves				
Weight lifting				
Arm strength				
Abdominal strength				

interfere with task learning or performance), the research involving MP has frequently not considered this phenomenon. Figure 2 illustrates that learning or performance gains occur with practice (MP or otherwise). However, as the length of practice becomes excessive, performance decreases. Reactive inhibition causes a decrease in the performance of the task to be learned. As with other types of practice it is likely that there is an optimal length for practice sessions. Ideally these practice sessions would not continue once reactive inhibition had begun (see Fig. 2). Harby's (1952) preliminary work suggests that an optimal length for MP sessions exists. However, his data are not convincing. Richardson (1967a,b) and Oxendine (1968) have reiterated Harby's contention, but they have not designed studies with the specific intent of investigating this contention. Twining (1949) has suggested that 5 minutes be the upper limit for length of MP sessions. A study by Shick (1969) revealed that extremely short practice sessions were not the most effective. Also, Shick's data indicated that 3-minute sessions were more effective in promoting improved skill performance than 1-minute sessions. The findings of the aforementioned investigations suggest that relatively short practice sessions are probably optimal. Investigators should keep this point in mind when designing MP studies.

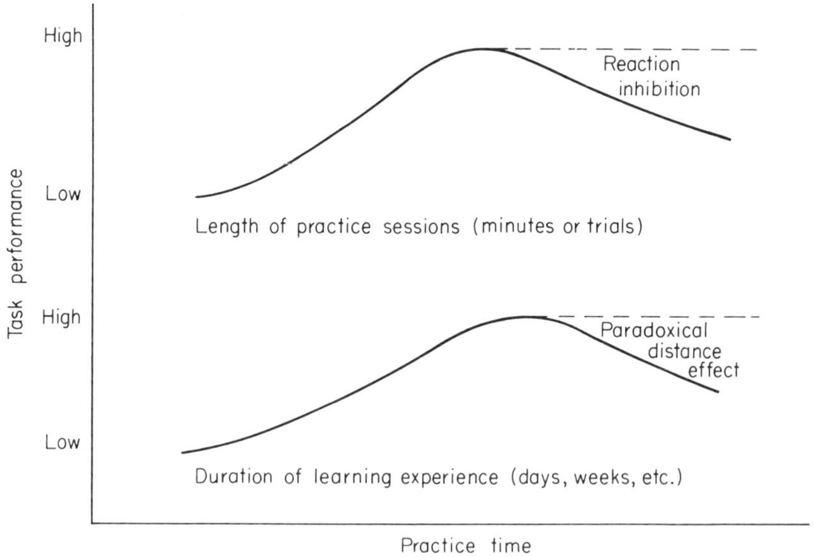

Fig. 2. Performance of a motor skill task improves with practice. However, too much practice may result in a decreased performance.

Closely related to length of practice is the duration of the learning experience. In other words, how long should the learner continue to practice (i.e., several days, weeks, months, years)? Whatever the length of sessions, the learner will repeat the sessions. Performance will improve with each successive session (see Fig. 2). As with length of practice, however, there may be an optimal number of practice sessions necessary to promote most effective skill learning. Additional practice sessions may cause no further increase in performance or learning. In fact, additional practice sessions may result in decreased performance (the paradoxical distance effect).

Investigators have ignored the matter of paradoxical distance effects, and MP sessions ranging from 1 day to several weeks have been used. Results from these studies are frequently compared just as though these studies had employed the same number of practice sessions. Further research must be done relating to this phenomenon, and controls must be made to consider this effect in future MP research.

B. Scheduling of Practice Sessions

Also of concern to the practitioner desiring to use MP as an ergogenic aid is the scheduling of practice. As in any learning situation, it is likely that some distribution of practice will lead to more effective learning than will massed practice. Research by Gilmore and Stolurow (1951) indicated that massed practice resulted in "motivation loss." Studies by Riley and Start (1960) and Luebke (1967) reported that alternate scheduling of MP and PP trials facilitated learning through MP. The dearth of research suggests this to be a fruitful area for future inquiry.

C. Type of Practice

Another condition that very likely could be related to the effective use of MP is the type of practice. Different studies have used undirected MP, reading with MP, observation of a performer, movies and loop films, and overt verbalization. It is entirely possible that each of these techniques could relate to a different theory of MP (see Section IV) and therefore evoke differential facilitation of overt performance.

Jones (1963) studied gymnastics performers and concluded that undirected MP was a better method of practice than MP accompanied by reading of specific skill instructions. The implication is that reading might actually interfere with conceptualization during MP.

The work of Brassie (1968) suggests that visual practice (observation of an overt performance) is more effective than reading a set of prepared instructions. However, Brassie also suggests both reading and visual practice to be better than overt verbalization. Overt verbalization was least effective of all MP techniques employed by Brassie. Also, Smith and Harrison (1962) reported that visual practice improved performance on a punchboard task.

Studies by Harby (1952), Hoban and Van Ormer (1950), and Beckow (1967) support the contention that loop films or moving pictures provide an extremely effective method of mental practicing. It was suggested that "nonmotivated" subjects might increase their attention span by watching movies.

Audio instructions in combination with MP were studied by Surburg (1968), who concluded that audio, visual, and audiovisual instructions all were effective when used in combination with MP. However, audio instructions used with MP were the most effective practice condition for improving skill in the forehand tennis stroke.

Wills (1970) studied various combinations of practice techniques including oral instructions, written instructions, and loop films. Wills concluded that the type of instruction given before MP may be as important, or more important, than the type of MP used.

D. Type of Task (Specificity)

As mentioned in Section III, the type of task to be learned may indeed be related to the extent to which MP promotes learning. Whether MP is effective in improving performance may well depend on whether the task to be performed is ideational, motor, or solely muscular.

Betts (1949) suggested that additional examples of task specificity may be associated with MP. For example, she speculates that specificity might be involved when projectiles are used, but not in other sport and physical activity tasks. Of related interest are the studies of Start (1964a). Jones (1963), McKeown (1967), and Maxwell (1968) using nonprojectile skills (sports skills), which revealed that MP did not evoke beneficial effects.

Brumbach (1968) has also suggested that MP effects are task specific, indicating that, in a study of performance of badminton skills, MP was more effective in improving a "restricted or precise" skill than in facilitating performance of more "gross and dynamic movements." The type of task must certainly be one consideration when MP is intended to serve as an ergogenic aid.

E. Performance Mechanics

The effective learning of any motor task requires sound performance mechanics. The physical principles that apply to movement must be considered if movement learning is to be effective. It seems logical to postulate that one of the conditions for the effective use of MP would be to employ established biomechanical principles.

VII. Mental Practice and the Consumer

There is little doubt that individual differences play a significant role in the learning process. Accordingly, innate or acquired differences in the consumer are likely to affect the consumer's ability to improve performance as a result of mental practicing. The following discussion of consumer characteristics might relate to the effective use of MP.

A. Previous Experience

Corbin (1967a,b) has argued that previous experience is a prerequisite for effective use of MP. In his initial study he intentionally selected a task in which subjects had no previous experience. The MP experience did not evoke improvement in overt performance. In a follow-up study, Corbin's subjects were administered controlled overt experience prior to receiving MP. Mental practice groups experienced significant improvements in overt skill performance following controlled practice.

Research by Phipps (1968) supports a "prerequisite experience" theory; however, he notes that the experience may be necessary when using MP to learn only complex skills. In other words, mental practice may facilitate the performance of simple tasks even without prerequisite experience, but experience is essential prior to MP designed to improve performance of complex skills.

A study by Schramm (1967) further supports the idea that performers must have prerequisite task experience if MP is intended to facilitate overt performance. Using an EMG to measure the muscle response to MP, Schramm noted that muscle activity (tentative movements) was highest during MP that was based on immediate prerequisite experience. It appears that the previous experience of the performer must be considered if MP results are to be used or studied.

B. Intelligence

Another characteristic of the performer that must be considered in discussing MP is intelligence. One might hypothesize that more intelligent performers would benefit most from MP because of greater abilities in abstract thinking. However, this hypothesis is not supported by the research. Studies by Clark (1960), Start (1960, 1964b). Whiteley (1962), and Oxendine (1968) indicate that the performer's intelligence is not related to his ability to use MP. The single exception to this view is the article by Perry (1939), which indicated MP to be more beneficial for performers of higher intelligence.

C. Conceptualizing Ability

Another characteristic of the consumer that might logically relate to effective use of MP is conceptualizing ability. Mental practice requires the subject to conceptualize or create a "mind's-eye view" of the task to be practiced. Cratty (1962) has established the need for mental imagery in skill learning, noting that sighted subjects rely heavily on mental imagery during blindfold tasks. It would seem logical to assume that persons with above-average ability to construct mental images or conceptualize would have above-average results from the use of MP. However, Johnson's (1967) work failed to reveal a correlation between ability on tests of verbal behavior and MP benefits. Also, Wilson (1960) reported a lack of relationship between skill improvement resulting from MP and spatial relationship.

Start and Richardson (1964) evaluated the hypothesis that persons with more vivid and controlled imagery might be better able to use MP than persons with less vivid and controlled imagery. Their tentative conclusions indicated that subjects with vivid, controlled imagery benefited most from MP. Next in their ability to use MP were subjects with the ability to conceptualize controlled, nonvivid images. Subjects with uncontrolled, nonvivid mental images were third in their use of MP, while subjects who had uncontrolled, vivid images were least able to benefit from MP. It appears that vividness of the mental image must be considered in combination with the subject's ability to control the image.

If, in fact, MP effects are enhanced by the ability to conceptualize, the results of Leuba and Dunlap (1951) are particularly significant. These investigators reported that subjects can increase their ability to create mental images through conceptualizing and/or MP experience.

D. Skill Level

Several investigations have been concerned with the extent to which skill level relates to a performer's ability to effectively use MP. Clark (1960) first investigated the relationship between mental practicing abilities and skill performance levels and noted that novice performers used MP more effectively than junior varsity and varsity performers while learning a one-handed basketball shot. Whiteley's (1962) results contradicted Clark's, indicating that performers of higher motor ability used MP more effectively than performers scoring low on a test of motor ability. The results of a study by Start (1962) supported the findings of Whiteley, indicating that performers scoring high in "games ability" used MP more effectively than subjects rated poor in "games ability." However, a later study by Start (1964b) revealed that motor ability was not related to mental practicing ability. Also, Doyle (1968) reported a lack of difference in MP benefits between high- and low-skill groups.

In view of the diverse tests used to measure skill level and the varying criterion tasks that were practiced mentally, it is difficult to interpret the literature in a meaningful context. At any rate, the relationship between skill ability and a performer's ability to benefit from MP remains unconfirmed.

E. Kinesthesis

Waterland (1956) has postulated that, in subjects encouraged to "feel" the kinesthetics of a skill while mentally practicing, the MP effect would be enhanced. Indeed, Waterland (1956) found that this kinesthetic MP improves bowling ability more than normal PP. On the basis of Waterland's study, it would seem that a performer's kinesthetic sense might relate to his ability to use MP. Start (1964b), using the Wiebe Test as a measure of kinesthesis, studied the relationships between kinesthetic ability and improvement of performance in subjects who mentally practiced a simple gymnastics task. The relationship between these variables was not significant.

F. Arousal State

Williams (1970) suggested that the MP effect might be attributable to the arousal (motivation) level of the performer. He implied that an increased arousal level in MP groups might simply reflect the "Hawthorne effect." If so, the MP effect might be a result of the increased arousal state rather than the actual MP. Furthermore, it would be possible that whatever MP effect really existed might be related to the arousal state of the performer. Williams used the EMG to establish an arousal index and concluded that arousal state is not a factor affecting a performer's ability to use MP.

G. Creativity

Although tests of creativity have been published and creativity is a variable that may be related to effective use of MP, no experiments have been reported relating these two variables. Therefore, speculation regarding the interaction of this psychometric property with MP must await empirical evidence.

H. Sex

While some studies have been conducted with male subjects only, some with female subjects only, and some with coeducational groups, little research has concerned itself with differences between men and women in their ability to use MP. A single study by Perry (1939) reported no significant differences when sexes were compared as to their ability to benefit from MP.

VIII. Methodology

The research on which the evaluation of MP is based must be taken into account before MP is considered by the practitioner. The practitioner must recognize that methodological problems may well limit the claims made for any ergogenic aid. The following methodological problems must be considered in evaluating the research that has dealt with MP.

A. Instructions

One major research problem is the nature of the instructions that precede MP. The time of administration of instructions (before or during MP) and the type of instructions (written, audio, none, visual, etc.) may affect the outcomes of research on MP. Also, as Wills (1970) has pointed out, it is entirely possible that instructions or directions may be responsible for performance gains rather than MP per se. The type of instructions that precede MP must be controlled in subsequent work.

B. The Hawthorne Effect

Hanson (1967) has noted that the Hawthorne effect can alter the performance of subjects performing motor tasks. He strongly suggests the consideration of the Hawthorne effect when designing experiments and interpreting findings involving skill learning. His warning seems especially pertinent when considering research dealing with MP. Comparison of control groups with MP groups is difficult if precautions are not taken to account for the "something" given to the MP group as opposed to the "nothing" given the control group.

C. Task Selection

As mentioned in Section III, the nature of the task may well be a factor relating to the facilitating effect of MP. Research indicates that varying results can be expected if the criterion skill is gross muscle as opposed to fine muscle, ideational as opposed to motor, familiar as opposed to unfamiliar, and simple as opposed to complex.

D. Design of Experiments

The design or model for experimentation is of vital importance if the results of a particular experiment are to be meaningful. One problem of experiment design has been the extensive use of the simple randomized model. In this design only one variable can be studied at a time, and this has usually been "type of practice" (i.e., mental practice versus physical practice or some combination of mental–physical practice). In as much as over 30 studies have been conducted using this design it seems appropriate to consider more sophisticated models for future research. As already discussed, there is a multitude of factors that must be studied if the ergogenic effects of MP are to be clearly understood. While the simple effects of each related variable must be studied, it is also important to study the interacting relationships of combinations of variables. For this reason multidimensional designs should be employed in future research. Figure 3 illustrates an example of an interaction between MP and a second variable. In this hypothetical example, subjects possessed

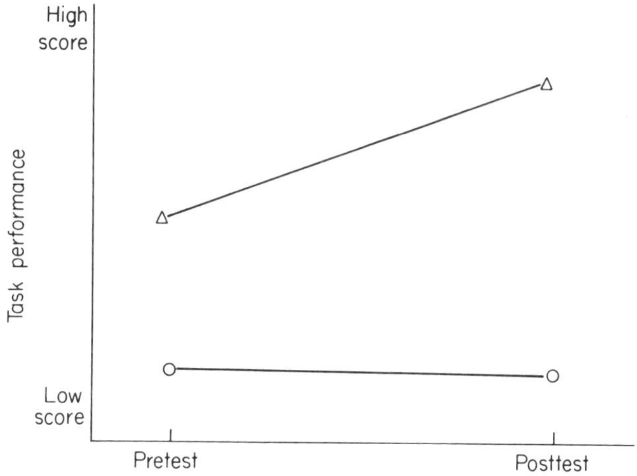

Fig. 3. Interaction between mental practice and second significant variable. The graph shows that MP is effective only for subjects with experience in the task that was practiced mentally (△, low-experience subjects; ○, high-experience subjects).

different amounts of previous experience in the experimental task. The subjects with previous experience showed a performance increase as a result of MP, while those without experience showed no gain in performance. The interaction between MP and experience is shown by the fact that subjects varied in their ability to use MP depending on the second variable, experience. Possible interactions between MP and other variables could be illustrated similarly. Any of the factors discussed in Sections VI and VII could be incorporated in a research project designed to study interactions between MP and other variables.

A second design problem associated with MP research is the tendency of investigators to combine treatments as experimental conditions. Frequently, studies have reported combined mental–physical practice to be superior to mental or physical practice alone (Trussell, 1952; Stebbins, 1968; Howe, 1967; Burns, 1953; Luebke, 1967; and Witker, 1968). The design of the experiment rarely allowed for the conclusion that combined mental–physical practice treatments were superior to other noncombined treatments. When practice conditions are combined there is no way of discovering to what extent either of the combined (mental or physical) conditions contributes to the total practice effect. Consider an experiment in which after 10 days one compares three groups having practiced (a) 20 mental repetitions a day, (b) 20 physical repetitions a day, and (c) 10 mental and 10 physical practices a day. To assume the combined-practice group to be superior because of a higher mean score would be hazardous. Since reactive inhibition and paradoxical distance effects may operate when using MP, it is possible that either the 10 mental or 10 physical practices alone could produce the greater performance by the combined-practice group. If it is theorized (and it is by many) that combined mental–physical practice is better than either PP or MP alone, then specific experiments must be designed to test this specific hypothesis.

IX. Summary

As early as 1916 theories existed which suggested imagined performance to be a technique that is in some way beneficial to improving skilled motor behavior. In the ensuing period more than 50 studies have dealt specifically with the phenomenon of MP. Classic studies (Vandell *et al.*, 1943; Twining, 1949) have indicated MP to be an effective ergogenic aid. At least 24 additional investigations have supported the view that MP evokes beneficial effects. Also, Steel (1952) and Harby (1952) have made positive conclusions concerning MP on the basis of questionable data. Other studies (Trussell, 1952; Gilmore and Stolurow, 1951; Corbin, 1967a,b) have indicated that skill facilitation is not evoked by MP. Reviews of the research (Buxton, 1942; Richardson, 1967a,b) noted more studies supporting than rejecting the view that MP is an ergogenic aid. While authors of certain popular publications (e.g., Maltz, 1960) have emphasized the efficacy and reality of MP, a careful perusal of the literature raises more questions than it answers. The purpose of this chapter has been simply to treat the topic of MP academically. While this author suggests that the advancement of meaningful conclusions regarding the effectiveness of MP must await controlled, rigorous experimental research, some generalizations seem to be justified.

There seems to be little doubt that mental practice can positively affect skilled motor performance, especially when practice conditions are "optimal." It is equally clear, however, that mental practice is not always an aid to performance and that factors such as the practice type, the skill task, and the nature of the performer ultimately reflect the extent of behavior change resulting from MP.

While we now know a great deal about MP as an ergogenic aid, there is a definite need to investigate the MP phenomenon directly. To date, research has dealt exclusively with the indirect assessment of MP. In other words, we have investigated behavior changes that accompany periods of alleged MP. Whether these behavior changes are a result of the MP or other treatment circumstances remains to be directly shown. This and evidence of the actual physiological mechanism involved in behavior change resulting from MP must be the subject of the creative efforts of tomorrow's researchers.

References

Beckow, P. A. (1967). "A Comparison of the Effectiveness of Mental Practice upon the Learning of Two Gross Motor Skills." Unpublished master's thesis, Univ. of Oregon, Eugene.

Betts, C. H. (1949). "The Distribution and Functions of Mental Imagery." Columbia Univ. Press, New York.

Bowdlear, C. W. (1927). *Amer. Phys. Educ. Rev.* **32,** 100.

Brassie, P. S. (1968). "Acquisition and Retention of a Motor Skill as a Function of Overt Self Verbalization and Physical or Mental Practice." Unpublished doctoral dissertation, Univ. of Iowa, Iowa City.

Brumbach, W. B. (1968). *Abstr. Res. Pap. AAHPER Conv.* p. 95.

Bruner, J. S. (1960). "The Process of Education." Random House, New York.

Burns, P. L. (1953). "The Effect of Physical Practice, Mental Practice and Mental–Physical Practice on the Development of a Motor Skill." Unpublished master's thesis, Pennsylvania State Univ., University Park.

Buxton, C. E. (1942). *Psychol. Rev.* **49,** 191.

Clark, B. J. (1960). *Res. Quart.* **31,** 560.

Corbin, C. B. (1967a). *J. Gen. Psychol.* **76,** 143.

Corbin, C. B. (1967b). *Res. Quart.* **38,** 534.

Cratty, B. J. (1962). *Calif. J. Educ. Res.* **14,** 36.

Cronk, J. M. (1967). "The Effects of Physical Practice, Mental Practice and Physical–Mental Practice on Development of Arm Strength." Unpublished doctoral dissertation, Florida State Univ., Tallahassee.

Doyle, J. F. (1968). "The Effect of Two Types of Practice on Motor Learning at Two Skill Levels." Unpublished master's thesis, Pennsylvania State Univ., University Park.

Eggleston, D. (1936). "The Relative Value of Actual vs. Imagery Practice in a Learning Situation." Unpublished master's thesis, Columbia Univ., New York.

Egstrom, G. H. (1964). *Res. Quart.* **35,** 472.

Freeman, G. L. (1931). *J. Gen. Psychol.* **5,** 479.

Gilmore, R. W., and Stolurow, L. M. (1951). *Amer. Psychol.* **6,** 295.

Hanson, D. L. (1967). *Res. Quart.* **38,** 723.

Harby, S. F. (1952). U.S. Naval Special Device Center Technical Report SDC, 269-7-25.

Hoban, C. F., and Van Ormer, E. B. (1950). Cited by Harby (1952).

Howe, D. P. (1967). "The Influence of Five Schedules of Mental Practice upon the Physical Performance of a Novel Gross Motor Skill after a Criterion Measure of Skill Had Been Attained." Unpublished doctoral dissertation, Texas Woman's Univ., Denton.

Jacobson, E. (1932). *Amer. J. Psychol.* **44,** 677.

Jacobson, E. (1944). "Progressive Relaxation." Univ. of Chicago Press, Chicago, Illinois.
Johnson, B. L. (1967). "An Examination of Some Factors Which Might Be Related to Effective Utilization of Mental Practice in Learning a Gross Motor Skill." Unpublished master's thesis, Univ. of Oregon, Eugene.
Jones, J. G. (1963). "Motor Learning without Demonstrations of Physical Rehearsal under Two Conditions of Mental Practice." Unpublished master's thesis, Univ. of Oregon, Eugene.
Kelsey, I. B. (1961). *Res. Quart.* **32**, 47.
Lawther, J. D. (1968). "The Learning of Physical Skills." Prentice-Hall, Englewood Cliffs, New Jersey.
Leuba, C., and Dunlap, R. (1951). *J. Exp. Psychol.* **41**, 352.
Luebke, L. L. (1967). "A Comparison of the Effect of Varying Schedules of Mental and Physical Practice Trials on the Performance of the Overarm Softball Throw." Unpublished master's thesis, Univ. of Wisconsin, Madison.
McKeown, B. C. (1967). "The Effect of Physical Practice, Mental Practice, and Mental–Physical Practice on the Learning of the Modified Triple Jump." Unpublished master's thesis, South Dakota State Univ., Brookings.
Maltz, M. (1960). "Psycho-Cybernetics." Prentice-Hall, Englewood Cliffs, New Jersey.
Maxwell, J. M. (1968). "The Effect of Mental Practice on the Learning of the Overhand Volleyball Serve." Unpublished master's thesis, Central Missouri State College, Warrensburg.
Morrisett, L. N. (1956). "The Role of Implicit Practice in Learning." Unpublished doctoral dissertation, Yale Univ., New Haven, Connecticut.
Morrison, A. J. (1932). "A New Way to Better Golf." Simon & Schuster, New York.
Morrison, A. J. (1940). "Better Golf Without Practice." Simon & Schuster, New York.
Oxendine, J. B. (1968). *Abstr. Res. Pap. AAHPER Conv.* p. 131.
Perry, H. M. (1939). *Arch. Psychol.* **34**, 5.
Phillips, J. (1955). *Reader's Digest* Vol. 66, April, 123.
Phipps, S. J. (1968). ""Effect of Mental Practice on Acquisition of Motor Skills of Varying Complexity." Unpublished master's thesis, Pennsylvania State Univ., University Park.
Richardson, A. (1964). *Physiotherapy* **50**, 148.
Richardson, A. (1967a). *Res. Quart.* **38**, 95.
Richardson, A. (1967b). *Res. Quart.* **38**, 263.
Riley, E., and Start, K. B. (1960). *Aust. J. Phys. Educ.* **20**, 13.
Rodriguez, G. J. (1967). "A Comparison of the Effects of Mental and Physical Practice upon Abdominal Strength in High School Girls." Unpublished master's thesis, Univ. of North Carolina, Greensboro.
Sackett, R. S. (1934). *J. Gen. Psychol.* **10**, 376.
Sackett, R. S. (1935). *J. Gen. Psychol.* **13**, 113.
Schramm, V. (1967). "An Investigation of EMG Responses Obtained During Mental Practice." Univ. of Wisconsin Press, Madison.
Shaw, W. A. (1939). *Newsweek* **14**, 30.
Shaw, W. A. (1940). *Arch. Psychol.* **35**, 5.
Shick, J. (1969). *Abstr. Res. Pap. AAHPER Conv.* p. 84.
Siipola, E. M. (1935). *Psychol. Monogr.* **44**, 66.
Smith, L. E., and Harrison, J. J. (1962). *Res. Quart.* **33**, 299.
Start, K. B. (1960). *Res. Quart.* **30**, 644.

Start, K. B. (1962). *J. Gen. Psychol.* **67**, 159.
Start, K. B. (1964a). *Res. Quart.* **35**, 316.
Start, K. B. (1964b). *Brit. J. Educ. Psychol.* **34**, 85.
Start, K. B., and Richardson, A. (1964). *Brit. J. Educ. Psychol.* **34**, 280.
Stebbins, R. J. (1968). *Res. Quart.* **39**, 714.
Steel, W. I. (1952). *J. Phys. Educ.* **44**, 101.
Steel, W. I. (1962). "Effect of Mental and Physical Practice on Endurance on a Bench Press Task." Unpublished research report, Univ. of Manchester, Manchester, England.
Surburg, P. R. (1968). *Res. Quart.* **39**, 728.
Trussell, E. M. (1952). "Mental Practice as a Factor in the Learning of a Complex Motor Skill." Unpublished master's thesis, Univ. of California, Los Angeles.
Twining, W. E. (1949). *Res. Quart.* **20**, 432.
Vandell, R. A., Davis, R. A., and Clungston, H. A. (1943). *J. Gen. Psychol.* **29**, 243.
Washburn, M. F. (1916). "Movement and Mental Imagery." Houghton, Boston, Massachusetts.
Waterland, J. C. (1956). "The Effect of Mental Practice Combined with Kinesthetic Perception When the Practice Precedes Each Overt Performance of a Motor Skill." Unpublished master's thesis, Univ. of Wisconsin, Madison.
Whiteley, G. (1962). "The Effect of Mental Rehearsal on the Acquisition of Motor Skill." Unpublished diploma in education dissertation, Univ. of Manchester, Manchester, England.
Williams, R. L. (1970). *N.C.P.E.A.M. Proc.* **73**, 43.
Wills, K. C. (1970). "Effect of Different Methods of Instruction and Practice on Skill Acquisition of a Motor Task." Unpublished doctoral dissertation, Texas A & M Univ., College Station.
Wilson, M. E. (1960). "The Relative Effect of Mental Practice and Physical Practice Learning the Tennis Forehand and Backhand Drives." Unpublished doctoral dissertation, Univ. of Iowa, Iowa City.
Witker, J. E. (1968). "The Relative Effect of Variations of Combined Mental and Physical Practice on Learning a Novel Task." Unpublished master's thesis, Illinois State Univ., Normal.

Chapter 5

Heat and Cold Applications

Harold B. Falls

I. Introduction

Before pursuing the subject of heat and cold as ergogenic aids, it is necessary to delimit the area to be covered by this presentation. The focus here will be specifically on the application of heat or cold as an attempt to improve the work performance of an individual or to lessen the fatigue associated with a particular work situation. The effects of environmental heat and cold on work performance have been adequately discussed elsewhere (Iampietro and Adams, 1968; Leithead and Lind, 1964; Lee, 1964; Folk, 1966). Also, it is not my intention in this review to touch on the broad area of heat and cold therapy in rehabilitation, although it is obvious that speedy healing of injury, etc., might be ergogenic in nature. This review is also limited primarily to the results of studies dealing with human subjects. Only in a few instances have the findings of work on other animals been cited and then only if it was felt that those results might have direct implications in the use of heat and/or cold applications on humans or if they might corroborate the results of human studies.

Many men have long been convinced that heat applications of various kinds could improve their health, work performance, and circulatory function if properly applied. However, it appears that the same kind of beliefs about the efficacy of cold applications is limited to this century (Wells, 1932). Research on both modalities as ergogenic aids has been meager and, to a certain degree, contradictory. A great deal of literature is available on the physiological effects of heat and cold, but relatively few studies have extended this knowledge to the use of the modalities as ergogenic aids. Even though a number of authors have previously summarized the physiological effects of heat and cold application, a brief review here seems essential for adequate interpretation and understanding of Section III.

II. Physiological Effects of Heat and Cold Applications

A. The Physical Transfer of Heat

Cooling or heating the body can be accomplished through one or more of three physical avenues. These are conduction, convection, and radiation. A fourth avenue, evaporation of sweat, is available for cooling. (For a detailed discussion of each of these avenues see Iampietro and Adams, 1968.) The usual procedure when temperature changes of an ergogenic nature are desired is to use topical applications involving convection and/or conduction, although some studies have investigated the ergogenic effects of radiative and evaporative temperature changes. Regardless of the modality, heat flow to or from the body or some specific part is involved in both cooling and heating. When the body or its segment(s) are to be heated, modalities with temperatures above the body or part temperature are used. Heat flows from the modality to the organism because of the temperature gradient. When cooling is desired a modality with a temperature lower than that of the body or its part is used. In this case heat flows in the opposite direction, away from the organism to the modality, thus cooling the body or the specific part. Modalities that are conductive in nature include hot and cold packs applied directly to the body surface and still hot or cold water baths in which the whole body or one of its parts is immersed. Modalities of a convective nature involve the streaming of air or water across the body surface. An example is the use of hot or cold showers. If the body or part is exposed to air less than fully saturated with water vapor, the evaporative avenue of body heat loss might also be invoked, and some heat could be removed from the body surface by sweat evaporation as well as simple conduction or convection.

B. Physiological Changes Mediated by Heat and Cold Applications

1. *Surface and Deep-Tissue Temperature Changes*

Application of heat or cold to the skin causes its temperature to change in a direction toward equilibrium with whichever modality is used. Skin temperature changes occur rapidly. Immersion in a cold bath at 4.4°–10°C causes skin temperature to drop below 15.5°C in less than 2 minutes. About 10 minutes is necessary in order to decrease it to 10°C (Behnke and Yaglou, 1951). Keatinge (1961) has shown even more rapid skin temperature drops. He repeatedly immersed men in water at 35°, 25°, 15°, and 5°C. The mean skin temperature fell to within 1.4°C of general water temperature within 2 minutes after the start of immersion, even at the lowest water temperature. A similar pattern of decline in skin temperature has been noted in individuals exposed nude to cool air temperatures (10°–21.1°C) for 1 hour (LeBlanc, 1954). Comparable rapid decreases have been observed in subjects exposed to cold showers. Mean skin temperatures of 23.8°–25.5°C were observed in five subjects immediately after showers varying in duration between 3 and 9 minutes at a mean temperature of 17.7°C (Falls and Humphrey, 1970). Conductive cooling by cold packs of various kinds also results in rapid reduction of skin temperature (Licht, 1965).

Freeze damage to the skin can occur upon brief exposure to modalities with temperatures slightly below 0°C. Prolonged exposures at temperatures in the range 1°–15°C can also cause damage (Licht, 1965). Maximal skin temperature tolerance to heat is approximately 44°–45°C (Millard, 1965; Downey *et al.*, 1968). Consequently, there is a wide range in the temperatures of heat and cold modalities that may be applied safely in the attempt to achieve an ergogenic effect.

Heat applications cause rapid rises in skin temperature. High levels of radiated heat elevate it at the rate of 0.5°–1.0°C/minute for the first 2–5 minutes of exposure. After a plateau period of 5–10 minutes, the mean skin temperature continues a gradual rise toward the maximal tolerable level. This later rise is at a slower rate than that seen initially

(Hasan *et al.*, 1966). Irregardless of whether the modality is heat or cold, efficient methods of conduction can achieve almost instantaneous changes in skin temperature (Rowell *et al.*, 1969). Figure 1 illustrates the effects that heating and cooling have on skin and core temperatures.

The rate at which skin temperature changes occur varies regionally within an individual and from one individual to another. At least three factors are responsible for these variations: (a) thickness of epidermis, dermis, fat, and muscle; (b) water content of the tissues; and (c) rate of blood flow (Licht, 1965). The degree to which skin temperature drops in relation to any standard cold exposure is especially related to the thickness of subcutaneous fat deposits. Subjects with larger skin-fold thicknesses exhibit skin temperatures on cold exposure that are lower than those of thinner individuals. Yet, these fatter subjects maintain their core temperature at a higher level than the thin subjects (Baker and Daniels, 1956; LeBlanc, 1954; Wyndham *et al.*, 1968; Keatinge, 1969). These relationships are illustrated in Fig. 2.

Muscle temperatures apparently do not change as rapidly nor to as

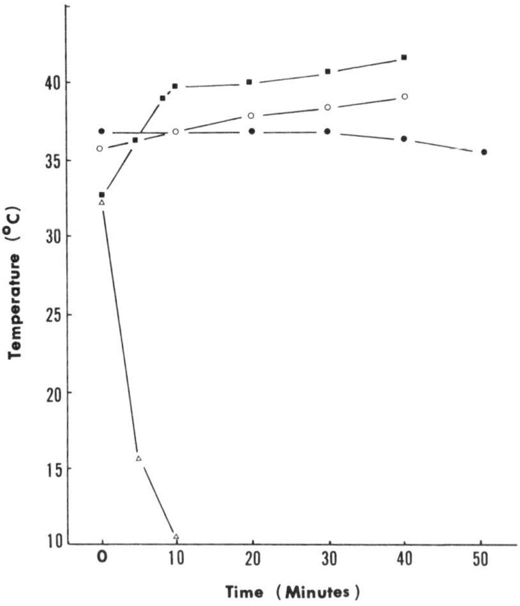

Fig. 1. Differential effects of heating and cooling on skin and core temperatures: ■, skin temperature (T_s) with radiant heat (sauna) 80°C, 5% relative humidity; ○, esophageal temperature in above exposure; △, T_s with water bath at 6.1°C; ●, rectal temperature in same water bath exposure. (Drawn after data presented by Behnke and Yaglou, 1951, and Hasan *et al.*, 1967.)

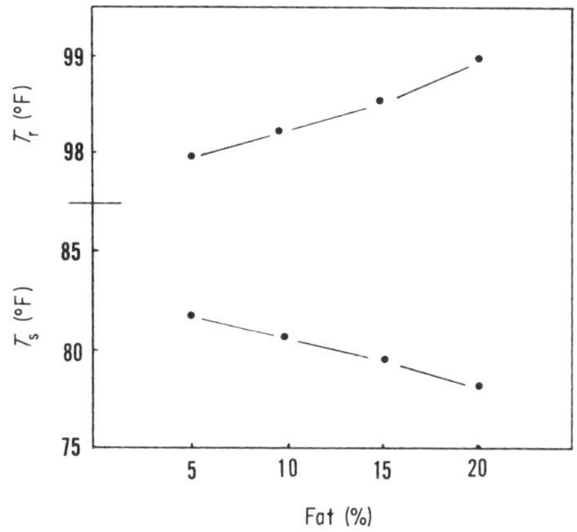

Fig. 2. Relative relationships between percent body fat (estimated from skin-fold thicknesses) and rectal (T_r) and skin (T_s) temperatures after a nude 2-hour exposure to air at 15°C. (Adapted from Baker and Daniels, 1956.)

great a degree as do skin temperatures when heat or cold is applied to the whole body or segment thereof. It has been shown that the temperatures of resting muscles are often 2°–3°C higher than skin temperatures in most regions of the body (Reader and Whyte, 1951). However, muscle temperatures are usually somewhat lower than deep-body (rectal) temperatures (Reader and Whyte, 1951; Saltin and Hermansen, 1966; Saltin *et al.*, 1968; Aikas *et al.*, 1962).

The degree to which deep-muscle temperature changes as a result of heating or cooling depends primarily on its distance from the surface of the body. Local heating of the skin to 43°C (by 20 minutes of exposure to infrared radiation) has very little effect on muscle tissue temperature 3–4 cm below the surface of the skin. Tissues at shallower depths are warmed in proportion to their proximity to the surface. Similar results have been obtained when conductive cooling with a water bath at 27°C was applied for periods ranging between 37 and 110 minutes. Even though the cold application was somewhat more effective than radiant heating in achieving temperature change, maximal temperature drop measured at a depth of 3 cm was only 1.1°C. Additional lowering of deep-tissue temperatures was achieved with conductive cooling from water baths at colder temperatures (down to 2.8°C), but the magnitude of changes was still only about 10% of that seen in skin temperatures (Reader and Whyte, 1951). The latter findings, obtained in studies on the lumbar region, have been corroborated by Waylonis (1967) in studies of ice massage effects on the thigh and calf. However, when the body part is immersed in very cold water (1°C) for long periods (up to

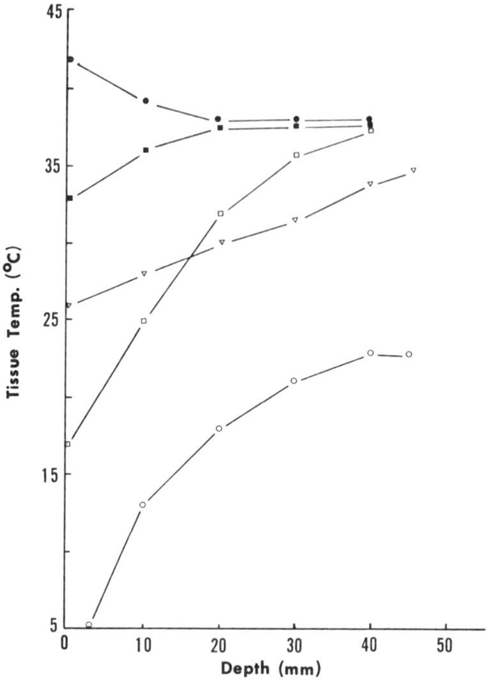

Fig. 3. Tissue temperatures at various depths after application of several forms of external heating or cooling: ●, radiant heat (20 minutes infrared), lumbar region; ■, control, lumbar region; ▽, water bath 26°C, 30-minute forearm; □, ice massage, posterior thigh, 10 minutes; ○, water bath 2°C, forearm, 30 minutes. (Drawn from data presented by Reader and Whyte, 1951; Waylonis, 1967; and Clarke *et al.* 1958b.)

40 minutes) muscle temperature can be decreased as much as 10°C. Noticeable drops in the muscle temperature are not achieved, however, until about 15 minutes of continuous exposure (Clarke *et al.*, 1958a). The effects of heat and cold applications on tissue temperatures at various depths are shown in Fig. 3.

2. *Core Temperature Changes*

Brief applications of external heat or cold do not appear to have pronounced effects on core temperatures. Local applications of heat or cold must be quite intense and continued for long periods of time before they will change core temperatures significantly by conduction through the more superficial tissues (Figs. 1 and 3). It is obvious that rapid changes must be achieved by thermal effects on blood flowing through the peripheral vessels. As it returns to the more central vessels, it warms or cools the body's core accordingly. The immediate reaction of peripheral vessels to thermal stimuli is to either conserve body heat or dissipate it. When cold is applied, general vasoconstriction reduces skin blood flow and conserves body heat, leading to a preservation of core temperature. Heat applications lead to vasodilatation, resulting in increased skin blood flow. This brings more heat to the body shell and enhances the possibility for its dissipation through conduction, convection, radiation, and evaporation. If the sweating mechanisms are functioning properly man can dissipate heat well at rest, even in the face of high heat loads, and can maintain a normal body temperature for relatively long periods of time. Men and women exposed in saunas at temperatures of 65°–90°C dry bulb, 40°–50°C wet bulb, exhibit rectal temperature increases approximating 1.0°–1.3°C during the first 30 minutes of exposure (Hasan *et al.*, 1966). A severe heat load of this nature would be rarely attempted as an ergogenic aid.

Men fully immersed in cold water show little change in deep-body temperature during the first 10 minutes of exposure, even when the temperatures are extremely cold. At 5°C in one study the mean fall was only 0.4°C (Keatinge, 1969). Men with relatively thick skin folds can maintain deep-body temperature at, or near, normal in these cold waters for as long as 30 minutes. Other investigators have shown that cold showers of the length usually employed in studies assessing their ergogenic qualities have no effect on rectal temperatures (Falls and Humphrey, 1970).

3. *Blood Flow Changes*

Application of cold to any part of the body surface causes a local vasoconstriction and, therefore, a reduction in blood flow (Fox, 1961; Downey, 1964; Murphy, 1960; Abdel-Sayed *et al.*, 1970). Full constriction of cutaneous vessels occurs when the local temperature reaches approximately 24°C (Downey *et al.*, 1968). Local heating results in cutaneous vasodilatation and an increased blood flow (Hasan *et al.*, 1967). An arm heated in water at 42°C exhibits a blood flow up to four or five times that of the resting level. The increased flow is confined almost entirely to the skin (Downey, 1964).

Because of the dilating and constricting effects that heat and cold have on local vessels, cutaneous blood flow is highly dependent on local skin temperature (Hertzman, 1953; Thauer, 1965). However, at any given local temperature, the absolute blood flow is highly related to the prevailing ambient temperature (Fig. 4).

When cold is applied to the skin, vasoconstriction is apparent until

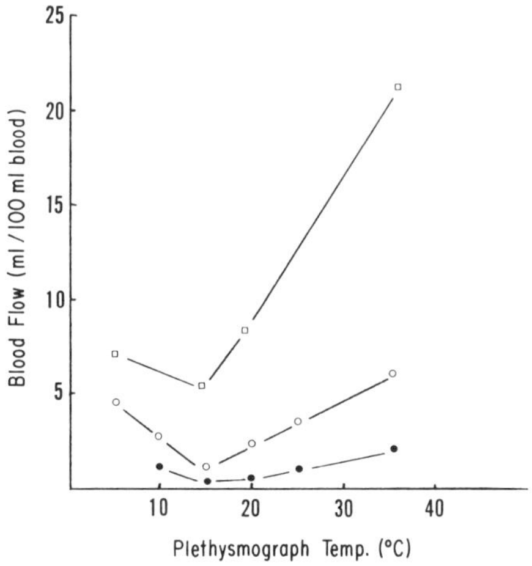

Fig. 4. Relation between blood flow in the human hand and plethysmograph water temperature at three different environmental temperatures, venous occlusion method: □, 32°C dry bulb (DB) temperature, 28°C wet bulb (WB) temperature; ○, 24°C DB, 19°C WB; ●, 16°C DB, 13°C WB. (Original data from Spealman, 1945. Redrawn from Thauer, 1965.)

the skin temperature drops to 10°–12°C. Temperatures below this point lead to periodic waves of vasodilatation in the skin vessels, thereby periodically increasing the local blood flow (Downey *et al.*, 1968; Fox, 1961; Clarke *et al.*, 1958a; Keatinge, 1969). Cold vasodilatation occurs in both local cooling situations and whole body immersion (Keatinge, 1969). The periodic vasodilatations at these low temperatures apparently result because temperatures below 10°–12°C cause a form of cold paralysis to occur in the vessels involved, leaving them incapable of responding to the constrictor influences of adrenaline and noradrenaline (Keatinge, 1969). As the vasodilatation allows increased blood flow, the blood raises the skin temperature above 10°–12°C. Secretion of adrenaline and noradrenaline again causes constriction. Thus, a cyclic rise and fall in blood flow is maintained as long as the exposure continues (Fig. 5).

Application of cold or heat to one part of the body, even though it may be only a small area, causes a reflex reaction in other areas of the body that is similar to the local effects at the point where the modality is applied. Heat causes reflex vasodilatation, and cold causes reflex vasoconstriction (Downey *et al.*, 1968; Murphy, 1960). The term consensual vasodilatation or consensual vasoconstriction, respectively, has been used to describe this phenomenon (Fischer and Solomon, 1965). The effect is illustrated in Fig. 6.

There is little evidence that local applications of heat and cold cause

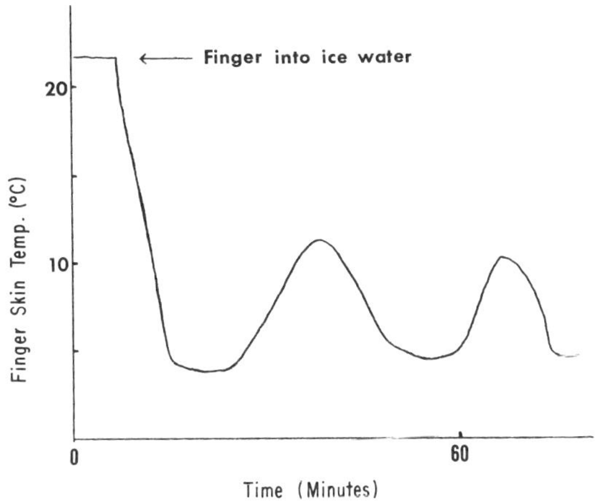

Fig. 5. Cold vasodilatation effects in finger. Readings from thermocouple on skin covered with three layers of adhesive tape. (Redrawn from Keatinge, 1969. Original from Lewis, 1930.)

changes in muscle blood flow similar to those in the skin (Downey, 1964). In fact, just the opposite may be true (Fox, 1961; Edholm *et al.*, 1956; Roddie *et al.*, 1956; Abramson *et al.*, 1958; Thauer, 1965). Figure 7 illustrates the effects that body heating and cooling have on total and local blood flow in contralateral limbs. As the body is heated, total limb blood flow increases while muscle blood flow decreases. With cooling the op-

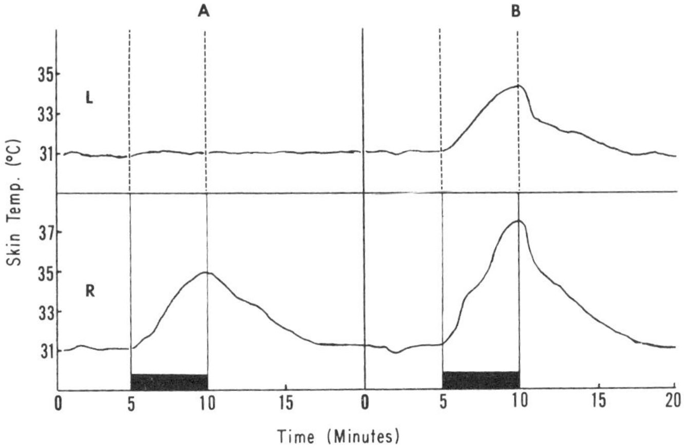

Fig. 6. Consensual temperature change in left foot (L) and direct temperature change in right foot (R) when the latter is irradiated for 5 minutes by infrared: A, a small intensity not producing a consensual reaction; B, twice the intensity producing a consensual reaction. (Redrawn from Fischer and Solomon, 1965.)

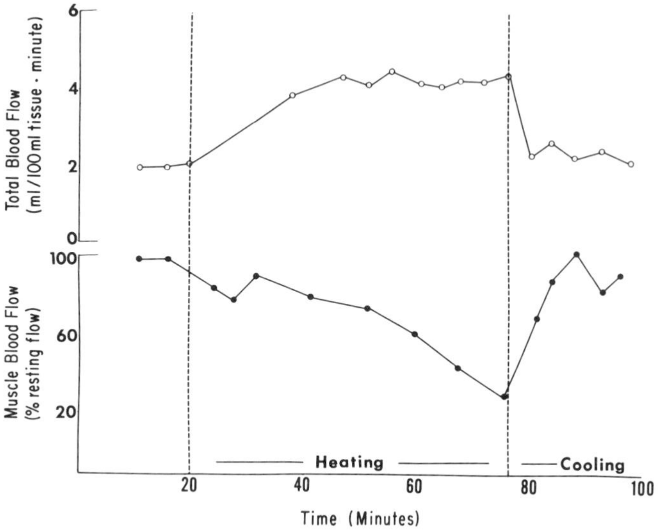

Fig. 7. Effect of body heating and cooling in a water bath on (●) muscle blood flow (left calf) and (○) total blood flow (right calf). (Adapted from Thauer, 1965. Original data from Barcroft *et al.*, 1955.)

posite effects are noted. These effects have been supported by recent investigations by Abdel-Sayed *et al.* (1970), who studied the effect of local cooling on the responses of muscular and cutaneous arteries and veins. Their results led them to conclude that cooling favors redistribution of blood flow away from cutaneous and into muscular vessels.

4. *Circulatory Changes Other Than Local Blood Flow*

It has already been noted that local application of cold to the body surface causes constriction of peripheral vessels (Section II,B,3). The veins as well as the arteries are affected (Wood *et al.*, 1958; Downey *et al.*, 1968; Rowell *et al.*, 1971). Constriction causes a decreased blood flow and increases the resistance to flow. The increased resistance is reflected in an elevated peripheral venous pressure (Rowell *et al.*, 1969; Wood *et al.*, 1958). There is evidence to support the occurrence of compensatory changes in the more central areas of the circulation (Murphy, 1960). For example, it has been noted that pulse wave velocities of the large central arterial vessels are slowed upon application of cold to the body surface. This has been accepted as a sign of vasodilatation within these vessels (Bazett *et al.*, 1937). Associated with these alterations are rises in systolic and diastolic blood pressures (Bazett *et al.*, 1937; Wells, 1932, 1933; Happ *et al.*, 1949; Keatinge *et al.*, 1964). Application of heat causes responses in opposition to those noted above for cold applications (Craig and Dvorak, 1966; Hasan *et al.*, 1967; Rowell *et al.*, 1971).

The peripheral circulatory changes favor shift of blood into the central circulation during cold application and shift to the skin vessels during heat application. As a result, a lower heart rate should be necessary in order to maintain a given cardiac output under cold application conditions compared to those of heat application. Several studies investigating heart rate and/or cardiac output responses to cold and heat applications present evidence in support of this adjustment. Bazett *et al.* (1937) observed that cooling a subject in water baths at a temperature of 32°C caused a reduction in cardiac output that was reflected in a reduced heart rate. There was no change in stroke volume. Warm baths up to 39.5°C resulted in an increased cardiac output that was a function of increases in both heart rate and stroke volume. Similar results have been obtained by Craig and Dvorak (1966), who immersed subjects in water baths at temperatures between 24° and 37°C for 1 hour. Favorable alterations in cardiovascular responses occurred in the midrange of water temperatures (35°–28°C). These changes, decreased heart rate and increased peripheral blood pressures, suggesting minimal flow of blood to the skin and minimal demands on cardiac output. At water temperatures above 35°C, an increased heart rate and reduced blood pressures were noted. These were suggestive of peripheral vasodilatation and increased demands on cardiac output. Heart rate was directly related to local temperature at water temperatures above 28°C. Heart rates had a tendency to increase toward control levels at water temperatures of 28°C and below, probably as a result of increased metabolic activity due to shivering, which occurred below 28°C.

Numerous investigators have consistently demonstrated lower pulse rates at rest (Happ *et al.*, 1949; Steinhaus and Wendhut, 1953; Keatinge and Evans, 1961; Robbins, 1942), during exercise (Falls and Wiebers, 1965; Falls, 1969; Falls and Humphrey, 1970; Muller, 1965), and during recovery (Michael, 1957; Walters *et al.*, 1960; Costill *et al.*, 1967; Falls, 1969; Falls and Wiebers, 1965; Falls and Richardson, 1967; Adee, 1953; Muller, 1965; Roundy and Cooney, 1968) as a result of various cold applications before, during, and/or after work. Similar results have been noted for work in water (Costill *et al.*, 1967; Muller, 1965). In the temperature range 17–34°C, a linear relationship between recovery pulse rate from endurance swims and pool water temperature has been noted by Adee (1953). Recovery pulse rates for 1500-m time trials and 20-minute paced swims were lowest in water at 17°C. The recovery rates increased 0.76 beats/minute for each 1°F increase in pool water temperature.

Heat applications in various forms have been shown to increase resting, exercise, and recovery pulse rates (Hasan *et al.*, 1967; Falls and Wiebers, 1965; Walters *et al.*, 1960; Dawson *et al.*, 1965; Wessman and Kottke, 1967).

Pulse rate changes during thermal application in the temperature range 24°–39°C occur before, or in the absence of, changes in core temperature and apparently are not a function of it. It is felt that average skin temperature plays a key role in effecting pulse rate changes, both at rest (Bazett *et al.*, 1937; Goff *et al.*, 1956) and during exercise (Falls and Humphrey, 1970). Reflex mechanisms elicited by thermal receptors are probably responsible (Bazett *et al.*, 1937). The recent work of Rowell *et al.* (1969) lends support to the hypothesis that skin temperature is the chief parameter involved in mediating changes in heart rate and cardiac output when heat or cold applications are made during exercise. With rapid changes in skin temperature between 26.9° and 40°C they were able to achieve coinciding changes in cardiac output and heart rate. Both rose and fell with skin temperature. Stroke volume responses were in the opposite direction. They fell with increases and rose with decreases in temperature of the skin. These responses are illustrated in Fig. 8. It is readily noted from the figure that changes in heart rate, cardiac output, and stroke volume were unrelated to rectal temperature. The circulatory changes shown in Fig. 8 are due to changes in tone of peripheral blood vessels. Heating the skin makes it more difficult to maintain a given blood flow to muscle tissue. Because of the peripheral vasodilatation, cardiac output must be increased in order to accomplish the task. These increases appear to be primarily due to increases in heart rate. When the skin is cooled some of the blood is shifted away from the peripheral vessels by vasoconstriction. As a result, a lower heart rate is required to pump the fraction of cardiac output that goes to the muscles and vital organs. These effects are well illustrated in tilt table experiments. When one is tilted from the recumbent to the erect posture, circulatory insufficiency occurs due to decreased venous return to the heart resulting from sudden pooling of blood in the extremities. Cardiac acceleration is called into play in an attempt to compensate for the decreased cardiac output. Horvath and Botelho (1949) demonstrated that the venous return is reduced still further because of vasodilatation when the subject is immersed for 20 minutes in a hot bath before tilting. In contrast, the vasoconstriction resulting from a bath of the same length at 18°C enables subjects to withstand tilting to upright with very little cardiac acceleration.

It thus seems reasonable to conclude from the evidence available that cold water application probably has an ergogenic effect on the circulation by shifting blood away from the periphery to the interior of the

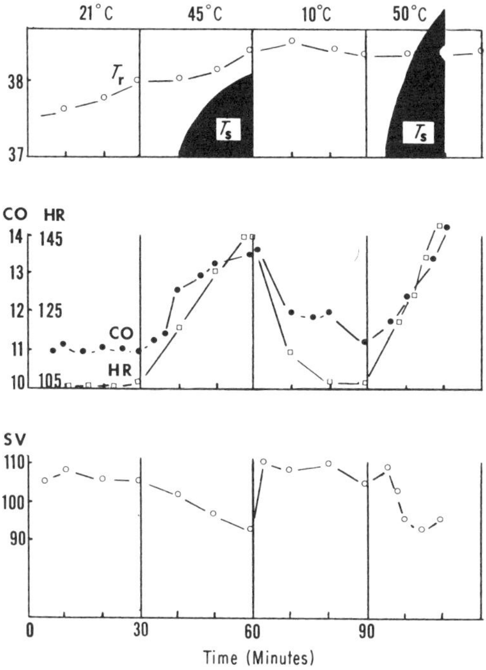

Fig. 8. Mean cardiac output (CO), heart rate (HR), and stroke volume (SV) in relation to changes in skin (T_s) and rectal (T_r) temperatures while a special garment was perfused with water at various temperatures (shown across top of graph). Data from six subjects working at 26.3–38.9% of maximal oxygen uptake. Similar results (not shown here) were obtained from four subjects working at 51.3–64.0% of maximal oxygen consumption. (Redrawn from data presented by Rowell *et al.*, 1969.)

body. The net effect would seem to be an increase in blood flow to muscle tissue without making necessary a corresponding increase in total cardiac output at any given work load.

It should be noted at this point that not all cold water temperatures elicit the desired ergogenic outcome of a reduced heart rate and favorable effects on cardiac output. Applications of water at extremely cold temperatures may cause increases in both heart rate and cardiac output. Keatinge and Evans (1961) found that subjects immersed in water at 15° or 5°C showed an elevation in heart rate at the beginning of exposure. The rates did drop after the initial rise, but it took 20 minutes for them to drop below the preexposure level in water at 15°C, and they were still considerably above preexposure levels after 20 minutes in water at 5°C. Extremely cold showers (2 minutes at 0°–2.5°C) have a similar effect on heart rate and also cause large increases in cardiac output (Keatinge *et al.*, 1964). It does appear possible, however, to habituate an individual to cold water exposure to such an extent that the initial heart rate increase at very cold temperatures is abolished. Keatinge and Evans (1961) were able to accomplish this at the end of eight immersions in water at 15°C. However, it would seem that, if an ergogenic effect is desired, immersion in water at this low temperature may be unnecessary since full vasoconstriction occurs at local temperatures above 20°C (see Section II,B,3).

5. *Metabolic and Respiratory Changes*

a. *Lung Ventilation.* The situation with regard to respiratory changes associated with heat and cold applications appears to be somewhat paradoxical. Minute volume of ventilation ($\dot{V}_E$), tidal air, and respiratory rate all increase with heat or cold applications. There is also a reduction in end-tidal P_{CO_2}. Keatinge *et al.* (1964) have shown that 2-minute showers at 0°–2.5°C on seated subjects increased pulmonary ventilation from 10.6 to 47.5 liters/minute, respiratory rate from 14.6 to 29.6 per minute, and tidal volume from 767 to 1677 ml/minute. There was a corresponding decrease in Pa_{CO_2} from 39.8 to 27.8 mm Hg. Keatinge and Nadel (1965) noted similar results from showers at considerably warmer temperatures (5°–25°C). The responses were also similar whether the showers covered mostly the trunk or mostly the extremities. However, the greatest response was elicited from trunk exposure. Although both tidal air and respiratory frequency showed increases, the tidal volume increase seemed to contribute most to the increased ventilation. The increase in ventilation and the inspiratory shift reached their maximal extent within 2–3 breaths after the start of a shower and then decreased. The decline was rapid during 25°C showers, respiration often returning to near normal within 20–30 seconds, but was less abrupt at colder temperatures. During cold water immersion ventilation shows a similar pattern over time. It increases immediately upon immersion but decreases rapidly toward normal values after about 1 minute into the exposure. If the exposure continues for a lengthy period of time, $\dot{V}_E$ again increases, probably as a result of shivering (Keatinge and Evans, 1961). The rapid decreases in ventilation after the initial rise are probably due to partial adaptation of the cutaneous cold receptors to the low skin temperature.

Showers in the range of 30°–40°C apparently do not cause changes in $\dot{V}_E$. Showers at temperatures above 40°C elicit responses similar to those below 30°C. The relationship of $\dot{V}_E$ to shower temperature is shown in Fig. 9. Exposures in hot baths (Bazett, 1924; Landis *et al.*, 1926) result

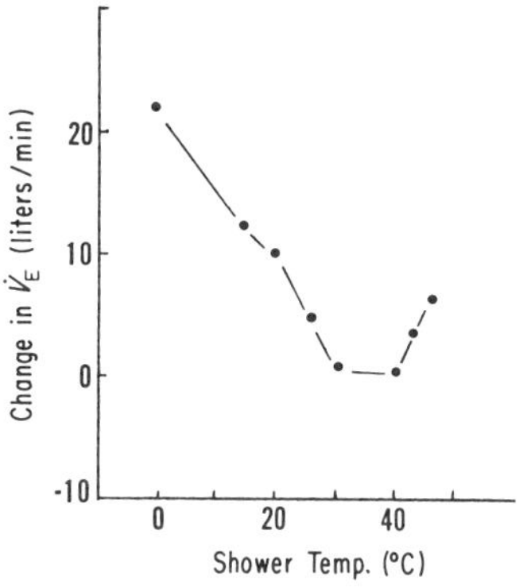

Fig. 9. Relationship of lung minute volume of ventilation ($\dot{V}_E$) to temperature (°C) of 2-minute showers over trunk and legs. (Redrawn from Keatinge and Nadel, 1965.)

in $\dot{V}_E$ responses similar to those noted above for hot shower exposures. Similar results have also been noted in individuals exposed to hot air (Bazett, 1924; Hasan *et al.*, 1966), but the magnitude of response is greater during water exposure when compared with that in air.

The increased $\dot{V}_E$ after cold and hot water exposures apparently mediates changes in both alveolar and arterial O_2 and CO_2 tensions (Keatinge and Evans, 1961; Keatinge and Nadel, 1965; Bazett, 1924); O_2 tensions are increased while those of CO_2 are decreased. Whether these changes might alter the volume of O_2 delivered to tissues during a work performance is unknown.

The increased $\dot{V}_E$ after cold and hot water exposures apparently medirespiratory centers directly through thermal receptors in the skin or indirectly through vascular pressure receptors (Keatinge and Evans, 1961; Keatinge and Nadel, 1965). The responses are too rapid to be caused by changes in temperature of deep tissues. Furthermore, it has been shown that lowering body temperature down to 1.1°C below normal has no effect on $\dot{V}_E$ (Whipp and Wasserman, 1970). Neither can the responses be attributed to changes in circulating catecholamines since these do not increase to any significant degree, at least during cold shower conditions (Keatinge *et al.*, 1964). Further support for the reflex hypothesis is based on the fact that the response can be significantly reduced by habituation (Keatinge and Evans, 1961) and, at least in hot water baths up to 39.5°C, does not even occur when temperature change is gradual rather than sudden (Bazett *et al.*, 1937).

b. *Metabolic Changes.* Early inferences about tissue utilization of oxygen at various temperatures were gained from studies of arterio-venous–oxygen differences measured in the forearm after it was immersed in cold, neutral, and hot water baths. The curve for O_2 saturation in forearm venous blood thus obtained by Goldschmidt and Light

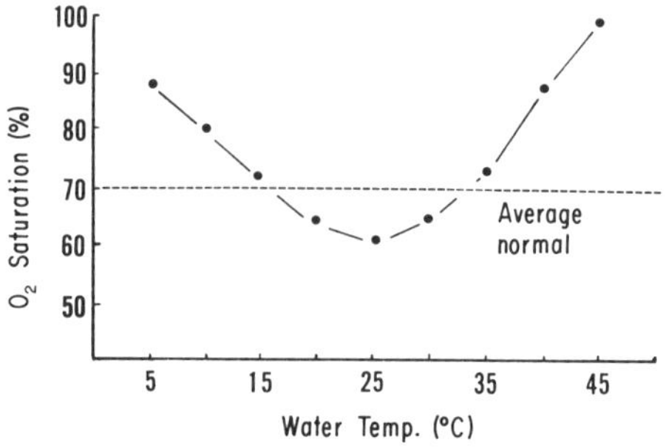

Fig. 10. Oxygen saturation of blood from veins of the forearm after immersion into water of various temperatures. (Redrawn from Goldschmidt and Light, 1925.)

(1925) is shown in Fig. 10. The curve shows the greatest arteriovenous difference at temperatures between 18° and 29°C. At both lower and higher temperatures, the arteriovenous–O_2 difference is smaller, suggesting a lower utilization of oxygen at these temperatures. The authors attributed the low utilization of O_2 at temperatures below 15°C to depression of metabolism by cooling of tissues and/or depression of dissociation of oxygen from hemoglobin. The former hypothesis was later confirmed by Bazett and Sribyatta (1928). However, the latter investigators did not feel that the decreased O_2 utilization at the lower temperatures could be due to failure of hemoglobin to release O_2 normally. This leaves operative the hypothesis that the decreased O_2 utilization is due to lower metabolism in the cooled tissue and is in agreement with the later interpretation of Clarke *et al.*, 1958b. The work of Goldschmidt and Light (1925) also suggests a lowered local oxygen consumption at temperatures above 35°C. Neither these authors nor Bazett and Sribyatta (1928) offer a satisfactory explanation for the results at higher temperatures, but it is quite unlikely that they are due to decreased local metabolism. Direct observations of local metabolism have identified a linear relationship between metabolism and local temperature (see Fig. 15 and Section III,A), with higher metabolism occurring at higher temperatures. It is more probable that the early results reflected vasodilatation in peripheral vessels as a consequence of the increased local temperature. This would result in a larger proportion of the venous flow being blood that had not passed through a capillary bed, and its oxygen content would be quite similar to that of arterial blood.

The literature on total metabolic responses to cold or hot applications indicates no change at rest when lower temperatures are applied unless shivering occurs (Craig and Dvorak, 1966). The increased O_2 consumption at or below the threshold for shivering is apparently due to the increased muscular activity associated with the shivering itself. Upon exposure to air or water at higher than normal body temperatures, oxygen consumption is increased, apparently as a result of accelerated chemical reactions due to increases in the mean temperature of the biological system (Hasan *et al.*, 1966). Hydrotherapy for 20 minutes at a temperature of 40°C causes a 16% increase in resting oxygen consumption (Dawson *et al.*, 1965). Similar increases have been noted for 15 to 20-minute hot air exposures at considerably higher temperatures in a sauna bath (Hasan *et al.*, 1966) and for hot exposures of 2½ hours at temperatures up to 50°C (Thauer, 1965).

It is unlikely that heat or moderate cold conditions have any effect on oxygen consumption levels during work. One group of investigators has claimed that energy expenditure during heat exposure is increased (Consolazio *et al.*, 1963). However, other workers have been unable to confirm their findings (Brouha *et al.*, 1963; Strydom *et al.*, 1966). Consolazio *et al.* (1963) based their conclusions on observed mean differences in O_2 consumption between work experiments in cool and warm environments. Strydom *et al.* (1966) later reworked the original data of the former group and were able to show by analysis of variance that the differences observed by them were not statistically significant.

Similarly, the volume of oxygen consumed is not different for standardized work loads when the individual is swimming in water at temperatures of 17.4°, 26.8°, and 33.1°C. However, the ventilatory equivalent ($\dot{V}_E/\dot{V}_{O_2}$) is lower during work at the intermediate temperature, indicating a more efficient respiration (Costill *et al.*, 1967).

6. *Connective Tissue and Joint Flexibility*

Joint flexibility is an important contributing factor in many areas of human performance. However, few studies of the effects of heat and cold applications on connective tissue extensibility and joint range of motion have been conducted.

It is known that heating of connective tissue increases its extensibility (Gersten, 1955), especially when combined with stretch during the heating and cooling process (Lehmann *et al.*, 1970). The type of heating modality employed appears to be a critical factor. Studies by Hollander and Horvath (1949) and Horvath and Hollander (1949) have shown that not all methods of "heating" are effective in raising intraarticular temperatures. Their work indicates that short-wave and microwave diathermy and paraffin are very effective in raising intraarticular temperature. Infrared radiation and hydrotherapy have little effect on these temperatures even though they raise skin temperature markedly. Paradoxically, hot packs decrease the intraarticular temperature as much as

2.2°F (a similar effect on muscle blood flow is discussed in Section II,B,3). Cold packs have opposite effects of the same magnitude.

Sechrist and Stull (1969) have compared mild activity (60 repetitions of joint flexion–extension), passive heating (10-minute immersion of joint in 45°C water), and passive cooling (10-minute immersion of joint in 10°C water) as to their effect on range of motion in the wrist, elbow, knee, and ankle joints. The authors concluded that mild activity and heating significantly increased joint range of motion but that cooling had no effect. However, it should be pointed out that the increases in range of motion were small, amounting to about 3%.

III. Effects of Heat and Cold Applications on Human Performance

A. Local Muscular Strength and Endurance

Because of the small number of studies that have investigated the effect of different levels of cold and heat applications on muscular strength and/or endurance, it is difficult to make conclusive statements. This problem is due mostly to the fact that significant differences exist among methods of investigation, range of temperatures studied, and duration of the cold and/or heat applications. The available evidence indicates that neither cold nor heat applications result in improved levels of strength. Work by Grose (1958) and Clarke and Royce (1962) wherein the forearm was immersed in water at 46°–48°C for 10 minutes indicated no significant change in strength expression of forearm muscles when compared with a control condition. In contrast, Clarke and Stelmach (1966), Robbins (1942), Sedgwick and Whalen (1964), Walters *et al.* (1960), and Hasan *et al.* (1967) reported decreases in muscle strength due to local and/or whole body heating. These decreases were in the range 4–7% of strength values exhibited under control conditions. The above results have been corroborated by studies on cats wherein moist heat was applied over the gastrocnemius muscle (Hall *et al.*, 1947). Strength reductions were attributed to reflex vasoconstriction within the muscle itself mediated through cutaneous receptors, since it was possible to abolish the effect by anesthetizing the skin with Butesin.

Cold apparently decreases contractile force when muscle temperature is below 27°C but is without effect above this temperature (Clarke *et al.*, 1958b). The muscle temperature of 27°C corresponds to a local water bath temperature of 18°C. Muscle temperature and not cutaneous temperature is the critical factor in force of contraction. In water at temperatures below 18°C the tension that can be exerted falls sharply with falling bath (and muscle) temperature to a value some 40% of the maximum at 2°C. Decreased contractile force at lower temperatures is believed to be a result of the more superficial and cooler fibers not contracting (Clarke *et al.*, 1958b). Fox (1961) has confirmed the above findings in a series of experiments assessing the effects of cold water immersion on typing speed. His subjects immersed their hands and forearms in water at various temperatures for 30 minutes. After removal they were rapidly dried and grip strength was measured before typing began. The grip strength levels as a percentage of control values are presented for various water temperatures in Fig. 11. The reduction in grip strength

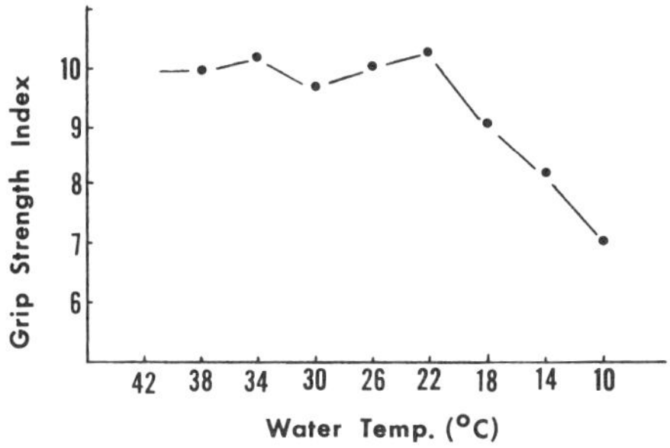

Fig. 11. The effect on grip strength of immersing both hands and forearms for half an hour in water of various temperatures. (Adapted from Fox, 1961.)

resulting from water bath applications at temperatures below 18°C has been further confirmed by Grose (1958), Clarke and Royce (1962), and Clarke and Stelmach (1966). They used water baths at 10°C and immersion was only for 10 minutes compared with 30 minutes in the studies previously cited. Strength reductions approximated 11–12% compared with a control condition. Grip strength force–time curves for control, hot water immersion, and cold water immersion are shown in Fig. 12. It is readily noted from Fig. 12 that the height of the force–time curve is reduced by the cold water immersion. In addition, the overall time of the release portion of the curve (not shown here) is increased by approximately 0.15 second. Similar results have been obtained from twitch tension curves recorded from the tibialis anterior muscle of cats (Maclagan and Zaimis, 1957). Earlier studies by Tuttle (1941) had demonstrated that latent time, contraction time, and relaxation time associated with involuntary contraction in the human gastrocnemius were all increased by packing the calf in ice for periods ranging between

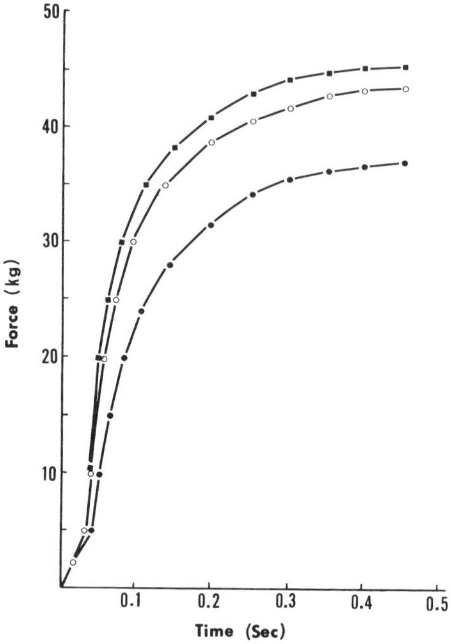

Fig. 12. Grip strength force–time curves for a control condition and after immersion of the forearm in hot (46°C) and cold (10°C) water for 10 minutes ($N = 31$): ■, hot; ○, control; ●, cold. (Adapted from Clarke and Royce, 1962.)

5 and 20 minutes. The degree of increase in the time of muscle response was proportional to the degree of cooling.

McGown (1967) has reported that 5 minutes of ice massage increases the isometric force exerted by the knee extensors. Since the ice massage would not be expected to lower deep-muscle temperature below 27°C (See Fig. 3), this result is not in conflict with the results of those studies utilizing water baths at temperatures below 18°C. It does seem to be in conflict with the work of Clarke *et al.* (1958b) and Fox (1961), who showed no strength change at muscle temperatures above 27°C. It could well be, however, that the different modality, ice massage, causes a greater psychological mobilization than does cold water immersion (McGown, 1967). A widely held thesis is that the expression of human strength is generally limited by psychologically induced inhibitions (Ikai and Steinhaus, 1961). If an enhanced psychological mobilization as postulated by McGown does occur, it could very well aid in overcoming some of the natural inhibitions to strength expression.

A muscle temperature of 27°C again assumes an important role when one examines the work on heat and cold effects on muscle endurance.

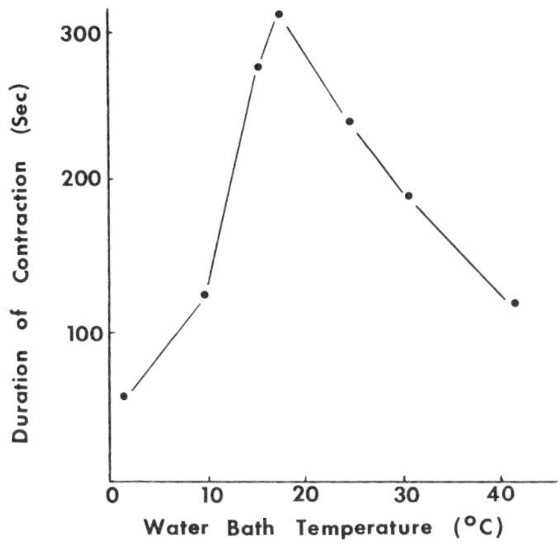

Fig. 13. Relation of water bath temperature and the duration of sustained contractions to fatigue in the forearm muscles. (Adapted from Clarke *et al.*, 1958b.)

Clarke *et al.* (1958b) have determined that a muscle temperature of 27°C (water bath 18°C) is optimal for sustained submaximal static contractions. At higher or lower temperatures, the time that the contraction can be held is reduced (Fig. 13). Investigations by Lind and Samueloff (1957) have confirmed that this temperature is optimal only if there is a relatively long interval between contractions (20 minutes). When the interval between contractions is reduced to 7 minutes, the sustained contractions can be held no longer at 18°C than at 34°C. Lind (1959) has concluded that the muscle temperature rises when the interval between contractions is short, thus abolishing the effect of the cold water bath. As with force of contraction, it appears that the muscle temperature itself is the critical determining factor. In the case of subjects with larger forearm diameters, longer endurance times are achieved at water bath temperatures somewhat below 18°C (about 14°C) probably because it takes the underlying muscle longer to cool to 27°C than in thinner arms (Clarke *et al.*, 1958b).

Earlier studies by Nukada (1955) and Nukada and Muller (1955) indicated that the endurance for both static and dynamic work could be increased by cold and decreased by hot applications. In the former study, subjects held a 5-kg weight at 90° of elbow flexion. With the elbow flexors precooled by water bath, the weight could be held for longer periods than when the same muscles were warmed by hot water baths or diathermy. This was true whether the circulation was free or occluded. In the second study, subjects worked a weight-loaded foot ergometer with the leg immersed in water. The temperature of the water varied from 10° to 40°C. The authors noted that the colder the skin temperature the longer the work output could be maintained.

Results similar to those of Clarke *et al.* (1958b) have been obtained by Clarke and Stelmach (1966), who investigated the effect of hot (46°C) and cold (10°C) water baths (10-minute duration) on maximal sustained static contraction. Hot water immersion resulted in a smaller total work output, while cold immersion seemed to have little, if any, effect. Neither hot nor cold water immersions during the subsequent 10-minute recovery period seemed to result in better recovery when compared with the control situation. Similarly, Clarke (1963) showed in an earlier study that immersing the arm in hot (46°C) or cold (10°C) water during a 10-minute recovery period after a 2-minute static contraction had no significant effect on strength of grip recovery curves.

The degree of postexercise hyperemia within a muscle group has been suggested as a relative measure of the fatiguing effect of a preceding muscle contraction (Andersen, 1968; Lind *et al.*, 1966). Higher levels of post exercise hyperemia are associated with a greater "blood debt" and, therefore, less efficient muscular contraction. Clarke and Hellon (1959) have shown that postexercise hyperemia is decreased after cooling in both sustained and slow rhythmic contractions, indicating a more efficient energy conversion. Cooling is ineffective in reducing the postexercise hyperemia associated with fast rhythmic contractions. Hyperemic responses to sustained and rhythmic contractions (both slow and fast) are illustrated in Fig. 14. Only in the case of sustained contraction is the postexercise hyperemia significantly reduced by bath temperatures that are below skin temperature (34°C). At the faster rates of rhythmic

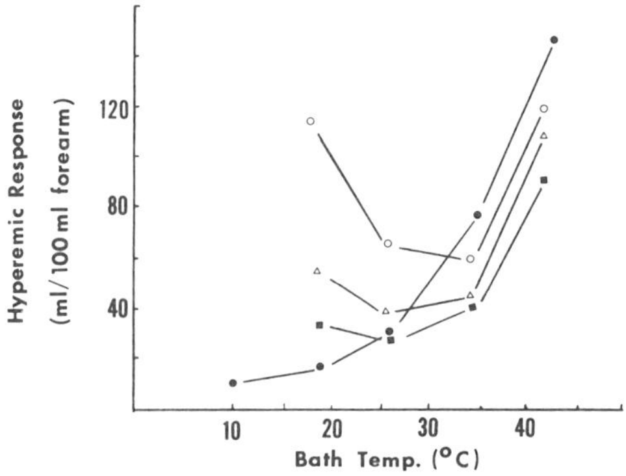

Fig. 14. Hyperemic responses after sustained and rhythmic contractions in the forearm at various water bath temperatures: ●, 1-minute sustained contraction; ■, rhythmic contractions for 1 minute at 30/minute; △, 45/minute; ○, 60/minute. (Redrawn from data presented by Clarke and Hellon, 1959.)

contraction, hyperemia at the colder temperatures is even increased, showing a trend similar to that of contractions in water above 34°C. These findings have been explained to be a result of increased viscosity in the muscles as a result of cooling. Therefore, more frequent contractions require a greater energy expenditure in order to overcome the viscosity. This leads to a greater demand for oxygen and, hence, a greater post-exercise blood flow associated with the muscular activity (Clarke and Hellon 1959).

Clarke *et al.* (1958b) have suggested that a 27°C muscle temperature is optimal for endurance because metabolism rises at muscle temperatures above 27°C, resulting in a more rapid accumulation of metabolites and leading to an earlier onset of fatigue. They further suggested that interference with neuromuscular transmission at temperatures below 27°C leads to a cessation of contraction in the cooler and more superficial fibers. This then results in a more rapid fatigue of the fibers that are still contracting. The results of several studies give at least partial support to the above hypotheses. It is known that muscle metabolism is directly related to local tissue temperature. Exposure of the tissues to local heat produces a definite rise in oxygen consumption, while cold has the opposite effect (Downey, 1964; Hasan *et al.*, 1966; Abramson *et al.*, 1957). The approximate O_2 consumption–temperature relationship for tissue temperatures between 24° and 40°C is shown in Fig. 15. Other workers have shown that motor nerve conduction can be either slowed or blocked by cooling (Abramson *et al.*, 1966; Bickford, 1939; Stevenson *et al.*, 1958). Interestingly enough, nerve conduction begins to fail at a temperature of approximately 27°C (Murphy, 1960).

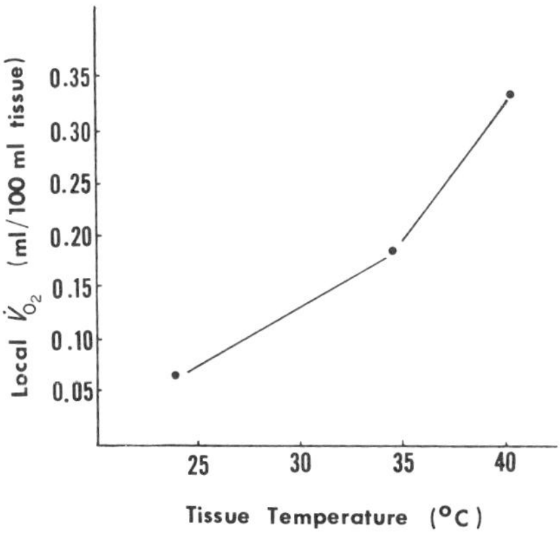

Fig. 15. Relationship between local tissue oxygen consumption and local temperature in 13 subjects. (Drawn from data presented by Abramson *et al.*, 1957.)

B. Work Output, Work Metabolism, and Circulatory Responses to Work Loads

Except for an early investigation by Asmussen and Bøje (1945), workers have been in agreement that hot applications generally reduce work output while cold applications increase it. The authors noted above claimed that the ability to do work was closely correlated with a rising internal temperature, especially within the muscles. They reported that "passive warming-up" by radiodiathermy and hot baths increased the capacity to do work in both a short, hard burst (12–15 seconds) and a more prolonged effort lasting 4–5 minutes. They also stated that a subject reached a higher maximal oxygen consumption when heated and that he needed less oxygen to perform a standard submaximal exercise.

These findings have not been confirmed to any extent by later investigators. In fact, there is general agreement that an elevated body temperature decreases physical performance, and most ergogenic studies have been aimed at keeping the body or various parts thereof cooled during work. It has already been noted that heat applications cause peripheral vasodilatation (Section II,B,3) leading to an increased skin blood flow. The increased flow to the skin vessels makes necessary an increased cardiac output in order to maintain adequate flow to the working muscles. If the environment is warm, sweating also begins. The dissipation of body heat through increased peripheral circulation and sweating places an extra burden on the circulatory system. When skin temperature is raised to 38.0–38.7°C cardiac output at a given oxygen consumption increases 14–19%, with a resultant reduction in stroke volume of 11–14% (Rowell *et al.*, 1969). These circulatory adjustments must, of necessity, lead to a lowered work output because a smaller volume of blood is available to the working muscles. Increased work output, decreased rectal temperature during work, decreased work heart rate, and decreased sweat production during work have been achieved with various forms of body cooling.

One popular ergogenic aid has been cold applications to the abdominal region by either cold pack or spray. It has been shown that abdominal cold packs applied for 10 minutes during a recovery period can increase the duration of a second bicycle ergometer ride (Happ *et al.*, 1949) or treadmill walk (Roundy and Cooney, 1968) immediately following the 10-minute recovery period. It has also been noted that the oxygen requirement for a given amount of work is reduced by applying abdominal cold packs before the work begins (Happ *et al.*, 1949).

Another form of ergogenic aid that has found wide use is the cold shower. It has been noted that repeat performances on the bicycle ergometer and treadmill can be prolonged by applying this modality during rest periods between exercise (Roundy and Cooney, 1968; Falls and Richardson, 1967). The use of showers as a form of cold application appears to be somewhat more thoroughly investigated than cold packs or other procedures of application. Falls (1969) has shown that pulse rates during a standard submaximal treadmill walk are significantly reduced by 10-minute cold showers even when the interval between shower and work is 20 minutes. Intervals of 30 minutes between shower and work resulted in exercise and recovery pulse rates that were lower than controls, but they were not significantly lower (Fig. 16). The level to which pulse rate is lowered during submaximal exercise appears to be related to the average skin temperature achieved as a result of the cold application (Falls and Humphrey, 1970). The same situation seems to hold for cold water immersion (Goff *et al.*, 1956).

Cooling the working muscles in water baths during rest pauses results in a large increment in work output due to the fact that fatigue is delayed. In one experiment, subjects performed 5-minute periods of heavy work on a leg ergometer with 10-minute rest pauses interspersed between them under a control condition and one in which the legs were

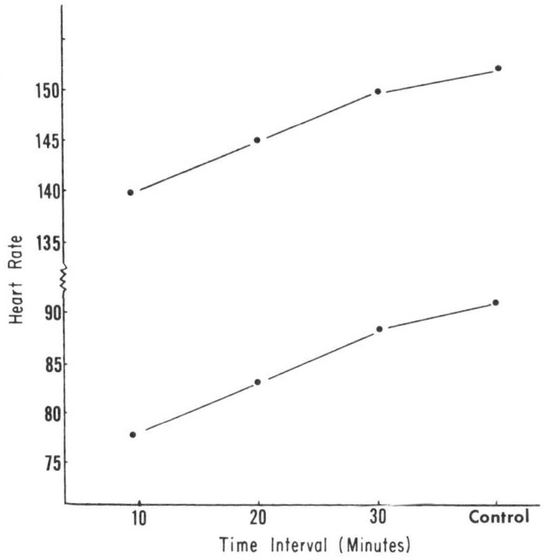

Fig. 16. Exercise (upper curve) and recovery (lower curve) heart rates after various time lapses between a cold shower (10 minutes at 68°F) and a 5-minute walk at 4 mph and 6% grade on a motor-driven treadmill. Recovery pulse rates were an average of the last 3 minutes of the 5-minute period immediately postexercise. (From Falls, 1969.)

immersed in water baths at 15°C during the rest pauses. Without cooling, the subjects were able to complete only two of the 5-minute work cycles because of the circulatory strain. With cooling they were able to complete five work cycles with very little evidence of circulatory strain (Muller, 1965). In the same series of studies it was further demonstrated that footwork in a water bath resulted in exercise and recovery pulse rates directly related to the temperature of the water bath in which the work was performed (Fig. 17).

The use of water bath immersions during or after work as an ergogenic aid is not feasible in many industrial situations or in space travel. However, rather high work loads must often be sustained in these situations. These problems have long been recognized, and the recent greater availability of federal funds has stimulated significant research on the effectiveness and feasibility of various types of water-cooled clothing. Most of this work has been concerned with cooling a portion of the individual's body by circulating cold water through tubing networks running through specially designed garments (Webb and Annis, 1968; Waligora and Michel, 1968; Rowell *et al.*, 1969). Other applications have included water cooled rectangular pads connected to a refrigerated tank and placed over the scapular, abdominal, and thigh regions (Byrne, 1968) and perforated suits containing dry ice (Petit *et al.*, 1970). Figure 18 illustrates the results of one experiment with a water-cooled suit. Sweat rate was restricted to less than 100 gm/hour. Rectal temperature (T_r),

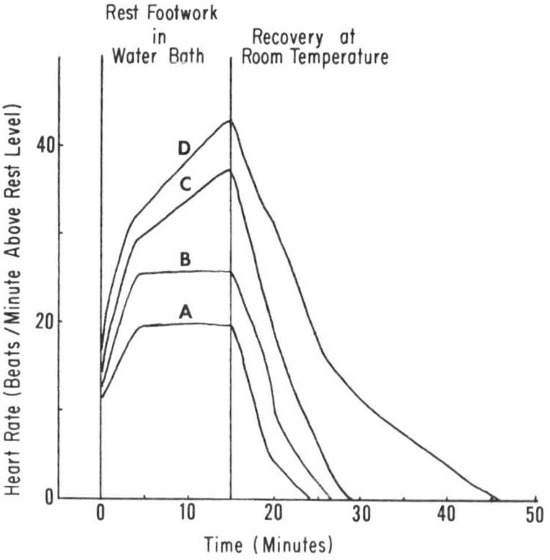

Fig. 17. Effect on exercise and recovery heart rates of doing 15 minutes of footwork in water baths at various temperatures. Bath temperatures were A, 16°C; B, 20°C; C, 30°C; and D, 40°C. (Redrawn from Muller, 1965.)

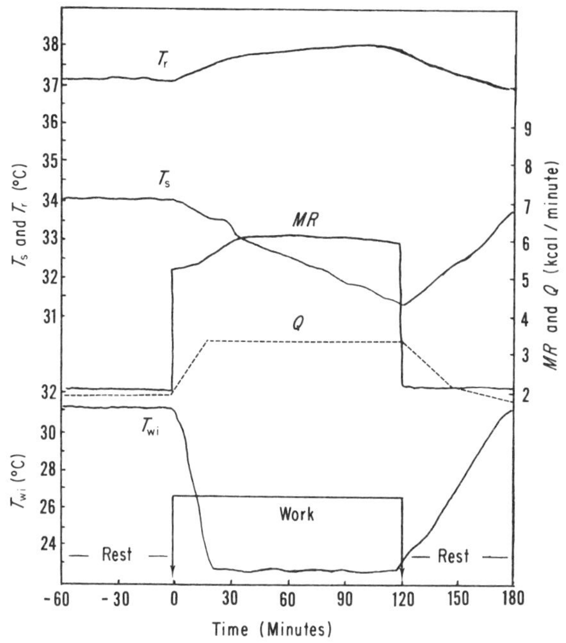

Fig. 18. Averaged data from six experiments in which subjects were cooled by controlling the water inlet temperature (T_{wi}) to a water-cooled suit while resting and while working at 5–6 kcal/minute for 2 hours. Heat loss (Q) is heat removed in the water-cooled suit plus a small evaporative heat loss; T_s and T_r are skin and rectal temperatures, respectively; MR is metabolic rate. Sweat loss was restricted to 100 gm/hour. (Redrawn from Webb and Annis, 1968.)

skin temperature (T_s), metabolic rate (MR) in kilocalories per minute, and heat loss (Q) in kilocalories per minute are shown in the upper portion of the figure. Water inlet temperature (T_{wi}) necessary to suppress the sweat rate below 100 gm/hour is shown in the lower portion of the figure.

The same type of cooling has been effective in reducing the physiological strain associated with exposure to hot environments (Petit *et al.*, 1970; Shvartz, 1970; Gold and Zornitzer, 1968; Shvartz and Benor, 1971). A water-cooled suit covering the chest, back, upper arms, and thighs reduced the modified Craig index of physiological strain* (I_s) 17–25% during short treadmill walks at 0 and 5% grade in environments with dry bulb temperatures of 40–50°C (Fig. 19) (Gold and Zornitzer, 1968).

* Modified Craig index of physiological strain (I_s): $I_s = HR/100 + \Delta T_r + \Delta Wt_n$, where HR is terminal heart rate (beats per minute), ΔT_r is increase in rectal temperature (degrees centigrade per hour), and ΔWt_n is sweat production (nude weight loss, kilograms per hour).

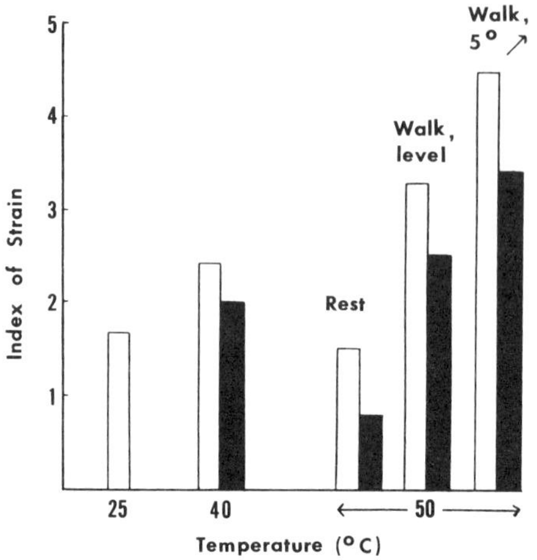

Fig. 19. Mean indices of physiological strain after 1 hour of work on a treadmill (30 minutes at 3 kph; 30 minutes at 5 kph) or rest with (solid bars) and without (open bars) partial body cooling. Environmental temperatures were 25°, 40°, and 50°C. (Redrawn from Gold and Zornitzer, 1968.)

The inlet temperature of the water was kept at 20°–21°C. The suit used in the work described here did not cool the abdominal area. It is quite possible that further reductions in physiological strain could have been achieved by cooling that part of the anatomy. It has been contended that cold applied to the abdomen is generally more effective as an ergogenic aid than applications to the back or thigh areas (Byrne, 1968). Adding a cooling hood to the type of suit described above results in additional reductions in physiological strain (Shvartz, 1970). In 2 hours of moderate work at 50°C dry bulb and 20% relative humidity, the hood portion of the apparatus, worn without the body garment, accounted for approximately 50% of the total reductions achieved in rectal temperature and heart rate (Fig. 20).

These results have been corroborated by Nunneley *et al.* (1971), who investigated the efficacy of a cooling cap consisting of a tygon tubing network that covered the scalp, cheeks, and neck. Cool water was forced through at various flow rate and temperature combinations. The authors found they could remove over 2 kcal/minute of metabolic heat with this device. The head apparently is an effective heat dissipation area due to the absence of vasoconstrictive innervation comparable to that in other areas of the body (Nunneley *et al.*, 1971).

The reductions in physiological strain noted in the foregoing discussion are undoubtedly a function of both central and peripheral effects of heat and are, therefore, highly related to both core and skin tempera-

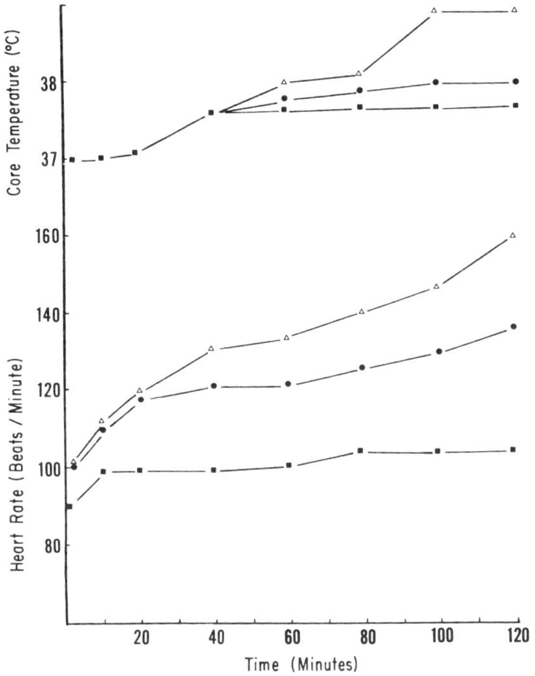

Fig. 20. Mean heart rate and core temperatures of six subjects during 2 hours of moderate work in cooling and no-cooling conditions. Environmental conditions were 50°C dry bulb and 20% relative humidity. No cooling, △; hood, ●; suit and hood, ■. (Redrawn from Shvartz, 1970.)

tures. Consequently, any cooling modality that reduces mean body temperature sufficiently would be expected to reduce the physiological strain of combined heat–exercise stresses. Water applications always appear so prominently because of the high heat capacity of water. The specific heat of water is approximately 1000 times that of air. In addition, the rate of transfer of heat by conduction in water is 25 times greater than in air (McNutt, 1966). It is small wonder that water is such an effective cooling medium. Nonetheless, successful reductions in physiological strain have been achieved by air cooling during moderate work (Webb and Annis, 1968), prior to exposure to high heat loads (Veghte and Webb, 1961), and during work in protective clothing while exposed to heat loads (Brown, 1965). Figure 21 shows the effect that wearing ventilated and nonventilated protective clothing has on working men exposed to heat load in an industrial setting. The air passing through the suit was only slightly cooler than normal skin temperature (26°–33°C).

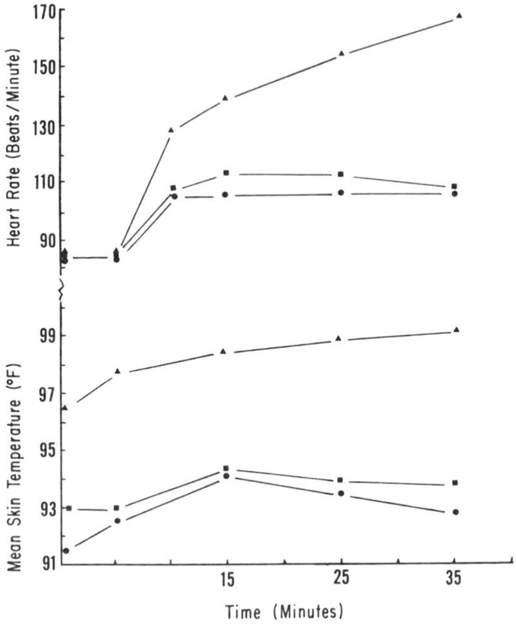

Fig. 21. Pulse rate and mean skin temperatures of men working in ventilated and nonventilated polyvinal suits. ▲, nonventilated; ■, suit only ventilated; ●, suit and hood ventilated. (Adapted from Brown, 1965.)

It has been shown that simply holding cold wet towels on the abdomen and draping them over the head during frequent rest pauses while a subject works in a hot, humid environment can reduce I_s significantly under its level during the same work without cooling. The towels were soaked in ice water at 1°C. Taking a 10-minute cold shower (14.8°C) 10 minutes prior to the exposure resulted in additional reductions (Falls and Humphrey, 1971). These effects are illustrated in Fig. 22. The reduction in physiological strain as a result of preexposure cooling is not a unique finding. Veghte and Webb (1961) cooled subjects with −1° and +7°C air and 16°C water for 30-, 60-, and 90-minute periods prior to exposures to high radiant heat loads (71°C). Air cooling increased tolerance times by at least 50% while water cooling increased them 50–80%. The tolerance times were highly related to mean body temperature prior to exposure. Mean body temperature was calculated as ⅓ skin + ⅔ rectal temperature. Similar effects of precooling have recently been noted by other investigators (Sinha and Verghese, 1969).

In regard to the application of ergogenic cooling during work, it appears that timing of the application is critical. Webb and Annis (1968)

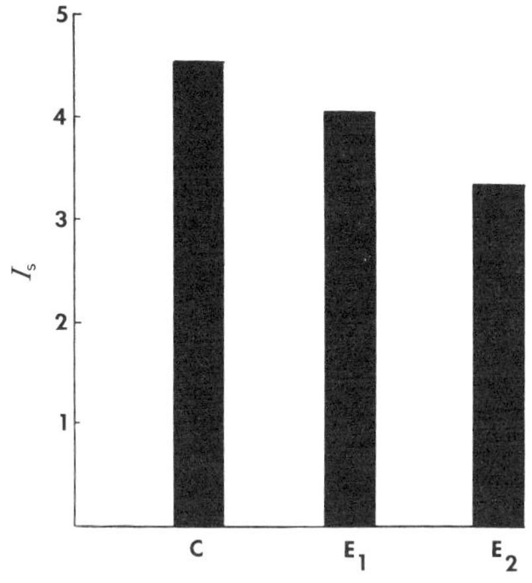

Fig. 22. Mean I_s (modified Craig index of physiological strain) values of six subjects working in a hot, humid environment (40.6°C dry bulb, 28.3°C wet bulb) for 1 hour. The subjects alternated 5 minutes of work with 1 minute of rest: C, control, no cooling; E_1, cold towel applications (1°C) to abdomen and head during the rest periods; E_2, same as E_1 except for a preexercise 10-minute cold shower at 14.8°C. (Drawn from data presented by Falls and Humphrey, 1971.)

and Nunneley *et al.* (1971) have presented evidence that cooling immediately at the beginning of work is less effective than cooling at a later time. Best results appear to be obtained when cooling is applied gradually along an exponential curve as work progresses (Nunneley *et al.*, 1971). This effect has been attributed to the fact that heat is not yet reaching the body surface and the resulting cold vasoconstriction limits later heat removal. It should be noted that the suppression of heat removal was observed coincidently with the application of very cold water cooling (5°C) and the effect may not be operative in cooling at more moderate temperatures.

C. Athletic Performance

Although very little research of this nature has been conducted, this section will deal with the effects of heat and cold applications on performance in athletic events or in events of an athletic nature, e.g., pedaling a bicycle ergometer for speed.

Arguments in favor of warm-up as an aid to performance are often supported by citing the study conducted by Asmussen and Bøje (1945). These authors observed improved sprint and endurance times on a bicycle ergometer in subjects who were "warmed up" in comparison with the same performances in a "cold" condition. Warming up consisted of, in addition to preliminary work on the bicycle ergometer, hot showers and application of short-wave radiodiathermy. The "cold" condition was one of exercise without warm-up and following a rest period. They reported decreases in sprint time (956 kg total work) ranging between 4.7 and 7.2% after both hot showers (10 minutes at 47°C) and radiodiathermy. Radiodiathermy increased endurance time (9680 kg total work) 3.9–7.6%. The authors, interestingly enough, did not report any results for the effect that hot showers might have had on endurance time. Since their study is very detailed, it seems unlikely that they did not investigate the effect. One must, therefore, conclude that this result was not in favor of the hot showers.

Similar results have been obtained in later studies on swimmers by Muido (1946) and Carlile (1956). Both authors observed improved times in swims ranging between 40 and 220 yd. In the former study, showers were 15–18 minutes at 40°–43°C, and in the latter study they were 8 minutes at 40.6°C. Both authors reported that these showers were too long and/or too hot for at least some subjects. Dizziness was reported and, in some cases, a rest period was necessary before swimming began. Reported improvements in time were in the range of 1–4%, mostly 1–2%. Muido (1946) also investigated the effect of cold water immersion (standing 12–15 minutes in pool water at 21°C) on performance and reported a decrement of 3.6–6.3%.

Although Asmussen and Bøje (1945), Muido (1946), and Carlile (1956) all reported improved performances after use of hot showers, they could not agree on whether core or muscle temperature was the predominating factor. Asmussen and Bøje (1945) presented a convincing argument favoring the level of muscle temperature being the major explanation for variations in performance between "warm" and "cold" conditions. Carlile (1956) was in agreement, while Muido (1946) felt that changes in blood temperature accounted for his findings. More detailed discussion of the performances of "warm" and "cold" muscles is provided in Chapter 6.

At least one study is available that contradicts the results of Muido (1946) and Carlile (1956). de Vries (1959), who experimented with 6-minute showers at as hot a temperature as the subject could withstand, found them to be without effect on 100-yd swim times.

The effect on performance of swimming in water at various temperatures has been investigated. Adee (1953) had subjects complete, in addition to a 20-minute paced swim, 50-yd and 1500-m time trials in water varying in temperature between 17° and 34.4°C. In both the dash and endurance events the best performances occurred when the rectal temperature after exercise was approximately 38°C. The 50-yd swim was best performed in the warmer water temperatures, while the 1500-m times were best at water temperatures between 23.3°–26.2°C. From his results, the author concluded that muscle stiffness associated with high muscle viscosity is a limiting factor when one works at lower rectal temperatures and that poor cardiovascular performance occurs in events where one works at higher rectal temperatures. His results suggest an optimal rectal tempeature near 38°C.

An investigation by Costill *et al.* (1967) lends further support to the possibility that for endurance swims best performances are likely to occur at intermediate water temperatures. These authors investigated metabolic and circulatory responses to standardized, submaximal 20-minute swims in water at 17.4°, 26.8°, and 33.1°C. Exercise and recovery heart rates were positively related to water temperature, while there was no significant difference in oxygen consumption at the three temperatures. Ventilatory efficiency ratio ($VE_{O_2} = \dot{V}_E/\dot{V}_{O_2}$) was about 2 liters/minute less during exercise in the 26.8°C water, suggesting, perhaps, a reduced stimulus to respiration from anaerobic metabolism. The 26.8°C is, of course, near the upper end of the optimal range of water temperatures obtained by Adee (1953).

Other investigators have been interested in the effect of cold applications on running performance. Sills and O'Riley (1956) reported that cold spray to the abdomen (6.6°–8.9°C for 8 minutes) during a rest pause between two bouts of spot running improved performance in the second bout when the number of steps achieved was the criterion of performance. Similarly, Rosen (1952) demonstrated improvements in a repeat performance of the 440-yard dash by applying cold abdominal spray during a 20-minute rest period between the sprints. The second 440 was on the average 1.4 second slower with rest only between the two races and only 0.8 second slower when the cold spray was used. Temperature of the water used for spraying started at 21°C and was gradually reduced to 7.2°C. The spray was maintained for 5 minutes. Kahler (1968), who investigated the effect of abdominal ice packs on performance in an initial 440 as well as a repeat performance, was unable to corroborate Rosen's results. Kahler found the abdominal ice packs to be without effect on performance. Packs were applied for a 10-minute period prior to each race.

Results of research on athletic performance after hot and/or cold applications are obviously, at best, contradictory—more so than research results utilizing physiological responses as a criterion of effect. The inconsistency of results can possibly be explained in part by the psychological impact of the situation on the research subject. First, athletic performance would be expected to vary widely from day to day because of general mental attitude, environmental factors, motivation, etc., especially in the case of untrained subjects. These fluctuations in performance inflate experimental errors and tend to mask real differences even where they may exist unless the research design is extremely sensitive. Second, the athlete himself may have a bias toward one experimental treatment versus another. If, for example, he is fully sold on the proposition that "warm-up" is beneficial to him and might prevent injury, it is unlikely that he would make a maximal effort in a "cold" condition out of fear of sustaining injury. In laboratory situations, the above problems are more easily controlled.

IV. Summary

The preponderance of literature related to the subject indicates that cold applications are more likely than hot applications to prove effective as an ergogenic aid to muscular performance and that cold water is the most effective means of application because of its high heat capacity. A cold application is most likely to be ergogenic if the performance is of an endurance nature and the effect of the application is at least partially dependent on circulatory function. Neither hot nor cold applications are likely to have an enhancing effect on the expression of human strength. However, application of hot or cold at extreme temperatures is likely to decrease the contractile force of a muscle (see Section III,A).

The potential benefit of cold and the detrimental effect of heat in regard to endurance performance reside in the fact that they are capable of altering the relationship between muscle and skin blood flow (Sections II,B,3 and 4). Cold causes a peripheral vasoconstriction and, apparently, at the same time a reflex vasodilatation within the muscle. The constriction of peripheral vessels and dilatation of muscle vessels causes a shift of blood from the skin to the muscles. As a result, a smaller overall cardiac output is required in order to perform a given amount of work. The external application of cold aids the central circulation (and hence muscle blood flow) still further because the cooler body surface enhances heat dissipation by simple conduction through body tissues. As a result, less peripheral blood flow is needed for this purpose.

Application of external heat produces effects opposite to those of cold application. Skin blood flow increases while muscle flow decreases reflexly. As a result, a greater cardiac output is required in order to maintain a given work rate under conditions of heat application. One specially complicating factor associated with external heat application is the effect it has on the body's thermoregulation. If adequate thermoregulation is to be maintained, skin temperature must remain at least 1.1°C (2°F) below core temperature. If this gradient is not maintained, the body will have increasing degrees of difficulty in transferring heat to the environment. As a result, core temperature will rise. This, in itself, often leads to fatigue and exhaustion, thereby decreasing performance or work output (Lind, 1964).

Even though cold applications appear to enhance work output, their indiscriminate use is not warranted. There appear to be optimal temperatures at which the beneficial effects occur. Full vasoconstriction in peripheral vessels has been reported to occur at 24°C (Downey *et al.*, 1968), and no beneficial effects of cooling have been reported to occur at surface temperatures below about 18°C. The concept of an adequately high muscle temperature is not to be ignored, and it is quite likely that extremely cold surface temperatures cause enough heat to be conducted away from the deeper-lying muscle that it cannot function properly. In the same sense, the muscle temperature can also apparently be too high for optimal function (Section III,A).

It should be borne in mind that the optimal levels of temperature vary among individuals. For instance, fatter persons show lower skin temperatures and higher core temperatures in response to standard cold exposures than do thinner subjects (Section II,B,1 and Fig. 2). Similarly, when partial body cooling is utilized, the applications required to attain optimal effects in individuals with thicker body segments are usually colder than those required for individuals with thinner segments (Clarke *et al.*, 1958b). In addition, there appears to be a differential effect of whole body cooling depending on the state of physical conditioning. It has been noted that conditioned men respond with greater heart rate decreases after cold showers than do poorly conditioned men (Michael, 1957). A conditioned individual would almost certainly respond better to heat applications (in the sense that there would be less adverse effect on his circulation and core temperature) than a nonconditioned person (Bass, 1971). Furthermore, it appears that the timing of a cold application is extremely important in certain work situations. It has been shown that, for some types of combined exercise–heat stress, cold applied gradually and at moderately cold temperatures is more effective in reducing the stress than when cooling begins immediately or is at extremely cold levels (Nunneley *et al.*, 1971).

Just as heat applications can cause increased peripheral circulation, body heat storage, and sweating—all imposing an additional burden on the central circulation—cold applications at temperatures that are too low may cause shivering and the associated extra metabolic activity that could abolish some or all of the ergogenic effects of a specific cold application. The onset of shivering varies directly with body composition, skin and core temperature, time of year, and length of exposure, but it usually occurs at a skin temperature of 25°–30°C (Carlson, 1964). Additionally, repeated use of a specific heat or cold application may cause habituation and abolish ergogenic effects that might be expected from future use of the modality (Section III,B,4 and Glaser *et al.*, 1959).

Even though thermal applications may mediate physiological changes that in certain instances are consonant with improved muscular performance, much more research is needed to identify the optimal levels of these applications for different individuals. Also, any interaction between commonly utilized physical warm-up procedures and thermal applications needs to be elucidated. On the surface, it would appear that physical warm-up and cold applications are diametrical opposites. However, closer examination reveals that both physical warm-up and cold application have as an objective increased muscle blood flow (Section II,B,3, Fig. 7, and Chapter 6). It has also been postulated that warm-up and cold water applications are similar in their cooling effect on the skin blood vessels (Muller, 1965). When an athlete "warms up" he begins to sweat. The movement of his body through the surrounding air causes rapid sweat evaporation. This has a cooling effect on the skin, and its temperature is lowered several degrees (Buskirk and Bass, 1960). As a consequence, peripheral blood vessels would be expected to constrict just as they do in cold application, forcing more blood into the muscle areas. Since external cooling and physical warm-up appear to have a similar effect on circulation in the muscle and skin, it is not unlikely that future research efforts will identify some combination of these procedures as having a maximal ergogenic effect on muscular performance.

References

Abdel-Sayed, W. A., Abboud, F. M., and Calvelo, M. G. (1970). *J. Appl. Physiol.* **219**, 1772.

Abramson, D. I., Kahn, A., Tuck, S., Turman, G. A., Rejal, H., and Fleischer, C. J. (1957). *J. Lab. Clin. Med.* **50**, 789.

Abramson, D. I., Kahn, A., Rejal, H., Turman, G. A., Tuck, S., and Fleischer, C. J. (1958). *J. Clin. Invest.* **37**, 1039.

Abramson, D. I., Chu, L. S. W., Tuck, S., Lee, S. W., Richardson, G., and Levin, M. (1966). *J. Amer. Med. Ass.* **198**, 156.
Adee, D. (1953). *Diss. Abstr.* **13**, 713.
Aikas, E., Karvonen, M. J., Piironen, P., and Ruosteenoja, R. (1962). *Acta Physiol. Scand.* **54**, 366.
Andersen, K. L. (1968). *In* "Exercise Physiology" (H. B. Falls, ed.), pp. 79–128. Academic Press, New York.
Asmussen, E., and Bøje, O. (1945). *Acta Physiol. Scand.* **10**, 1.
Baker, P. T., and Daniels, F. (1956). *J. Appl. Physiol.* **8**, 409.
Barcroft, H., Bock, K. D., Hensel, H., and Kitchin, A. H. (1955). *Arch. Gesamte Physiol. Menschen Tiere* **261**, 199.
Bass, D. E. (1971). *In* "Encyclopedia of Sports Sciences and Medicine" (L. A. Larson, ed.), pp. 1581–1585. Macmillan, New York.
Bazett, H. C. (1924). *Amer. J. Physiol.* **70**, 412.
Bazett, H. C., and Sribyatta, L. (1928). *Amer. J. Physiol.* **86**, 565.
Bazett, H. C., Scott, J. C., Maxfield, M. E., and Blithe, M. D. (1937). *Amer. J. Physiol.* **119**, 93.
Behnke, A. R., and Yaglou, C. P. (1951). *J. Appl. Physiol.* **3**, 591.
Bickford, R. G. (1939). *Clin. Sci.* **4**, 159.
Brouha, L., Maxfield, M. E., Smith, P. E., and Stopps, G. J. (1963). *J. Appl. Physiol.* **18**, 1095.
Brown, J. R. (1965). *Med. Ser. J. Can.* **21**, 518.
Buskirk, E. R., and Bass, D. E. (1960). *In* "Science and Medicine of Exercise and Sports" (W. R. Johnson, ed.), pp. 311–338, Harper, New York.
Byrne, T. G. (1968). U.S. Aeromedical Research Lab Report AMRL-TR-66-188.
Carlile, F. (1956). *Res. Quart.* **27**, 143.
Carlson, L. D. (1964). *In* "Medical Climatology" (S. Licht, ed.), pp. 196–228. Elizabeth Licht, New Haven, Connecticut.
Clarke, D. H. (1963). *Arch. Phys. Med. Rehabil.* **44**, 565.
Clarke, D. H., and Royce, J. (1962). *Int. Z. Angew. Physiol. Einschl. Arbeitsphysiol.* **19**, 330.
Clarke, D. H., and Stelmach, G. (1966). *Res. Quart.* **37**, 468.
Clarke, R. S. J., and Hellon, R. F. (1959). *J. Physiol. (London)* **145**, 447.
Clarke, R. S. J., Hellon, R. F., and Lind, A. R. (1958a). *Clin. Sci.* **17**, 165.
Clarke, R. S. J., Hellon, R. F., and Lind, A. R. (1958b). *J. Physiol. (London)* **143**, 454.
Consolazio, C. F., Matoush, L. O., Nelson, R. A., Torres, J. B., Issac, G. J. (1963). *J. Appl. Physiol.* **18**, 65.
Costill, D. L., Cahill, P. J., and Eddy, D. (1967). *J. Appl. Physiol.* **22**, 628.
Craig, A. B., and Dvorak, M. (1966). *J. Appl. Physiol.* **21**, 1577.
Dawson, W. J., Kottke, F. J., Kubicek, W. G., Olson, M. E., Harsted, K., Bearman, J. E., Canner, P. L., and Canterbury, J. B. (1965). *Arch. Phys. Med. Rehabil.* **46**, 605.
de Vries, H. A. (1959). *Res. Quart.* **30**, 11.
Downey, J. A. (1964). *J. Amer. Phys. Ther. Ass.* **44**, 713.
Downey, J. A., Darling, R. C., and Miller, J. M. (1968). *Arch. Phys. Med. Rehabil.* **49**, 308.
Edholm, O. G., Fox, R. H., and Macpherson, R. K. (1956). *J. Physiol. (London)* **134**, 612.
Falls, H. B. (1969). *Res. Quart.* **40**, 45.

Falls, H. B., and Humphrey, L. D. (1970). *Res. Quart.* **41**, 353.
Falls, H. B., and Humphrey, L. D. (1971). *Res. Quart.* **42**, 21.
Falls, H. B., and Richardson, R. D. (1967). *Res. Quart.* **38**, 550.
Falls, H. B., and Wiebers, J. E. (1965). *Res. Quart.* **36**, 243.
Fischer, E., and Solomon, S. (1965). *In* "Therapeutic Heat" (S. Licht, ed.), pp. 127–169, Elizabeth Licht, New Haven, Connecticut.
Folk, G. E. (1966). "Introduction to Environmental Physiology." Lea & Febiger, Philadelphia, Pennsylvania.
Fox, R. H. (1961). *Brit. Med. Bull.* **17**, 14.
Gersten, J. W. (1955). *Amer. J. Phys. Med.* **34**, 362.
Glaser, E. M., Hall, M. S., and Whittow, G. C. (1959). *J. Physiol.* (*London*) **146**, 152.
Goff, L. G., Brubach, H. F., Specht, H., and Smith, N. (1956). *J. Appl. Physiol.* **9**, 59.
Gold, A. J., and Zornitzer, A. (1968). *Aerosp. Med.* **39**, 944.
Goldschmidt, S., and Light, A. B. (1925). *Amer. J. Physiol.* **73**, 146.
Grose, J. E. (1958). *Res. Quart.* **29**, 19.
Hall, V. E., Munoz, E., and Fitch, B. (1947). *Arch. Phys. Med. Rehabil.* **28**, 493.
Happ, W. P., Tuttle, W. W., and Wilson, M. (1949). *Res. Quart.* **20**, 153.
Hasan, J., Karvonen, M. J., and Piironen, P. (1966). *Amer. J. Phys. Med.* **45**, 296.
Hasan, J., Karvonen, M. J., and Piironen, P. (1967). *Amer. J. Phys. Med.* **46**, 1226.
Hertzman, A. B. (1953). *Amer. J. Phys. Med.* **32**, 233.
Hollander, J. L., and Horvath, S. M. (1949). *Arch. Phys. Med. Rehabil.* **30**, 437.
Horvath, S. M., and Botelho, S. Y. (1949). *J. Appl. Physiol.* **1**, 586.
Horvath, S. M., and Hollander, J. L. (1949). *J. Clin. Invest.* **28**, 469.
Iampietro, P. F., and Adams, T. (1968). *In* "Exercise Physiology" (H. B. Falls, ed.), pp. 173–197. Academic Press, New York.
Ikai, M., and Steinhaus, A. H. (1961). *J. Appl. Physiol.* **16**, 157.
Kahler, R. W. (1968). *Quart. Rev. U. S. Track Coaches Ass.* p. 56.
Keatinge, W. R. (1961). *Quart. J. Exp. Physiol.* **46**, 69.
Keatinge, W. R. (1969). "Survival in Cold Water." Blackwell, Oxford.
Keatinge, W. R., and Evans, M. (1961). *Quart. J. Exp. Physiol.* **46**, 83.
Keatinge, W. R., and Nadel, J. A. (1965). *J. Appl. Physiol.* **20**, 65.
Keatinge, W. R., McIlroy, M. B., and Goldfien, A. (1964). *J. Appl. Physiol.* **19**, 1145.
Landis, E. M., Long, W. L., Dunn, J. W., Jackson, C. L., and Meyer, U. (1926). *Amer. J. Physiol.* **76**, 35.
LeBlanc, J. (1954). *Can. J. Biochem. Physiol.* **32**, 354.
Lee, D. H. K. (1964). Public Health Monograph 72. U.S. Department of Health, Education, and Welfare, Washington, D. C.
Lehmann, J. F., Masock, A. J., Warren, C. G., and Koblanski, J. N. (1970). *Arch. Phys. Med. Rehabil.* **51**, 481.
Leithead, C. S., and Lind, A. R. (1964). "Heat Stress and Heat Disorders." Davis, Philadelphia, Pennsylvania.
Lewis, T. (1930). *Heart* **15**, 177.
Licht, S. (1965). *In* "Therapeutic Heat" (S. Licht, ed.), pp. 538–563. Elizabeth Licht, New Haven, Connecticut.
Lind, A. R. (1959). *J. Physiol.* (*London*) **147**, 162.
Lind, A. R. (1964). *In* "Medical Climatology" (S. Licht, ed.), pp. 164–195. Elizabeth Licht, New Haven, Connecticut.
Lind, A. R., and Samueloff, M. (1957). *J. Physiol.* (*London*) **136**, 12P.

Lind, A. R., McNicol, G. W., and Donald, K. W. (1966). *In* "Physical Activity in Health and Disease" (K. L. Andersen, ed.), pp. 38–63. Oslo Univ. Press, Oslo.

McGown, H. L. (1967). *Phys. Ther.* **47,** 185.

Maclagan, J., and Zaimis, E. (1957). *J. Physiol.* (*London*) **136,** 89P.

McNutt, D. (1966). *J. Sports Med. Phys. Fitness* (*Italy*) **6,** 134.

Michael, E. D. (1957). *Res. Quart.* **28,** 38.

Millard, J. B. (1965). *In* "Therapeutic Heat" (S. Licht, ed.), pp. 240–251. Elizabeth Licht, New Haven, Connecticut.

Muido, L. (1946). *Acta Physiol. Scand.* **12,** 102.

Muller, E. A. (1965). *Ergonomics* **8,** 409.

Murphy, A. J. (1960). *Phys. Ther. Rev.* **40,** 112.

Nukada, A. (1955). *Int. Z. Angew. Physiol. Einschl. Arbeitsphysiol.* **16,** 74.

Nukada, A., and Muller, E. A. (1955). *Int. Z. Angew. Physiol. Einschl. Arbeitsphysiol.* **16,** 61.

Nunneley, S. A., Troutman, S. J., and Webb, P. (1971). *Aerosp. Med.* **42,** 64.

Petit, J. M., Hausman, A., Pirnay, F., and Deroanne, R. (1970). *Arch. Environ. Health* **20,** 274.

Reader, S. R., and Whyte, H. M. (1951). *J. Appl. Physiol.* **4,** 396.

Robbins, A. C. (1942). *Res. Quart.* **13,** 373.

Roddie, I. C., Shepherd, J. T., and Whelan, R. F. (1956). *J. Physiol.* (*London*) **134,** 444.

Rosen, M. (1952). *Res. Quart.* **23,** 226.

Roundy, E. S., and Cooney, L. D. (1968). *Res. Quart.* **39,** 690.

Rowell, L. B., Murray, J. A., Brengelmann, G. L., and Kraning, K. K. (1969). *Circ. Res.* **24,** 711.

Rowell, L. B., Brengelmann, G. L., Detry, J.-M. R., and Wyss, C. (1971). *J. Appl. Physiol.* **30,** 64.

Saltin, B., and Hermansen, L. (1966). *J. Appl. Physiol.* **21,** 1757.

Saltin, B., Gagge, A. P., and Stolwijk, J. A. J. (1968). *J. Appl. Physiol.* **25,** 679.

Sechrist, W. C., and Stull, G. A. (1969). *Amer. Correct. Ther. J.* **23,** 120.

Sedgwick, A. W., and Whalen, H. R. (1964). *Res. Quart.* **35,** 45.

Shvartz, E. (1970). *J. Appl. Physiol.* **29,** 36.

Schvartz, E., and Benor, D. (1971). *J. Appl. Physiol.* **31,** 24.

Sills, F. D., and O'Riley, V. E. (1956). *Res. Quart.* **27,** 217.

Sinha, K. C., and Verghese, C. A. (1969). *Aero Med. Soc. India J.* **12,** 25.

Spealman, C. R. (1945). *Amer. J. Physiol.* **145,** 218.

Steinhaus, A. H., and Wendhut, G. (1953). *J. Appl. Physiol.* **5,** 677.

Stevenson, G. C., Collin, W. F., Randt, C. T., Saurwein, T. D. (1958). *Amer. J. Physiol.* **194,** 423.

Strydom, N. B., Wyndham, C. H., Williams, C. G., Morrison, J. F., Bredell, G. A. G., Von Rahden, M. J., and Peter, J. (1966). *Fed. Proc. Fed. Amer. Soc. Exp. Biol.* **25,** 1366.

Thauer, R. (1965). *In* "Handbook of Physiology—Circulation" (W. F. Hamilton, ed.), Vol. III, pp. 1921–1966. Amer. Physiological Soc., Washington, D. C.

Tuttle, W. W. (1941). *J. Lab. Clin. Med.* **26,** 1913.

Veghte, J. H., and Webb, P. (1961). *J. Appl. Physiol.* **16,** 235.

Waligora, J. M., and Michel, E. L. (1968). *Aerosp. Med.* **39,** 485.

Walters, C. E., Garrison, L., Duncan, H. J., Hopkins, F. V., and Snyder, J. W. (1960). *Phys. Ther. Rev.* **40,** 266.

Waylonis, G. W. (1967). *Arch. Phys. Med. Rehabil.* **48,** 37.
Webb, P., and Annis, J. F. (1968). *J. Appl. Physiol.* **25,** 489.
Wells, G. (1932). *Res. Quart.* **3,** No. 4, 108.
Wells, G. (1933). *Res. Quart.* **4,** No. 1, 162.
Wessman, H. C., and Kottke, F. J. (1967). *Arch. Phys. Med. Rehabil.* **48,** 567.
Whipp, B. J., and Wasserman, K. (1970). *Resp. Physiol.* **8,** 354.
Wood, J. E., Bass, D. E., and Iampietro, P. F. (1958). *J. Appl. Physiol.* **12,** 357.
Wyndham, C. H., Williams, C. G., and Loots, H. (1968). *J. Appl. Physiol.* **24,** 282.

Chapter 6

Physical Warm-up

B. Don Franks

I. Introduction

A. Overview

Many of the "aids" to performance presented in this book have been controversial since their inception. Physical activity prior to muscular performance, on the other hand, has been widely practiced and accepted until recently (Miller, 1951; Mellerowicz and Hansen, 1971). Although warm-up is still used widely, the value of warm-up itself has become a worthy research problem (Karpovich, 1971; Sessoms, 1971). Perhaps more importantly, comparisons of different types and amounts of warm-up are being made in controlled studies. Although the optimum warm-up cannot be defined at this time, numerous studies have been reported during the last two decades.

B. Purpose

This chapter will review studies concerned with different types of warm-up on different kinds of physical performance. It will emphasize the effects of the use of physical activities as warm-ups. The main form of passive warm-up (heat) is covered in Chapter 5. Although the longitudinal effect of different types of warm-up is one of the factors that can be studied in training programs (e.g., Brose and Hanson, 1967; Harvill, 1966; Webb, 1963), this chapter will include only the acute effects of warm-up. These short-term effects are temporary and relate only to the immediate performance. Further, this chapter will review only studies that used actual performance as the criterion; thus, the effects of warm-up on physiological functions will not be considered. Also, single group studies concerned only with differences over trials or days are not included in this review.

II. Type of Warm-up

Many types of physical activities have been used prior to performance and can be called "physical warm-up" or "active warm-up." Classification of the type of activity used in warm-up is based on its relationship to the task to be performed. The three types of physical warm-up are activities that are identical to the performance, directly related to the performance, or indirectly related to the performance. Passive methods of warming up have included baths, showers, short-wave diathermy, and massage.

A. Identical Activities

One form of preperformance activity almost universally used in performances of short duration is the exact activity to be performed. This has been one of the activities listed under formal or related warm-up. For example, a tennis player will normally attempt several serves prior to a match.

B. Directly Related Activities

Another type of preperformance activity used widely includes activities that use similar but not identical skills (e.g., distance or speed may vary from those used in the performance). Direct warm-up also includes components of the performance done separately. An example of this type of activity is a discus thrower working only on his release.

C. Indirectly Related Activities

Indirect warm-up activities are different from the task to be performed but are aimed at making changes that will influence the performance. Calisthenics using the same muscle groups to cause an increase in muscle or core temperature are commonly used as indirect warm-up. These activities are sometimes called general, informal, or unrelated warm-up.

D. Passive Warm-up

Both indirect and passive warm-up are aimed at bringing about better performance by influencing factors that are thought to affect performance. For example, there is some basis for believing that muscles perform better when the temperature is increased (within limits). Indirect warm-up would attempt to raise the temperature with running or other vigorous activity, whereas passive warm-up would attempt to accomplish the same goals with hot baths, showers, or massage.

E. Examples

1. *Baseball Throw*

Examples of the types of warm-up for a baseball pitcher in which accuracy and velocity are involved follow. Identical warm-up would involve throwing a baseball under the same conditions as found in the game (distance, mound, plate, etc.). Direct warm-up might consist of pitching with less than maximum velocity. Indirect warm-up would involve activities such as running, flexibility, and strength exercises. A hot shower or massage are examples of passive warm-up.

2. *Running*

If the 100-m dash were the criterion, identical warm-up would consist of running 100-m dashes in the same manner as the race, i.e., factors such as the start and finish would be identical to the performance. Direct warm-up would include running different distances and/or speeds. It would also include working on elements of the performance such as the start. Indirect warm-up would include stretching and strength exercises. Passive warm-up might consist of hot baths or massage.

F. Combination

Although it is necessary to separate the types of warm-up in trying to understand their relative effects on performance, most performers recommend and use a combination of warm-ups. Many of the "how to" coaching articles deal primarily with the sequence and duration of different forms of warm-up. Many coaches have shared their experiences concerning the types of warm-up that have seemed to aid their athletes (e.g., Homola, 1968; Messina, 1965; Moss, 1966; O'Connor, 1955; Owens, 1970; Van Buren, 1964; Warner, 1954).

III. Types of Performance

Many different types of performance have been investigated. These can be grouped into the following: cycling, jumping, movement of selected parts of the body, running, sports skills, and swimming.

A. CYCLING

The studies using cycling as the criterion performance (dependent variable) are summarized in Table I. Endurance on the bicycle ergometer was enhanced by direct warm-up (Asmussen and Bøje, 1945; Sucec, 1967), indirect warm-up (Schmid, 1947), and passive warm-up (Asmussen and Bøje, 1945; Schmid, 1947), but rest was better than direct warm-up in two studies (Allen, 1962; Karpovich and Pestrecov, 1941). Carter (1958) found 1 minute of direct warm-up to be no different from rest, but both of these conditions were better than 5 minutes of direct warm-up. Nonsignificant differences were found between indirect warm-up and rest by Massey *et al.* (1961) in a study in which the Ss did not know which experimental treatment (independent variable) had been received since the warm-up or no warm-up was done in a hypnotic trance. The assumption that the Ss would have performed better with warm-up if they had been aware of the experimental conditions leads to interesting conclusions concerning the psychological component of warm-up. Unfortunately, there is no evidence that these Ss would have had a better performance if they had been conscious of the warm-up.

Speed on the bicycle ergometer was enhanced by direct warm-up (Asmussen and Bøje, 1945; Powers, 1960), indirect warm-up (Powers, 1960), and passive warm-up (Asmussen and Bøje, 1945). In the study by Powers (1960), direct was found to be better than indirect warm-up, which was in turn better than rest. Schutz (1966) found rest to be better than direct warm-up, even though the speed (4 or 6 mph), duration (1, 6, 11 minutes), and rest period (1, 6, 11 minutes) were systematically varied. All of the studies finding warm-up to be favorable, and those observing no significant differences, employed college Ss with the exception of Schutz, who used 12 to 14-year-old boys.

It would appear that direct warm-up can either aid or hinder cycling endurance. There is slight evidence that ergometer speed can be increased with direct or passive warm-up in college-age Ss and by rest in junior high school Ss.

B. JUMPING

One study (de Vries, 1960) found that ballistic stretching was superior to static stretching and relaxation or rest in the standing long jump. The vertical jump has served as the dependent variable in other investigations involving jumping performance (Table II). No studies found rest to be

TABLE I

CYCLING

Subjects	Warm-up		Criterion	Findings[a]	Investigator
			ENDURANCE		
6 ♂ physical education majors	1. 5-minute ergometer ride, 10 lb resistance, 15 mph	2. Same, 2½ minutes 3. Rest	Time to reach HR[b] = 180 beats/minute; ergometer ride, 15 lb resistance, 15 mph	3 better than 1, 2	Allen (1962)
4 ♂ athletes (age 25–31)	1. 30-minute ergometer ride, 660 mkg/minute 2. 10-minute hot shower, 47°C	3. Short-wave diathermy 4. 15-minute massage 5. Rest	Ergometer, time for 35 revolutions, time for 450 revolutions	1, 2, 3 better than 4, 5[c]	Asmussen and Bøje (1945)
15 ♂ physical education track classes	1. 1-minute ergometer, 10 mph, 0 load	2. 5 minutes, same 3. Rest	All-out ergometer, 15 mph, 10-lb load	1, 3 better than 2	Carter (1959)
12 ♂ prisoners (age 22–50)	1. 15 to 20-minute ergometer ride, 0 load	2. Rest	Time for all-out ergometer, moderate intensity	2 better than 1	Karpovich and Pestrecov (1941)
15 ♂ college athletes and physical education majors	1. 10-minute jog + calisthenics[d]	2. Rest[d]	Time for 100 revolutions	NS[e]	Massey *et al.* (1961)
5 ♂, ♀ athletes, non-athletes	1. 12 to 15-minute walk–run 2. Massage	3. Hot bath 4. Rest	All-out ergometer ride	1, 2, 3 better than 4	Schmid (1947)
36 ♂ college	1. 10-minute light ergometer, 250 kpm/minute	2. Same, 500 kpm/minute 3. Rest	All-out ergometer ride, 500 kpm/minute	1, 2 better than 3	Sucec (1967)

			SPEED[f]		
5 ♂ college	1. Calisthenics 2. Run, 220 yd/minute 3. Hot shower	Warm-ups, 1 minute 1st week; additional 1 minute each week	Rate for 1-minute ergometer	NS;[e] 2 minutes was best duration	Ihm (1956)
3 ♂ college experienced ergometer riders	1. 5-minute ergometer, 5.5 lb, 60 rpm	2. Rest	Time for 35 revolutions on ergometer	NS[e]	Karpovich and Hale (1956)
29 ♂ college physical education classes	1. 5-minute ergometer, 0 load	2. 5-minute run + calisthenics 3. Rest	Speed for riding 100 yd	1 better than 2; 2 better than 3	Powers (1960)
13 ♀ college physical education majors	1. 8 revolutions on ergometer	2. Rest	Ergometer, 0.1 mile	NS[e]	Skubic and Hodgkins (1957)
66 ♂ (age 12–14)	Three factors on ergometer ride: 1. 4 or 6 mph 2. 1, 6, 11 minutes duration	3. 1, 6, 11 minutes rest 4. Rest	25-second ergometer ride, total no. of revolutions; max. no. per second; time for 4 revolutions	4 better than 1, 2, 3; 6 mph better than 4 mph; factors 2, 3, NS[e]	Schutz (1966)
20 ♂ college (age 19–34)	1. 2-minute run with arm movement	2. Same, 4 minutes	Rate of arm crank, 2 days	NS,[e] 1, 2; 2nd day better	Lotter (1959)[g]

[a] In this and the following tables, 3 better than 1, 2, for example, means that warm-up 3 was significantly better than 1 and 2, and there was no significant difference between 1 and 2.

[b] Heart rate.

[c] Muscle temperature appeared to be related to performance.

[d] Done under hypnosis; *Ss* unaware of treatment.

[e] NS means no significant differences among the warm-up conditions used.

[f] For the work of Asmussen and Bøje (1945) and Massey *et al.* (1961) see under Endurance.

[g] All studies in Table I used a bicycle ergometer for the legs except Lotter, who used an arm crank.

TABLE II

JUMPING

Subjects	Warm-up	Criterion	Findings[a]	Investigator
21 ♂ college	1. Static stretch + relaxation 2. Ballistic stretch 3. Rest	Standing long jump	2 better than 1, 3	de Vries (1960)
16 ♂ college varsity track	1. 5-minute run and calisthenics 2. Placebo 3. Rest	Vertical jump	1 better than 2, 3	Esper (1966)
	1. Active stretching 2. Passive stretching 3. Rest Different durations of warm-up	Vertical jump	1 better than 2, 3; duration, NS	Graw (1959)
10 ♂, 1 ♀ college and graduate students	1. Stretch 2. Deep knee bends 3. Run in place 4. Rest	Vertical jump, 6 trials, 5 days	1, 2, 3 better than 4; NS, trials, days	Pacheco (1957)
166 ♀ junior high school	1. 3-minute run in place 2. Rest	Vertical jump, 5 trials, 2 days	1 better than 2; 2nd day better; 5th trial better than 1st.	Pacheco (1959)
80 ♀ high school	1. 1 minute step (25 steps/minute); 15 in. 2. 2 minutes same 3. 4 minutes same 4. 6 minutes same 5. Rest	Vertical jump	1, 2 better than 3; 5 better than 4	Richards (1968)
19 ♀ college basketball players	1. Direct calisthenics 2. Run 4 laps 3. Rest	Vertical jump	1, 2 better than 3	Steacy (1960)
44 ♂ college	1. Practice with 10% body wt overload 2. 5% overload 3. 0% overload	Vertical jump	Decrease with 3	Stockholm and Nelson (1965)
15 ♂ high school athletes and nonathletes	Different amounts of calisthenics	Vertical jump	Longer duration better	Van Grundy (1963)

[a] NS means no significant differences among the warm-up conditions used.

better than physical warm-up, except for mixed results by Richards (1968). This study found that 1 and 2 minutes of bench stepping aided jumping; 6 minutes of bench stepping was detrimental to jumping; and 4 minutes of bench stepping was nonsignificantly different from rest. Most forms of indirect warm-up were beneficial to jumping, except that two studies (de Vries, 1960; Graw, 1959) found ballistic stretching superior to static or passive stretching. Pacheco's (1957, 1959) design determined not only the effect of indirect warm-up, but also day-to-day and trial-by-trial improvement. She found that indirect warm-up aided the performance of college Ss (1957) and junior high school girls (1959). There was no significant effect of identical warm-up (trials) or day-to-day improvement in the college Ss, but the junior high school girls showed improvement in all three (indirect, identical, and day-to-day).

One investigator (Esper, 1966) attempted to increase performance psychologically in college varsity track men. A bogus news article about a new pill that had the same effects as warm-up was placed on the bulletin board 1 month prior to the study. This study then compared the effects of an indirect warm-up (running and calisthenics), taking a placebo (the "new pill"), and rest. The indirect warm-up was superior to the pill and rest, with no significant differences between the placebo and rest. Some of the Ss did report "physiological" changes after taking the placebo. Others reported no change. Their performance was not highly related to the "reactions" to the pill.

Indirect warm-up appears to facilitate jumping performance, and active stretching seems to be better than passive.

C. Movement of Parts of the Body

Several studies have dealt with accuracy, response time, range of motion, and strength of various limbs and/or joints (Table III). Various novel tasks have been used to determine the effects of warm-up on accuracy. In no study was rest found to be better than warm-up for accuracy. Identical (Baumgarten, 1965), direct (Catalano and Whalen, 1967), and indirect (Barch, 1963; Baumgarten, 1965) warm-ups were found to be beneficial to rotary pursuit and the Minnesota Manual Dexterity Tests. No differences were found for indirect (Burke, 1957; Thompson, 1958) or direct warm-up (Thompson, 1958) on a novel task using the foot or typing accuracy, although Elbel (1940) found that basketball practice and competition increased performance on a matching task to a greater extent than did rest.

No significant differences were found in studies using reaction time, except that basketball practice and competition were better than bench

TABLE III Movement of Part of the Body

Subjects		Warm-up	Criterion	Findings[a]	Investigator
			ACCURACY		
45 ♂, ♀ college	1. Practice with nonpreferred hand	2. Rest	Rotary pursuit, preferred hand	1 better than 2	Barch (1963)
64 ♂, ♀ college nonathletes	1. Trace pattern with load, preferred hand 2. Load, nonpreferred hand	3. Load, preferred hand opposite direction 4. No load	Rotary pursuit, warm-up done between trials	1, 2, 3 better than 4	Catalano and Whalen (1967)
40 ♀ college	1. Practice on test 1 minute 2. 1 minute arm and hand calisthenics	3. 1 minute jumping jacks 4. Rest	Minnesota Manual Dexterity Tests, 3 trials, 4 days	1, 2 better than 3, 4; NS, trials; day 4 better than day 3 and day 2 better than day 1	Baumgarten (1965)
72 ♂ college freshmen nonathletes	Two factors—bench step: 1. Intensity, 55, 81, 108 steps/minute	2. Duration, 2, 5, 8 minutes 3. Rest	Push disk with foot to target	NS	Burke (1957)
50 ♂, ♀ high school, Typing II	1. 5 minutes typing	2. Rest	Typing speed and accuracy	NS	Powers (1960)
13 ♀ college, Typing II	1. 3 minutes typing 2. 3 minutes finger calisthenics	3. Rest	Typing speed and accuracy	NS	Thompson (1958)
			Response time[b]		
129 ♂ college athletes and nonathletes	1. Bench step + max push-ups 2. 1½ hours basketball	3. Fencing 4. Rest	Reaction, finger Reaction, palm Response, body Fencing lunge Matching task	NS 2 better than 1, 4 2 better than 1, 4 3 better than 4 2 better than 4	Elbel (1940)
24 ♂ junior high school	1. Calisthenics with weight 2. Heat (blankets)	3. Cold (ice) 4. Rest	Movement time; reaction time	NS[c]	Glidewell (1964)
30 ♂ college	1. Calisthenics 2. 2-minute ergometer ride (15–20 mph) 3. 4-minute ergometer ride (15–20 mph) 4. 6-minute ergometer ride (15–20 mph)	5. Ergometer ride to exhaustion 6. 3 minutes cooling 7. No warm-up	Reaction time, finger; reaction time, foot	NS	Hoogendoorn (1963)
17 ♂ college	1. Intensity a. Low b. High	2. Warm-up type a. Related b. Unrelated 3. 7-minute hot shower 4. Rest	Speed of movement; 1, 2 feet tapping; leg circles	1b better than 1a; 1b, 2b best; 3 showed some improvement	McGavin (1968)

19 ♂ college students and faculty (age 21–37)	1. Overload prior	2. Overload during	Arm speed	NS[d]	Nelson and Lambert (1965)
135 ♂ college (age 18–26)	1. 6-minute stretch 2. 9 curls, 9 presses, 25 lb	3. Rest	Movement time, right and left elbow extension	1 better than 2, 3	Paseltiner (1957)
75 ♂ college	1. $2\frac{1}{2}$ minutes moderate arm calisthenics 2. 10 minutes heavy stepping	3. Rest	Reaction time Movement time 60 trials	NS 2 better than 1, 3 NS	Phillips (1963)
			Range of motion		
33 ♂ college	1. 1 practice trial 2. 4 related calisthenics 3. 6 related calisthenics	4. 8 related calisthenics 5. Rest	Toe touch, distance from floor	2, 3, 4 better than 1, 5	Fieldman (1968)
19 ♂ high school and adults	Calisthenics, ankle, knee, hip, trunk, shoulder, elbow, wrist		Change from pre- to posttest	Increased range of motion after warm-up	Lukes (1954)
14 ♂ college physical education majors	1. 10 squat thrusts 2. General calisthenics	3. Rest	Shoulder and trunk, range of motion	1, 2 better than 3	Teague (1966)
			STRENGTH		
72 ♂ college freshmen nonathletes	Two factors—bench stepping: 1. Low, moderate, high intensity	2. 2, 5, 8 minutes 3. Rest	Knee flexor strength	Moderate and high intensity and duration better than low intensity and rest	Burke (1957)
16 ♂ college	1. 2-minute treadmill run between trials, 6 mph, 0% grade	2. Rest	Knee extension strength, 10 trials	1 better than 2	Kaye (1967)
24 ♂ junior high school	1. Calisthenics with overload 2. Passive heating	3. Passive cooling 4. Rest	Strength/leg; power/leg	NS[e]	Glidewell (1964)
20 ♂ college physical education majors (age 18–23)	1. Calisthenics + 2-minute run in place	2. Rest	Leg extension strength	NS	Thompson (1958)
90 ♂ (age 18–55)	1. All-out ergometer ride, 7000 ft-lb/minute; between trials		Right and left grip and forearm flexion strength	Post better than pre	Dohrmann (1956)
21 ♂ college	1. 9 minutes arm and hand calisthenics 2. Rest		Grip endurance	NS[f]	Sedgwick (1964)

[a] NS means no significant differences among the warm-up conditions used. [b] For the work of Thompson (1958) see under Accuracy.
[c] 3 inferior to 1, 2, 4. [d] Although perceived as faster after overload.
[e] 3 worse than 1, 2, 4. [f] 1 did increase muscle temperature.

TABLE IV RUNNING

Subjects	Warm-up	Criterion	Findings[a]	Investigator
		AGILITY		
81 ♀ college	1. Identical; 2. Jumping jacks; 3. 1 + 2; 4. Rest	4-part shuttle run	2, 4 better than 1, 3	Emerson (1968)
86 ♀ college	1. 3 minutes calisthenics; 2. Rest	Obstacle run, 2 trials	1 better than 2; all *S*s with favorable attitude, 1 better than 2; NS in *S*s with less favorable attitude	Smith and Bozymowski (1965)
14 ♂ college physical education majors	1. 10 squat thrusts; 2. General calisthenics; 3. Rest	Shuttle run	NS	Teague (1966)
551 ♀ junior high school	1. 2-minute run in place; 2. Rest	Illinois Agility Run	2 better than 1	Zieger (1964)
		ENDURANCE		
Athletes	1. 5- to 30-minute run and calisthenics; 2. Sauna bath; 3. Rest; 4. Rest period, 0, 15, 30, 45 minutes	800 m, 400 m, 100 m	1 better than 2, 3; 0-, 15-minute rest better than 30-, 45-minute	Högberg and Ljunggren (1947)
13 ♂ college non-athletes	1. 5-minute jog and calisthenics; 2. Same + 0.1-mile sprints; 3. Rest	1-mile run	2 better than 1, 3[b]	Grodjinovsky and Magel (1970)
2 ♂ college cross-country runners	1. 23-minute run and rest; 2. Rest	All-out treadmill run	1 better than 2	Lynch (1959)
12 ♂ college physical education majors	1. 10 squat thrusts; 2. General calisthenics; 3. Rest	All-out treadmill run	NS	Teague (1966)
11 ♂ college varsity cross-country runners	1. Warm-up, 6-minute rest; 2. Warm-up, 14-minute rest; 3. Warm-up, 22-minute rest; 4. Rest	1-mile run	1, 2 better than 3, 4	Blohm (1969)
		SPRINT[c]		
22 ♂ college sprinters	1. Combination warm-up; 2. Rest	60-yd dash	NS	Tremble (1962)
20 ♂ junior high track	1. 2-minute direct; 2. Warm shower; 3. Hot shower; 4. Rest	5 yd at max speed with running start	NS	Smith (1960)
9 ♂ college	1. Sprint; 2. Stretch; 3. Vigorous calisthenics; 4. Rest	100 yd	1, 2, 3 better than 4	Malan (1960)
♂ high school athletes and nonathletes	Different duration of calisthenics	100 yd	Longer duration better	Van Grundy (1963)
7 ♂, ♀ moderate and well trained	1. 12- to 14-min run + calisthenics; 2. Breathe 50% O_2; 3. Rest	100 m	1 better than 2, 3	Simonson *et al.* (1936)

14 ♂, ♀ athletes and nonathletes	1. 12- to 15-min walk–run 2. Massage	3. Hot bath 4. Rest	100 m	1, 2, 3 better than 4	Schmid (1947)
54 ♂ track and field athletes	1. Walk, run, calisthenics	2. Walk, min stretching	120 yd (athletes); 100 yd (nonathletes)	1 better than 2	Blank (1955)
11 ♂ college track	1. Run 2. Static stretch	3. Ballistic stretch 4. Relaxation	220 yd	NS	de Vries (1960)
13 ♂ college non-athletes	1. 5-minute jog + calisthenics 2. Same + 0.1-mile sprints	3. Rest	60 yd 440 yd	1, 2 better than 3	Grodjinovsky and Magel (1970)
16 ♂ high school	1. 30 minutes calisthenics and run	2. Rest	440 yd	1 better than 2 for both athletes and non-athletes	Buresh (1967)
12 ♂ college athletes	1. Calisthenics + sprints + massage	2. 5-minute massage	440 yd	NS	Hale (1949)
6 ♂ college freshmen and varsity track	1. 10-minute run + calisthenics 2. Same + 5-minute cold shower	3. Fast walk, 220 yd	440 yd, 20-minute rest between run	1 better than 2 better than 3 on 1st run; NS on 2nd run	Hansen (1959)
48 ♂ college non-athletes	1. Calisthenics + jog + sprints	1-, 4-, 10-minute rest interval	440 yd	NS	Hutterly (1967)
50 ♂ high school non-athletes	1. Jog, calisthenics, sprints	2. Rest	440 yd	NS	Mathews and Snyder (1959)
7 ♂ college freshmen and varsity track	1. 10-minute jog calisthenics + sprints 2. Deep massage (5 minutes/leg)	3. Digital stroking (5 minutes/leg)	440 yd	NS	Karpovich and Hale (1956)
5 ♂ college freshmen and varsity track	1. Digital stroking	2. Rest	440 yd	NS	Karpovich and Hale (1956)
16 ♂ college track	1. Continuous movement between trials	2. Cold spray + movement	440 yd; 2 trials, 10 minutes between	2 better than 1	Rosen (1952)
			STATIONARY		
72 ♂ college non-athletes	Two factors—bench step: 1. Low, moderate, high intensity 2. 2-, 5-, 8-minute duration	3. Rest	Run in place, speed and endurance	NS	Burke (1957)
15 ♂ (age 18–36)	1. 1- to 10-minute step test, 30 steps/minute, 13-in. bench 2. Same + cold shower	3. Ice pack 4. Hot shower	Run in place; rate of stepping, 30 seconds	1, 2 better than 3, 4	Raines (1952)
18 ♂ (age 19–28)	1. 10-minute walk–jog 2. Cold spray	3. Rest	No. of steps, 10 seconds, run in place; 5 trials	2 better than 1, 3	Sills and O'Riley (1956)

[a] NS means no significant differences among the warm-up conditions used. [b] Maximum $\dot{V}_{O_2}$, NS. [c] For work of Högberg and Ljunggren (1950) see under Endurance.

stepping and push-ups or no warm-up on reaction time with the palm of the hand. However, nonsignificant differences were observed in the same study using finger reaction time (Elbel, 1940). Indirect warm-up (Elbel, 1940; Paseltiner, 1957; Phillips, 1963) was found to improve movement time. In no study was rest found to be better than warm-up, although some studies found no significant differences.

Direct and indirect warm-up were beneficial to range of motion in every study reviewed. Indirect warm-up improved measures of strength in several investigations. Burke (1957) found that low-intensity and short-duration warm-ups were inferior to longer and more intense warm-ups. Sedgwick (1964) found nonsignificant differences between the effects of 9 minutes of arm and hand calisthenics and rest on grip endurance, although the warm-up did increase the muscle temperature.

In general, there is evidence that direct and indirect warm-up are beneficial for accuracy, movement time, range of motion, and strength of various parts of the body. There is only slight evidence that reaction time is affected.

D. Running

Those investigators who have employed running as the dependent variable have used agility, endurance, sprint, and stationary tasks (Table IV).

Smith and Bozymowski (1965) found that 3 minutes of calisthenics was better than rest on an agility run ($N = 86$). When the Ss with more favorable ($N = 23$) and less favorable ($N = 23$) attitudes toward warm-up were analyzed separately, the Ss with favorable attitudes showed a significant difference favoring warm-up (0.01 level), whereas the Ss with less favorable attitudes toward warm-up had nonsignificant differences (0.11 level). Also, Zeiger (1964) found rest to be better than an indirect warm-up in junior high school girls on the Illinois Agility Run, and Teague (1966) found no significant differences among indirect warm-ups and rest on a shuttle run task.

Several types of direct and indirect warm-up have been found to be better than rest and other types of warm-up for distance runs (Högberg and Ljunggren, 1950; Grodjinovsky and Magel, 1970; Lynch, 1959). Rest was not superior to warm-up in any of the investigations reviewed. However, Teague (1966) reported that warm-up did not differ significantly from a rest condition on performance of an all-out treadmill run.

In sprints up to and including 440 yd, rest was not better than various forms of warm-up in any study reviewed. Some types of direct and indirect warm-up were better than rest on the short (less than 120 yd) sprints (Malan, 1960; Van Grundy, 1963; Simonson *et al.*, 1936; Schmid, 1947; Blank, 1955; Högberg and Ljunggren, 1950; Grodjinovsky and Magel, 1970). Several of the studies on the longer dashes (mainly 400 m and 440 yd) found nonsignificant differences, although combination warm-ups were found to be better than rest for the 400-m run (Högberg and Ljunggren, 1950) and 440-yd run (Buresh, 1967; Grodjinovsky and Magel, 1970; Hansen, 1959). Hansen (1959) administered two 440-yd runs with a 20-minute rest between runs. He found that a combination of running and calisthenics was superior to the application of a cold pack, which was better than simply walking (control) on the first run. There were nonsignificant differences on the second trial. It appears from this study that warm-up is beneficial; however, there is no evidence that a combination of direct, indirect, and identical warm-up is better than the identical warm-up alone in the 440-yd dash.

No significant differences between active warm-up and rest were found in studies using running in place, although bench stepping warm-up with and without cold was found to be better than just cold or heat (Raines, 1952). A cold spray was found by Sills and O'Riley (1956) to be better than indirect warm-up or rest.

There is some evidence that sprint and distance running are enhanced by some forms of direct and indirect warm-up. Agility running and running in place have not been studied extensively enough to warrant general conclusions.

E. Sports Skills

Overload warm-up has been demonstrated to increase velocity but not accuracy of a baseball throw (Table V). Accuracy has been observed to be slightly worse immediately following overload (Creek, 1964; Straub, 1968; Van Huss *et al.*, 1962). It has been hypothesized by Van Huss *et al.* (1962) that overload might cause continued firing of motor units, thus increasing velocity and improvement in some kinds of neuromuscular tasks. Direct and indirect warm-up were found to be better than rest on a softball throw for distance task by Michael *et al.* (1957) and Rochelle *et al.* (1960) even when Ss in the no-warm-up condition were motivated by money. Identical warm-up (trials) caused improvement only when not preceded by direct warm-up in the study by Rochelle *et al.* (1960). There were no significant differences among identical, indirect, or rest conditions in the investigation of Skubic and Hodgkins (1957).

Identical and direct warm-up were better than indirect warm-up and

TABLE V

SPORTS SKILLS

Sport	Subjects	Warm-up		Criterion	Findings[a]	Investigator
Baseball/ softball	74 ♂ nonathletes	1. Heavy softball	2. Regular softball	Accuracy, 10 trials	2 better than 1	Creek (1964)
	77 ♂ (age 17–20)	1. Play catch 2. Calisthenics + run	3. Rest	Softball throw for distance, 3 trials	1, 2 better than 3; NS, trials	Michael *et al.* (1957)
	46 ♂ (age 18–22)	1. 5 minutes catch	2. Rest[b]	Softball throw for distance, 3 trials	1 better than 2; increase within trials for 2 only	Rochelle *et al.* (1960)
	13 ♀ college physical education majors	1. 8 revolutions on ergometer 2. 5 softball throws	3. Free throws 4. 12 jumping jacks 5. Rest	Softball throw; basketball free throws, 10 trials	NS	Skubic and Hodgkins (1957)
	60 ♂ college	1. 20 throws, 15-oz ball	2. Same, 20-oz ball 3. Same, regular ball	Accuracy, velocity, baseball throw	NS	Straub (1968)
	50 ♂ varsity baseball players	1. 11-oz ball	2. Regular ball	Accuracy Velocity, baseball throw	NS 1 better than 2	Van Huss *et al.* (1962)
	561 ♀ junior high school skilled and unskilled	1. Jumping jacks + running, 5, 10, 20 bouts		Softball accuracy	NS	Witte (1962)
	27 ♂ high school baseball players	1. 1 minute 45 seconds, regular bat (34 oz) 2. Same with 27-oz weight on bat	3. Calisthenics 4. Rest	Velocity of bat, best of 3 trials	NS	Kracik (1969)
	20 ♂ elementary grades 6 and 7	1. Batting practice, 15 swings	2. Rest	Batting average for season	1 better than 2	Williamson (1959)

Basketball[c]	34 ♂ high school and college basketball players	1. 25 free throws 2. Jog + calisthenics	3. Rest	Free throws, 25 trials	NS	Bailin (1964)
	10 ♂ college varsity basketball players	1. 5 shots 2. 1 minute jumping	3. Rest	Free throws, 10 trials	1 better than 2, 3	Benedict (1966)
	18 ♂ college freshmen and intramural basketball players	1. 30 free throws 2. 20 minutes practice	3. 5 minutes mental practice 4. Rest	Free throws	1, 2 better than 3, 4	Powers (1960)
	19 ♀ college basketball players	1. Basketball skills 2. 4 laps	3. Rest	Basketball pass accuracy; free throws	1 better than 2; 2 better than 3	Steacy (1960)
	20 ♂ college freshmen basketball players	1. Shooting, passing, free throws	2. Rest	Free throws, 20 trials	1 better than 2	Thompson (1958)
Bowling	30 ♂ college bowling class	1. 6 frames 2. Mental practice	3. Rest	4 games total	NS	Powers (1960)
Football	20 ♂ college non-athletes	1. 3 minutes passing (30 passes same distance) 2. 3-minute run and calisthenics	3. Mental practice 4. Rest	Accuracy, football passing	NS	Severino (1966)
	6 experienced football quarterbacks	1. Calisthenics of throwing arm and shoulder	2. General calisthenics 3. Rest	Football passing, 5 trials at 10, 20, 35 yd	1, 2 better than 3	Swan (1968)
Gymnastics		1–6 Six different methods of warm-up	7. Rest	Gymnastic performance	1–6 better than 7; NS among 1–6	Morgenegg and Jensen (1966)
Hammer throw	9 college experienced hammer throwers (age 19–24)	1. Light calisthenics 2. Heavy calisthenics	3. Rest	Hammer throw, 6 trials	NS[d]	Myers (1967)

[a] NS means no significant differences among warm-up conditions used.
[b] Money offered for good performance; more for first trial.
[c] For work of Skubic and Hodgkins (1957) see under Baseball/softball.
[d] Fewer fouls after 1.

rest in basketball shooting and passing (Benedict, 1966; Powers, 1960; Steacy, 1960; Thompson, 1958). Direct warm-up and mental practice were not different from rest in affecting bowling performance. Accuracy of football passing was better after involving the throwing arm and shoulder than general calisthenics or rest in six experienced quarterbacks (Swan, 1968). Using college nonathletes, Severino (1966) found no significant differences in football-passing accuracy. Although different types of warm-up were better than rest in gymnastics performance, there were no significant differences among the types of warm-up (Morgenegg and Jensen, 1966). Indirect warm-up had no significant effect on the hammer throw (Myers, 1967).

In general, warm-up appears to benefit throwing velocity and distance in baseball. Also, basketball shooting and passing are enhanced by warm-up, and there is slight evidence of improvement in the football-passing accuracy of experienced passers. In addition, gymnastics performance is facilitated by warm-up.

F. Swimming

Direct, indirect, and combination warm-ups have caused improved swimming performance in distances ranging from 50 to 200 m (Table VI). de Vries (1959) found that direct warm-up was better than indirect, passive, or no warm-up in experienced swimmers. When Ss were divided into freestyle or breaststroke swimmers, he found that calisthenics aided the breaststrokers and hindered the freestylers. He noted that the breaststrokers did better with calisthenics even though they believed the calisthenics would hinder their performance. Lueft (1958) determined which Ss had a positive, negative, or indifferent attitude toward warm-up. When compared with performance, there was little relationship between attitude and best performance. Overall, he found nonsignificant differences, even though 32 Ss had favorable attitudes, 12 negative attitudes, and 5 were indifferent. Several types of warm-up were not significantly different from rest, but rest was not found superior in any study.

IV. Injury

One of the benefits claimed for warm-up is the prevention of injury. Numerous coaches, trainers, performers, physical educators, and physiologists have advanced the opinion that lack of warm-up might lead to

TABLE VI
SWIMMING

Subjects	Warm-up	Criterion	Findings[a]	Investigator
49 ♂ college advanced swimming class	1. 30-second shower, calisthenics, 50-yd swim; 2. 30-second shower + rest	30 yd (crawl)	NS	Lueft (1958)
16 ♂ college advanced swimming class	1. 8-minute stretch and relax; 2. 6-minute hot shower + 100-yd swim; 3. Rest	50 yd	NS	de Vries (1960)
14 ♂, ♀ athletes and nonathletes	1. 20-minute swim; 2. Massage; 3. 15-minute hot bath; 4. Rest	50 m (breast)	1, 2, 3 better than 4	Schmid (1947)
13 ♂ college swimmers: 7 freestyle, 5 breast and dolphin	1. 500-yd swim; 2. Kiphuth calisthenics, 300 movements; 3. 10-minute massage; 4. 6-minute hot shower; 5. Rest	100 yd (various styles)	All swimmers, 1 better than 2, 3, 4, 5; free, 2 worse; breast, 2 better[b]	de Vries (1959)
12 ♂ college varsity swimmers	1. Calisthenics, flutter kick; 2. Rest	100 yd (crawl)	NS	Filipponi (1951)
10 ♂ college varsity swimmers	1. Moderate or heavy warm-up; 2. 2-, 15-, 30-minute interval; 3. Rest	100 yd (crawl)	NS	Scogin (1969)
25 ♂ college freshmen and varsity swimmers	1. Calisthenics, swim, rest; 2. 8-minute hot shower,; 3. 4-minute hot whirlpool; 4. Rest	100 yd (crawl)	1 better than 4 better than 2, 3	Twardowski (1962)
60 ♂ college (age 17–28)	1. 2- to 3-minute hot shower, calisthenics, and swim; 2. Calisthenics; 3. Rest	30 yd (crawl)	1 better than 2, 3	Thompson (1958)
3 ♂ athletes (age 30–32)	1. 10-minute jog; 2. 10-minute ergometer ride (1080 mkg/minute); 3. 15-minute hot shower; 4. Diathermy; 5. 15-minute cold bath; 6. Rest	50 m (crawl), 400 m (crawl), 200 m (crawl)	1, 2, 3, 4 better; 6 better than 5[c]	Muido (1946)
12 ♂ college experienced swimmers	1. 1½- to 2-minute swim; 2. Rest	100 yd, 500 yd	NS	Middlebrooks (1966)

[a] NS means no significant difference among warm-up conditions used.
[b] Subjects thought it would hinder.
[c] Warm-up lasted 60–80 minutes; core temperature appeared to be related to performance.

injury (e.g., Mellerowicz and Hansen, 1971), but the problem is quite difficult to approach. For example, Karpovich (1971) has pointed out that researchers would not try to induce injury as a part of their experimental design. However, there has been some interesting indirect evidence concerning injuries. Start (1962) reported that out of several hundred maximum contractions at the ankle, knee, and hip, and with respect to total leg strength in 38 college male athletes and nonathletes, there was only one injury reported even though there was no warm-up prior to these efforts (the one injury was in a S who had concealed an earlier injury in order that he could participate in the study). The only discomfort reported by the Ss related to the belt rubbing the skin during the hip extension test. It is interesting to note that, in all the studies reviewed, only one (de Vries, 1966) mentioned any injury occurring even though most of these studies employed a no-warm-up condition. The exception involved injuries to two sprinters in the 100-yd dash. Four studies specifically mentioned that there were no reports of injury in the 440-yd dash (Mathews and Snyder, 1959), softball throw for distance (Michael *et al.*, 1957), and cycling (Massey *et al.*, 1961; Sucec, 1967). Sucec (1967) reported no difference between warm-up and no warm-up on muscle soreness, but there was less soreness after longitudinal training. It is possible, of course, when athletes are not in peak condition that level of condition is more important than whether there is warm-up. For example, Delforge (1966, 1969) found that more injuries were reported early in the season.

The testimony of trainers and coaches, as well as the opinions of many physical educators and physiologists, cannot be completely ignored. However, there is little experimental evidence at this time to justify warm-up on the basis of prevention of injury. This may be simply an academic question, since there appears to be adequate experimental support for warm-up in most tasks and almost no support for the no-warm-up position.

V. Factors Influencing Effects of Warm-up

There are many possible factors that affect the presence or absence of a warm-up effect. Some of these factors can be divided into two categories: (a) factors related to the warm-up, which can be applied to all types of warm-up, and (b) factors related to certain characteristics of the participant.

A. Factors Related to Warm-up

Various authors have speculated about the physiological bases for a warm-up effect (e.g., Stansbury, 1942; Van Grundy, 1965; de Vries, 1966; Jensen, 1966; Morehouse and Miller, 1967; Karpovich, 1971). These have included various circulatory, metabolic, respiratory, and neurological adjustments made as a result of warm-up. Although various physiological changes with warm-up are sometimes included in studies, the relative importance of these measures to typical physical performances is unclear. For example, two studies that recorded different temperatures along with warm-up and performance disagree concerning whether core temperature (Muido, 1946) or muscle temperature (Asmussen and Bøje, 1945) was more directly related to performance. Sedgwick (1964) found an increase in muscle temperature with warm-up but no significant difference between warm-up and rest on muscular endurance. None of the studies reviewed was designed to determine whether specific changes in physiological functions caused changes in performance, and the few studies that measured physiological function and performance could only discuss relationship, not infer cause and effect. The appropriateness of applying the results of studies on isolated muscle to physical performance involving the whole person is not clear. It does seem probable that changes in some physiological functions influence subsequent muscular performance. More definitive statements do not appear to be possible at this time.

To the extent that physiological changes resulting from warm-up do influence performance, several aspects of the warm-up must be considered, namely, amount of work, duration, intensity, and rest period between warm-up and performance. None of these factors can be considered in isolation since they most likely interact with each other in producing the effects of a particular warm-up.

1. *Amount of Work*

The total amount of work done during the warm-up depends on the duration, intensity, and number of muscles involved in the warm-up. Some of the physiological adjustments, as well as possible fatigue effects, vary according to the energy expenditure during a warm-up.

2. *Duration*

The duration of the warm-up is limited by rules and practical considerations in many cases. The duration of warm-up in the studies reviewed has varied from one practice trial (Fieldman, 1968) or 8 revolutions on the bicycle ergometer (Skubic and Hodgkins, 1957) to a 30-minute ergometer ride (Asmussen and Bøje, 1945) or 1½ hours of basketball practice (Elbel, 1940). It is interesting to note that, in these extremes, Fieldman (1968) and Skubic and Hodgkins (1957) found non-significant differences, whereas Asmussen and Bøje (1945) and Elbel (1940) found that the warm-up caused improvement. Most of the studies ranged from 2 to 10 minutes, which represents a less than normal warm-up time for athletes. In general, the longer durations seemed more beneficial, although that was not always the case, especially in nonathletes (e.g., Carter, 1959; Karpovich and Pestrecov, 1941; Richards, 1968).

3. *Intensity*

The intensity of warm-up in the studies reported has ranged from very mild to maximum effort. A few studies have varied this aspect of the warm-up, but the intensities have been determined arbitrarily rather than in relation to the individual's own maximum. Phillips (1963) and McGavin (1968) found that high intensity was better than low intensity for speed of movement. Burke (1957) found that moderate- and high-intensity warm-ups were better than low-intensity warm-up in knee flexor strength but found no differences in speed and endurance. Sucec (1967) found that increasing the intensity (and total amount of work) did not increase the effect of the warm-up on an all-out ergometer ride. Grodjinovsky and Magel (1970), on the other hand, found that the addition of sprints to jogging and calisthenics caused significant improvement on the mile run when compared with 5 minutes of jogging and calisthenics or rest. It is not possible to determine whether it was the increased intensity of the sprints or the amount of work that caused the difference. Two studies that have attempted to systematically vary some of the factors such as intensity have not found significant differences between the rest and warm-up conditions (Burke, 1957; Scogin, 1969). Schutz (1966) found that rest was better than warm-up in young boys, although within the warm-up condition, the higher intensity was better.

4. *Rest Interval*

The rest interval between warm-up and performance cannot always be controlled because of procedures associated with various performances. However, to the extent that the effects of warm-up are due to temporary physiological adjustments and changes, it would appear necessary to perform soon after the warm-up. The rest intervals in the studies reported varied from 0 to 20 minutes, with most of the performances being 30 seconds to 5 minutes after the warm-up. Unfortunately, several studies failed to report the rest period (e.g., Asmussen and Bøje, 1945; Karpovich and Hale, 1956). Högberg and Ljunggren (1947) and Blohm (1969) found shorter rest intervals after warm-up to be better in runs ranging from 100 m to 1 mile. Although Muido (1946) tested his Ss 20 minutes after warm-up, he reported warm-up effects lasting 60–80 minutes. Hutterly (1967) and Schutz (1966) found nonsignificant differences with rest intervals ranging from 1 to 11 minutes.

B. Factors Related to the Participant

Certain factors that might be related to the effects of warm-up deal with the participant. These factors include age, sex, physical condition, skill, attitude toward warm-up, and motivation.

1. *Age*

There are few data on young children and older adults. Most of the available data are on college Ss, although there are some data on teenagers and middle-aged adults. With one exception (Allen, 1962), all of the studies that found rest to be superior were conducted on non-college-age Ss. Richards (1968) found that shorter warm-ups were beneficial and that longer warm-ups were not different from rest in high school girls. Glidewell (1964) noted large individual differences and found cooling to be detrimental to junior high school boys. Karpovich and Pestrecov (1941) found that warm-up decreased performance in older Ss (male prisoners, 22–50 years old), and Simpson (1968) found greater changes with warm-up in older subjects. Pacheco (1957, 1959) reported warm-up effects for both junior high school girls and college Ss. However, the girls also showed trial-by-trial and day-to-day improvements, which has not been found in other studies. The studies reviewed suggest that younger untrained subjects might be more variable and less affected by warm-up. Final conclusions concerning the effects of age must await systematic study of this factor.

2. *Sex*

Most of the studies reviewed used males or both sexes together, and there does not seem to be any observable trend for differential effects due to sex. However, the influence of sex cannot be determined until there are studies conducted in which sex serves as one of the independent variables.

3. *Physical Condition*

It is interesting to note that all of the studies that found rest superior to warm-up used nonathletes, although some studies using untrained Ss did find a warm-up effect. Wells (1908) reported that strenuous warm-up may be more beneficial to those in better physical condition. This would seem reasonable since strenuous activities that might cause desirable physiological adjustments would cause more fatigue in those in poorer physical condition. However, Kaye (1967) reported that unfit Ss exhibited a greater increased rate of strength gain following indirect warm-up than did fit Ss. Although some studies have used both trained and untrained subjects, this factor has not been included as a separate independent variable.

4. *Level of Skill*

Subjects with a lower skill level benefit more from identical warm-up (practice) since they are still learning the skill. It is questionable whether the studies that demonstrate basically learning in the unskilled have any direct application to the effect of warm-up in the skilled performer. Larger absolute differences may be possible in the unskilled and have little practical importance. However, very small differences can be important to the highly skilled.

5. *Attitude toward Warm-up*

It is difficult to find any study that does not mention the possibility of a "psychological" component of warm-up (or any other "aid" to performance); however, systematic studies of which psychological components interact with which type of warm-up to benefit various performances are yet to come. It might be hypothesized that state anxiety (see Chapter 2) increases with warm-up activities since various physiological concomitants of state anxiety such as heart rate, systolic blood pressure, and catecholamine excretion increase with physical activity. This being the case, it might be reasoned that optimal warm-up would evoke a desirable level of state anxiety. This, of course, is simply speculation.

One psychological aspect of warm-up that has received some attention is the S's attitude toward an awareness of warm-up. Several studies (e.g., Asmussen and Bøje, 1945) have tried to control for this factor by keeping the subjects naïve concerning the purpose of the study. Massey *et al.* (1961) administered either indirect warm-up or no warm-up while the Ss were under hypnotic trance. The Ss performed not knowing which previous treatment was administered to them. Nonsignificant differences were found. This study has been widely quoted to "show" that the effects of warm-up are psychological. Unfortunately, whether these particular Ss would have had increased performance with the particular warm-up had they been aware of the warm-up is mere conjecture. Another study found that most of the Ss had a favorable attitude toward warm-up (Smith and Bozymowski, 1965). The authors found that the total group, and those Ss most favorable toward warm-up, performed significantly better after warm-up than after rest (0.01 level). They also found that the Ss with the least favorable attitude toward warm-up had nonsignificant differences after warm-up and rest (0.11 level). This confirms the logical assumption that a favorable attitude toward warm-up enhances its value. Esper (1966) found that indirect warm-up was superior to taking a pill, which was falsely described as having the same benefits as warm-up, or rest. Several of the Ss did have "physiological" responses to the placebo, but there did not seem to be a substantial relationship between the reaction to the pill and performance. de Vries (1959) found that an indirect warm-up was beneficial to some swimmers who had a negative attitude toward that warm-up. He later (1960) found that Ss' subjective feelings about readiness to perform had little relationship to their actual performance. Lueft (1958) found that 32 Ss preferred warm-up, 12 preferred no warm-up, and 5 were indifferent to warm-up. He found no significant difference between warm-up and rest. When looking at an individual's best performance, he found that 22 out of 29 who had their best performance after warm-up preferred warm-up and that 5 out of 12 who had their best performance after rest preferred no warm-up. This would hardly indicate that the major factor in the effectiveness of warm-up is attitude toward warm-up. It does appear that most Ss have a favorable attitude toward warm-up and that warm-up is beneficial in many performances. However, there is little evidence that would allow one to infer that positive attitude toward warm-up is the factor that causes increased performance. The conclusions in this area, too, must await systematic study.

6. *Motivation*

The incentive to perform well is normally present in athletic events (albeit at different levels according to the nature of the contest). However, when a performance is attempted in a controlled experimental setting and/or with coerced "volunteers," as is the case in many studies, the problem of obtaining maximum performance is a constant one. In addition, as Karpovich (1971) has pointed out, the motivation may be related to one's attitude toward warm-up and it is difficult to obtain a maximum effort in the no warm-up condition by Ss who believe warm-up is important. Verbal encouragement, grades, money (Rochelle *et al.*, 1960), and other incentives have been used to encourage maximum performance in all experimental conditions, but it is difficult to "prove" that the incentives were effective. This issue is confounded in that "good" subjects may try to "help the experimenter prove" what they perceive he believes, and "bad" subjects may try to prevent such results. In either case, the true conditions are thwarted. These points are pursued in detail in Chapter 1.

VI. Summary and Implications

A. Summary

The short-term effects of identical, direct, and indirect warm-up and rest on muscular performance have been reviewed. There is evidence that some types of warm-up are beneficial and some types are detrimental to cycling endurance and speed. Warm-up is strongly supported for jumping performance, with ballistic stretching better than passive stretching. Warm-up assists accuracy, movement time, range of motion, and strength in movements of selected parts of the body, but there is little evidence that it affects reaction time. In running, warm-up appears to enhance the sprints and distance runs, but there is little evidence that it improves agility or stationary running. Warm-up causes increased velocity of the baseball throw (using overload), increased distance in the softball throw, and produces a higher batting average for children, but there is no evidence that accuracy of throwing is improved. Basketball shooting and passing accuracy are enhanced by warm-up, and there is some evidence that football-passing accuracy in experienced passers and gymnastic performance are improved by warm-up. There was no significant effect of warm-up or rest in the one study on the hammer throw.

There is slight evidence that some forms of warm-up can be detrimental to jumping, agility running, sprinting, baseball throwing for accuracy, as well as the cycling endurance and speed tasks mentioned above. There are several studies using various performances that did not find evidence to support either warm-up or no warm-up as being advantageous to performance in that nonsignificant differences were observed.

Although it is widely claimed that warm-up prevents injury, there is little direct evidence to support that contention. In all the studies reviewed, most of which included maximum performance without warm-up as one of the experimental treatments, only one mentioned an injury during a no-warm-up condition. Several studies reported no soreness and/or injury resulting from performances done with and without warm-up.

The effects of factors related to warm-up and the participant cannot be determined until these factors are systematically studied. There is some indirect evidence from the studies reviewed suggesting that warm-up is more likely to benefit college-aged, trained persons with positive attitudes toward warm-up. It also appears that vigorous warm-ups with fairly short rest intervals between warm-up and performance are desirable. There are probably physiological and psychological aspects of warm-up. However, the individual components of each, their relative importance, and interaction with type of S, warm-up, and performance cannot be determined from the information available at present.

B. Implications

1. *General*

Table VII summarizes the frequency with which some type of warm-up was found to be either significantly better or worse than rest. It must

TABLE VII

Frequency of Performances Aided and Hindered by Warm-up

Results[a]	Number of performances ($N = 143$)	Percent
Active warm-up[b] better than no warm-up	76	53
No warm-up better than warm-up	10	7

[a] Fifty-seven performances (40%) did not support either warm-up or no warm-up in that there were no significant differences between some type of warm-up or no warm-up (see Section VI,B,1 for comment).

[b] Studies that used only passive warm-up were not reviewed. However, in the studies that included both passive and active warm-up, the passive warm-up was better than rest in 44% of the cases, worse than rest in 8% of the cases, and nonsignificant differences between warm-up and rest were observed in 48% of the cases.

be emphasized that the value of this type of "scorecard" has obvious limitations; e.g., each study reviewed was not equally well designed or conducted. This summary is included primarily because of the type of comparison that is made. Most reviewers have compared (a) studies finding significant differences in favor of warm-up over rest with (b) studies finding no significant differences between warm-up and rest (e.g., Howell, 1971; Jensen, 1966; Karpovich, 1971; Neuberger, 1969; Van Grundy, 1965). Finding about equal numbers of each, these reviewers have erroneously concluded that the value of warm-up compared to rest is an open question. The fault of such an analysis is that the wrong comparison has been made, based on illegitimately "accepting the null hypothesis" from nonsignificant differences. The comparison to determine value of warm-up generally should be between the two groups of results shown in Table VII, namely, (a) those studies that have found warm-up to be better than rest compared with (b) those studies that have found rest to be superior to warm-up. When this comparison is made, there is substantial evidence indicating that some types of warm-up are better than rest and little evidence that the types of warm-up used in the studies reviewed are worse than rest. On the basis of the studies reported, it is concluded that there is strong evidence that some kinds of warm-up are beneficial to performance, some evidence that a few types of warm-up are detrimental to performance, and many studies that do not find any evidence to support the benefit of either warm-up or no warm-up.

It would seem appropriate to make further comment about nonsignificant differences because of the wide misinterpretation of these studies. It is not possible to determine why the performances were not significantly different after warm-up and rest. Some of the possible reasons would be large errors, variance, and/or low reliability in tests used and small number of subjects (some of the studies finding no significant differences were almost certain to get those results because of the size and type of sample and the test). It is possible that these studies chose ineffective types, durations, and/or intensities of warm-up. Another possibility (the one normally selected by reviewers without regard to the others) is that there is no difference between warm-up and no warm-up prior to performance. The last possibility is highly unlikely in view of the numerous studies finding otherwise.

On the basis that some types of warm-up have improved performance, the logical question is not whether warm-up is beneficial, but rather which types of warm-up are beneficial for the various types of performances and participants. There would seem to be three main factors involved that should be considered in future research designs, either studied as separate independent variables, or controlled: (a) type of warm-up—identical, direct, indirect, or passive, with lack of warm-up as a control; (b) factors related to warm-up—amount of work, duration, intensity, and rest period; and (c) factors related to the participant, such as age, sex, physical condition, level of skill, attitude toward warm-up, and incentive to perform. It is further believed that none of these factors can be studied in isolation in that they interact with one another and with the specific type of task to produce the observed performance.

2. *Specific*

Although further research can (and should) define further the relative importance and contribution of the types of warm-up for various Ss and performances, this information will be a beginning rather than a final solution for the participant. Each individual will have to determine the optimal warm-up for his performance. A thorough understanding of the findings of prior research studies will provide a good starting point. The utilization of systematic methods of varying different factors involved with warm-up to determine the best combination will assist the participant in finding his own best warm-up regime.

References

Allen, T. R. (1962). "A Study of the Effects of Warm-up on Endurance." Unpublished master's thesis, Univ. of Toledo, Toledo, Ohio.

Asmussen, E., and Bøje, O. (1945). *Acta Physiol. Scand.* **10,** 1.

Bailin, S. (1964). "The Effect of Formal, Informal, and Lack of Warm-up upon the Accuracy of the Basketball Free Throw." Unpublished master's thesis, Univ. of Massachusetts, Amherst.

Barch, A. M. (1963). *Percept. Mot. Skills* **17,** 723.

Baumgarten, N. R. (1965). "The Effect of Warm-up on the Performance of a Simple Task Involving Speed of Gross Movements of the Hand and Arm." Unpublished master's thesis, Temple Univ., Philadelphia, Pennsylvania.

Benedict, G. E. (1966). "Comparative Effects of Three Experimental Warm-up Conditions upon Accuracy." Unpublished master's thesis, Univ. of British Columbia, Vancouver.

Blank, L. B. (1955). *Athletic J.* **35,** 104.

Blohm, F. (1969). "Running Endurance Performance as Affected by Warm-up and Varied Rest Intervals." Unpublished doctoral dissertation, Univ. of Arkansas, Fayetteville.

Brose, D. E., and Hanson, D. L. (1967). *Res. Quart.* **38,** 528.

Buresh, D. A. (1967). "The Effect of Warm-up on the Running Performance of Trained and Untrained Subjects." Unpublished master's thesis, Univ. of Wyoming, Laramie.

Burke, R. K. (1957). "Relationships between Physical Performance and Warm-up Procedures of Varying Intensity and Duration. Doctoral dissertation microcards, Univ. of Southern California, Los Angeles.
Carter, L. F. (1958). "The Effect of Warm-up Activities upon Fatigue and Endurance." Unpublished master's thesis, Univ. of California, Los Angeles.
Catalano, J. F., and Walen, P. M. (1967). *Percept. Mot. Skills* **24**, 1223.
Creek, R. E. (1964). "The Effect of Overload Warm-up on the Accuracy of Throwing a Twelve-inch Softball." Unpublished master's thesis, Eastern Illinois Univ., Charleston.
Delforge, G. (1966). "An Analysis of Selected Factors related to the Occurrence of Athletic Injuries with Implication for Prevention." Unpublished master's thesis, Kent State Univ., Kent, Ohio.
Delforge, G. (1969). *Athletic J.* **49**, 108.
de Vries, H. A. (1959). *Res. Quart.* **30**, 11.
de Vries, H. A. (1960). "Warm-up Effects of Relaxation and Stretching Techniques upon Gross Motor Performance." Doctoral dissertation microcards, Univ. of Southern California, Los Angeles.
de Vries, H. A. (1966). "Physiology of Exercise in Physical Education and Athletics." W. C. Brown, Dubuque, Iowa.
Dohrmann, P. F. (1956). "The Effect of Strenuous Exercise of the Lower Extremities upon the Strength of the Hands and the Forearms." Unpublished master's thesis, State Univ. of Iowa, Iowa City.
Elbel, E. R. (1940). *Res. Quart.* **11**, 86.
Emerson, M. H. (1968). "The Relationship of Formal, Informal, and Lack of Warm-up Exercises to Performance Involving Speed of Movement." Unpublished master's thesis, Smith College, Northampton, Massachusetts.
Esper, R. E. (1966). "Effects of Physical and Psychological Warm-up on the Vertical Jump." Unpublished master's thesis, Univ. of Florida, Gainesville.
Fieldman, H. (1968). *Res. Quart.* **39**, 518.
Filipponi, M. L. (1951). "The Effect of Warming-up upon Speed of Swimming 100 yds." Unpublished master's thesis, Springfield College, Springfield, Massachusetts.
Glidewell, W. F. (1964). "An Investigation of Various Warm-up Procedures in Relation to Physical Performance." Unpublished doctoral dissertation, Univ. of Texas, Austin.
Graw, H. (1959). "The Effect of Preliminary Muscular Stretching on Jumping Performance." Unpublished master's thesis, Univ. of California, Berkeley.
Grodjinovsky, A., and Magel, J. R. (1970). *Res. Quart.* **41**, 116.
Hale, C. J. (1949). "Effect of Preliminary Massage on the 440 Yard Run." Unpublished master's thesis, Springfield College, Springfield, Massachusetts.
Hansen, G. F. (1959). "Relationship of Different Types of Warm-up on Performance in the 440-yard Run." Unpublished master's thesis, Univ. of Iowa, Iowa City.
Harvill, A. H. (1966). "The Relative Effects of Selected Warm-up Experiences on Strength, Agility, Flexibility, and Power." Unpublished doctoral dissertation, Indiana Univ., Bloomington.
Högberg, P., and Ljunggren, O. (1947). *Sv. Idrott* **40**; quoted in P. O. Åstrand and K. Rodahl (1970). "Textbook of Work Physiology," p. 524. McGraw-Hill, New York.
Homola, S. (1968). *Scholastic Coach* **37**, 38.
Hoogendoorn, R. H. (1963). "The Effects of Cooling and Various Intensities of

Preliminary Exercise on Reaction Time." Unpublished master's thesis, Univ. of Toledo, Toledo, Ohio.
Howell, M. L. (1971). *In* "Encyclopedia of Sport Sciences and Medicine" (L. Larson, ed.), pp. 1578–1579. Macmillan, New York.
Hutterly, W. U. (1967). "Effects of Varied Intervals of Rest between Warm-up and Performance on 440-yard Dash Times." Unpublished master's thesis, North Texas State Univ., Denton.
Ihm, J. A. (1956). "A Comparison of the Effectiveness of Three Methods of Warm-up." Master's thesis microcards, State Univ. of Iowa, Iowa City.
Jensen, C. R. (1966). *Athletic J.* **47,** 24.
Karpovich, P. V. (1971). *In* "Encyclopedia of Sport Sciences and Medicine," pp. 166–171. Macmillan, New York.
Karpovich, P. V., and Hale, C. (1956). *J. Amer. Med. Ass.* **162,** 1117.
Karpovich, P. V., and Pestrecov, K. (1941). *Amer. J. Physiol.* **134,** 300.
Kaye, G. E. (1967). "The Effect of Standard Rate Warm-up on Static Knee Extension Strength." Unpublished master's thesis, Michigan State Univ., East Lansing.
Kracik, C. J. (1969). "The Effect of Selected Preliminary Activities on Bat Speed." Unpublished master's thesis, Illinois State Univ., Normal.
Lotter, W. S. (1959). *Res. Quart.* **30,** 57.
Lueft, R. J. (1958). "The Effect of Warm-up on Swimming Speed." Unpublished master's thesis, Pennsylvania State Univ., University Park.
Lukes, H. J. (1954). "The Effect of Warm-up Exercise on the Amplitude of Voluntary Movement." Master's thesis microcards, Univ. of Wisconsin, Madison.
Lynch, R. M. (1959). "The Circulatory and Metabolic Effects of Preliminary Work on an 'All-out' Performance." Unpublished master's thesis, Univ. of Illinois, Urbana.
McGavin, R. J. (1968). *Res. Quart.* **30,** 125.
Malan, E. (1960). *Proc. Coll. Phys. Educ. Ass.* **36,** 45.
Massey, B. H., Johnson, W. R., and Kramer, G. F. (1961). *Res. Quart.* **32,** 63.
Mathews, D. K. and Snyder, A. H. (1959). *Res. Quart.* **30,** 4.
Mellerowicz, H., and Hansen, G. (1971). *In* "Encyclopedia of Sport Sciences and Medicine" (L. Larson, ed.), pp. 1585–1587. Macmillan, New York.
Messina, V. (1965). *Athletic J.* **45,** 97.
Michael, E., Skubic, V., and Rochelle, R. (1957). *Res. Quart.* **28,** 357.
Middlebrooks, G. H. (1966). "The Effect of Warming-up upon Swimming Performance." Unpublished master's thesis, Springfield College, Springfield, Massachusetts.
Miller, R. (1951). *Athletic J.* **31,** 28.
Morehouse, L. E., and Miller, A. T., Jr. (1967). "Physiology of Exercise," 5th ed. Mosby, St. Louis, Missouri.
Morgenegg, B., and Jensen, C. R. (1966). "The Relative Effectiveness of 6 Methods of Warm-up on Gymnastic Performance." Unpublished study. Quoted by Jensen (1966).
Moss, D. (1966). *Scholastic Coach* **35,** 17.
Muido, L. (1946). *Acta Physiol. Scand.* **12,** 102.
Myers, D. G. (1967). "The Effects of Varied Intensities of Informal Warm-up upon Performance in Throwing the Hammer." Unpublished master's thesis, Springfield College, Springfield, Massachusetts.
Nelson, R. C., and Lambert, W. (1965). *Res. Quart.* **36,** 296.
Neuberger, T. (1969). *JOHPER* **40,** 75.

O'Connor, W. R. (1955). *Scholastic Coach* **25**, 48.
Owens, J. (1970). *Athletic J.* **50**, 39.
Pacheco, B. A. (1957). *Res. Quart.* **28**, 55.
Pacheco, B. A. (1959). *Res. Quart.* **30**, 202.
Paseltiner, L. R. (1957). "The Immediate Effect of Light Warm-ups and Heavy Resistance Exercise on Speed of Movement of Arm Extension." Doctoral dissertation microcards, Pennsylvania State Univ., University Park.
Phillips, W. H. (1963). *Res. Quart.* **34**, 370.
Powers, J. H. (1960). "The Effects of No Warm-up, Review of Skill, Informal Warm-up, and Mental Practice on Physical Performance in Selected Activities." Unpublished master's thesis, Pennsylvania State Univ., University Park.
Raines, P. A. (1952). "The Effect of Warm-up, a Cold Pack, and a Hot Shower upon Performance on the Step Counter." Unpublished master's thesis, State Univ. of Iowa, Iowa City.
Richards, D. K. (1968). *Res. Quart.* **39**, 668.
Rochelle, R. H., Skubic, V., and Michael, E. D. (1960). *Res. Quart.* **31**, 499.
Rosen, M. (1952). *Res. Quart.* **23**, 226.
Schmid, L. (1947). *Cas. Lek. Cesk.* **26**, 950.
Schutz, R. W. (1966). "The Effects of Various Warm-up Procedures on Acceleration, Velocity, and Muscular Endurance." Unpublished master's thesis, Univ. of Alberta, Edmonton.
Scogin, H. D. (1969). "A Comparison of Swimming Performances Following Selected Intensities of Warm-up with Varied Rest Intervals." Unpublished master's thesis, Univ. of Arkansas, Fayetteville.
Sedgwick, A. W. (1964). *Res. Quart.* **35**, 532.
Sessoms, H. D. (1971). *In* "Encyclopedia of Sport Sciences and Medicine" (L. Larson, ed.), pp. 13–20. Macmillan, New York.
Severino, W. R. (1966). "The Effect of Warm-up upon Accuracy in Football Passing." Unpublished master's thesis, Illinois State Univ., Normal.
Sills, F. D., and O'Riley, V. E. (1956). *Res. Quart.* **27**, 217.
Simonson, E. N., Teslenko, W., and Gorkin, M. (1936). *Arbeitsphysiologie* **9**, 152.
Simpson, E. L. (1968). "The Influence of Warm-up Exercise Heart Rate at Three Age Levels." Unpublished master's thesis, Univ. of Arkansas, Fayetteville.
Skubic, V., and Hodgkins, J. (1957). *Res. Quart.* **28**, 147.
Smith, J. L., and Bozymowski, M. F. (1965). *Res. Quart.* **36**, 78.
Smith, L. H. (1960). "A Study on the Effect of Warm-up on Speed of Running." Unpublished master's thesis, Univ. of Iowa, Iowa City.
Stansbury, E. (1942). *Athletic J.* **22**, 18; **22**, 33.
Start, K. B. (1962). *Archiv. Phys. Med. Rehabil.* **43**, 284.
Steacy, G. B. (1960). "Relationships between Warm-ups and Physical Performance." Unpublished master's thesis, Woman's College of the Univ. of North Carolina, Greensboro.
Stockholm, A. J., and Nelson, R. C. (1965). *Res. Quart.* **36**, 337.
Straub, W. F. (1968). *Res. Quart.* **39**, 370.
Sucec, A. (1967). "The Effects of Preliminary Exercise on Endurance Performance." Doctoral dissertation microcards, Univ. of California, Berkeley.
Swan, R. B. (1968). "The Effect of Warm-up on the Passing Accuracy of Quarterbacks." Unpublished master's thesis. Sacramento State College, Sacramento, California.
Teague, E. (1966). "The Relative Effectiveness of No Warm-up, Squat Thrusts and

Conventional Warm-ups on Endurance, Flexibility, and Speed and Agility." Unpublished master's thesis, Univ. of Washington, Seattle.

Thompson, H. (1958). *Res. Quart.* **29,** 231.

Tremble, N. C. (1962). "The Influence of Warm-up on Injury to the Hamstring Muscles in College Sprinters." Unpublished doctoral dissertation, Colorado State College, Greeley.

Twardowski, E. T. (1962). "The Effect of Warm-up upon 100-yard Swimming Performance." Unpublished doctoral dissertation, Temple Univ., Philadelphia, Pennsylvania.

Van Buren, E. G. (1964). *Athletic J.* **45,** 16.

Van Grundy, W. F. (1963). "Relation of Amount of Warm-up to the Effectiveness of Motor Performance." Unpublished master's thesis, Univ. of California, Berkeley.

Van Grundy, W. (1965). *Scholastic Coach* **34,** 44.

Van Huss, W. D., Albrecht, L., Nelson, R., and Hagerman, R. (1962). *Res. Quart.* **33,** 472.

Warner, J. F. (1954). *JOHPER* **25,** 12.

Webb, B. (1963). "The Effectiveness of Two Methods of Warm-up on Physical Fitness." Unpublished master's thesis, Arkansas State Univ., Jonesboro.

Wells, F. L. (1908). *Amer. J. Psychol.* **19,** 437.

Williamson, K. R. (1959). "The Effects of Batting Warm-up on Performance." Unpublished master's thesis, Univ. of California, Los Angeles.

Witte, F. (1962). *Res. Quart.* **33,** 308.

Zieger, P. C. (1964). "Influence of Warm-up, Running Surface and Different Types of Obstacles on Performance of the Illinois Agility Run." Unpublished master's thesis, Univ. of Washington, Seattle.

Chapter 7

Hypnosis and Muscular Performance

William P. Morgan

I. Introduction

A. Overview

The popular literature contains countless examples of superhuman feats following hypnotic suggestion. As a matter of fact there seems to be little doubt that significant increments in muscular performance can be elicited in certain Ss following hypnotic suggestion. The fact remains, however, that a review of the experimental literature does not justify the view that performance in the hypnotic or posthypnotic states will necessarily surpass performance in the motivated waking state. The transcendence of normal capacity following hypnotic suggestion represents a very complex issue.

In order to assert that the hypnotic transcendence of normal capacity has occurred, it is imperative that authentic rather than pseudo-base-line measures of physical working capacity be obtained initially. This, of course, is a thorny measurement problem. While human-performance researchers speak of maximal tests of physical capacity, there is strong evidence to support the view that maximal performance is not possible without severe physical damage to the S (e.g., broken bones, torn ligaments, heat exhaustion, etc.). Maximal effort in the research laboratory should probably be regarded as "all-out" work, and this should be viewed operationally within the context of functional limitations. Such concessions can be tolerated when rigorous research design and statistical control are imposed. It must be reiterated, however, that valid base-line data must be available in order to meaningfully assess the effect of hypnotic suggestion.

B. Purpose

Reviews dealing with hypnosis and muscular performance have been presented by Hull (1933), Gorton (1959), Johnson (1961a), Weitzenhoffer (1963), and Barber (1966). The primary purpose of the present chapter is to update these earlier reviews and examine the efficacy of hypnosis as an ergogenic aid.

C. Earlier Reviews

One of the earliest critical reviews of the literature dealing with hypnotic suggestibility and the transcendence of voluntary capacity was written by Hull (1933). He concluded that the available evidence was contradictory, and he explained the conflicting findings in terms of design inelegancies.

Following a review of neuromuscular functioning in the hypnotic state, Gorton (1959) suggested that the enhanced muscular performance commonly reported might result from disinhibition of inhibitory phenomena. For example, he pointed out that ". . . the full contractile power of human muscle is known to be greater than is normally apparent as demonstrated by the fractures due to muscular contraction observed as complications in electric shock therapy" (p. 266). He suggested that reserves of muscular power probably exist but are not available under normal conditions. Also, he proposed that hypnotic suggestion is possibly capable of mobilizing these reserves.

Johnson (1961a) reported that under certain conditions direct suggestions designed to enhance muscular performance may work, but such suggestions cannot be counted upon to facilitate muscular strength and endurance. He emphasized, however, that negative suggestions to decrease muscular performance are much more likely to be effective.

Weitzenhoffer (1963) reviewed a series of studies dealing with hypnosis and muscular strength, and he emphasized that few of the investigations were comparable in procedure. This led him to suggest that the apparent contradictions among studies might simply reflect dissimilar designs. In general, his review does not support the view that hypnosis improves muscular performance.

More recently, Barber (1966) presented a critical review of research studies dealing with the effects of hypnosis and motivational suggestions on muscular strength and endurance. He concluded that the hypnotic state, without suggestions for enhanced muscular performance, does not produce increments in muscular strength and endurance. In addition, he reported that motivational suggestions are generally capable of augmenting muscular strength and endurance in both the waking and hypnotic states, and he emphasized the necessity of not confounding hypnosis and suggestion.

Actually, one of the most serious methodological problems that has characterized hypnosis research involving muscular performance has been the confounding of suggestion and state. Typical experimental paradigms have involved the comparison of muscular performance following suggestions of enhanced or decreased capacity in the hypnotic state with no suggestions in the waking state. It seems that several alternative approaches might be employed. First, if the investigator is concerned with the influence of hypnosis per se on muscular performance, then Ss should be tested under identical circumstances in both the hypnotic and waking states. This strategy was employed by Eysenck (1941), who found that hypnosis per se resulted in facilitation of grip endurance. A second approach would be to present task-motivating instructions to the same S in both the hypnotic and waking states (Nicholson, 1920) or to present the same suggestions to different groups of Ss (Barber and Calverley, 1964). While Nicholson (1920) observed that suggestions given during hypnosis were much more effective than the same suggestions in the waking state, Barber and Calverley (1964) found that motivational instructions in the waking state were just as effective as the same suggestions presented under hypnotic conditions. These, of course, are simply selected examples chosen to illustrate two preferred approaches. The important point is that investigators should not compare task-motivating instructions in the hypnotic state with no suggestion in the waking state. As pointed out earlier, this represents confounding of suggestion and state.

The necessity of not confounding such variables is illustrated by Manzer's (1934) nonhypnotic study. He tested 50 males and 50 females between the ages of 18 and 25 on a strength of grip task. Manzer (1934) did not employ hypnosis, but his investigation is cited here because the findings support the view that suggestion in the waking state is capable of both increasing and decreasing muscular strength. Twenty-five males and 25 females served as experimental Ss, while a like number of both sexes served as controls. The experimental Ss were requested to perform maximal contractions and they were informed that the dynamometer spring would be adjusted to easy, medium, and hard loads, which would be compared to a standard load. The S was told which resistance he was squeezing against prior to each test, but the load was actually of uniform resistance under all conditions. The control Ss performed all trials against the "standard" resistance.

The male Ss experienced reductions of 7.24 and 4.82% following suggestions of easy and medium resistance, respectively, while the suggestions of hard resistance evoked an increment of 4.66% above the control suggestions. Also, the difference between the suggestions of easy and hard was significant. While suggestions of easy and medium resistances did not reduce the performance of the female Ss, suggestion of the hard load evoked a 7% increase. In addition, the reliability coefficients for the task ranged from 0.93 to 0.94 under the control conditions, whereas these reliabilities were much lower for the experimental trials, ranging from 0.69 to 0.89. Furthermore, the suggestion of easy resistance increased variability the most while the suggestion of hard resistance increased it the least.

Manzer's (1934) investigation demonstrates that muscular strength can be increased and decreased significantly under waking conditions. Therefore, it is imperative that investigations involving hypnotic suggestion include appropriate waking controls in order to prevent confounding of independent variables.

D. Summary

An examination of earlier reviews dealing with the enhancement of muscular performance by means of hypnotic suggestion is generally not favorable, but these reviews emphasize that many questions remain unanswered. The only point of agreement seems to be that negative suggestions are almost always effective.

II. Review of Literature

A. Overview

The effect of hypnotic suggestion on muscular activity has been examined from several vantage points. The majority of such research has dealt with the effect of various forms of suggestion on variables that physical educationists have historically regarded as muscular strength and endurance. Additional research has been concerned with human-performance variables such as oxygen uptake and physical working capacity. These studies have been experimental and conducted in research laboratories for the most part. In addition, a number of clinical reports have been presented regarding the hypnotic investigation and treatment of motor problems in athletes. These topics are considered separately in the following review.

B. Muscular Strength and Endurance

One of the earliest experiments was conducted by Rieger (1884), who evaluated the arm endurance of one female S. In this investigation the S held a pin between her extended fingers, and her arm was maintained in a horizontal position. The pin's shadow was cast on the drum of a moving kymograph, and a permanent record was made by simply making dots where the shadow fell. Rieger (1884) emphasized that hypnotic catalepsy of the extended arm greatly facilitated the S's performance. In view of the fact that only one S was employed, there was no mention of tremor under the two conditions, reference was not made to whether the S's arm was visible for the two treatments, quantitative data were not presented, and suggestions were different for the two states, it would seem reasonable to conclude that Rieger's (1884) investigation does not support the view that muscular endurance is enhanced by hypnosis. Also, single-S designs should not be employed when extensive normative data do not exist for the dependent variable; that is, meaningful interpretation of performance is not possible in such a case. This problem characterizes much of the hypnosis research to be reviewed in the present chapter.

In a related investigation Charcot (1889) measured arm tremor as the S held his arm extended with the palm down. One "hystero-epileptic" patient served as the hypnotic S, and his performance was compared to that of a control S. A pressure chamber was placed on the back of the S's hand, and the chamber's rubber membrane supported a weight. Air pressure in the chamber changed with vertical arm movement, and this enabled an attached marking lever to record tremor. The tremors recorded for the hypnotic S were perfectly smooth, whereas the control S's record reflected a great deal of agitation. Also, Charcot reported that the hypnotic S had shallow and regular breathing, whereas the control S's breathing was deep and irregular. These findings are difficult to evaluate since it is not clear whether they reflect an effect due to hypnosis or the psychological state of the patient. Also, the patient may have possessed superior physical ability in the waking state as well. Indeed, psychiatric patients have been found to decrease on standard tests of muscular performance as they improve psychologically.

While Moll (1913) apparently conducted similar experiments, he did not present an actual description of his studies. However, he reported that a hypnotic S can hold a weight in his outstretched hand longer and more steadily than a control S in the waking state. The reports of Reiger (1884), Charcot (1889), and Moll (1913) are frequently cited as evidence that hypnosis facilitates muscular performance. The evidence from these studies, however, is certainly not convincing.

In a number of investigations attempts have been made to facilitate performance on the hand dynamometer task by means of hypnotic suggestions. In one of the earliest studies, Hadfield (1924) reported that the mean strength of grip was 101 lb for three male Ss in the control waking state. The Ss were then tested following hypnotic suggestion that they would be very strong, and their mean performance increased to 142 lb. The Ss were aware of the experiment's purpose, and therefore it is conceivable that the Ss actually suppressed their performances in the waking state. While this is certainly a possibility, it is not likely that the mean gain of 41 lb under the hypnotic condition completely represents an elevation over a pseudo-base line since 126 lb would be the highest predicted value for any age (Kellor *et al.*, 1971). In other words, it would seem reasonable to suggest that approximately 25 lb of the 41-lb increment might be attributable to initial suppression. In either case, the hypnotic performance is considerably higher than one would anticipate on the basis of published norms (Toews, 1964; Kellor *et al.*, 1971). Of course, Hadfield (1924) confounded state and suggestion, and he did not counterbalance the treatments.

One of the most frequently cited investigations was conducted by Nicholson (1920), who exercised seven Ss with a Mosso ergograph. The

Ss flexed the middle finger every 2 seconds in time with a metronome,* and the weight employed on the ergograph was 3 kg. All Ss were capable of entering a deep trance characterized by cataleptic rigidity. The ergograph performance of each S was first assessed in the waking state. Work capacity was then assessed (a) during hypnosis with suggestions of increased ability throughout work, (b) in the waking state immediately following hypnosis, (c) in the hypnotic state immediately following the preceding treatment, (d) in the hypnotic state that was induced when the waking S worked almost to the point of fatigue, and (e) in the waking state with motivational suggestions given when the working S almost reached the point of fatigue. Nicholson (1920) concluded that ". . . a very definite increase in muscular efficiency can be obtained by suggestion in the hypnotic state and that suggestions given even while the subject is fully awake influence muscular efficiency to some extent" (p. 90). He emphasized, however, that suggestions given during hypnosis were much more effective than the same suggestions administered in the waking state.

Young (1925) assessed strength of grip in 12 hypnotic Ss under control and hypnotic conditions, and compared their performance with that of three nonhypnotic Ss under pseudohypnotic and waking conditions. Seven hypnotic Ss did better under the hypnosis condition, four did worse, and one equaled his record. Young interpreted the findings as follows. "These results seem to indicate that the capacity of the muscles brought into play is about equal in the two states (p. 220)." It is unfortunate that he did not present the actual values for the various conditions. At any rate, these findings were not treated statistically and it is difficult to accept Young's conclusion in view of the fact that seven of his twelve Ss improved in the hypnotic state.†

Wells (1928) reported a case study dealing with a 27-year-old male. The S was administered an "achievement capacity" test in which he was required to stand on his toes as long as possible, and he stood on a mechanism that provided a visual display pointer for self-evaluative purposes. The S was first tested in the waking state (apparently without suggestion), and 12 days later he was tested in the hypnotic state. Suggestions of immunity to fatigue and of maximal endurance were administered in the hypnotic state. The S scored 8 minutes and 30 seconds in the waking state as compared with 9 minutes and 30 seconds in the hypnotic state. Wells concluded that ". . . there is not much reason to

* See Williams (1929) for a thorough critique of Nicholson's paper. In retrospect there can be little question about the heuristic value of Nicholson's report (1920). Unfortunately, Nicholson died while his article was in press.

† In a later report Eysenck (1941) critically discussed Young's work (1925) in light of his own observations.

believe that the latter results would have been different if the suggestions had been given to the patient without any hypnotic preliminaries" (p. 275). Case studies of this nature are difficult to assess unless repeated measures are performed in counterbalanced fashion. At any rate, an increase of 1 minute on a muscular endurance task would generally be regarded as a significant increment.

Five Ss were tested by Williams (1929) on a modified Mosso ergograph in which finger flexion was performed at a rate of 80 times/minute to the beat of a metronome. The resistance consisted of a 5-kg weight for all cycles except two in which a 3-kg weight was employed. Four of the five Ss were somnambules and the fifth, while having no amnesia for the trance period, experienced all forms of catelepsy. The five Ss were tested in both the trance and waking states. Williams (1929) concluded that there was an increase in the amount of work done in the trance state as compared with the waking state even though equivalent suggestions were employed in each state. Inspection of the data reveals that one S accounted for much of the average gain observed during the trance state. For example, the average percent increase was 16.08 in the trance state, and this average increase drops to 6.87% when the one extreme score is eliminated. At any rate, a gain of only 7% would also be regarded as significant for such a task. Furthermore, it should be emphasized that comparable suggestions were employed in both the hypnotic and waking states.

Nevski and Sryashchich (1930) reported a study dealing with the influence of hypnosis on muscular strength. These investigators evaluated muscular strength with a dynamometer in the waking state, during hypnosis, and following posthypnotic suggestion. An insignificant decrease in muscular strength was observed during weak hypnosis where special instructions regarding muscular strength were not given. However, a total adynamy was observed during deep hypnosis. Also, a special suggestion in mild hypnosis was found to decrease muscular performance from 50% to complete adynamy, whereas a corresponding suggestion was unable to improve performance. Furthermore, posthypnotic suggestions had practically no effect on muscular strength.

Williams (1930) evaluated arm-holding endurance in eight Ss (two male and six female). In this task the S's arm was rotated outwardly with the arm horizontal to the floor and the palm forward. A string was attached to the S's wrist, extended over a pulley, and attached to a kymograph. The dependent variable was arm oscillation and vertical descent. The Ss were given two practice trials and then tested four times in the trance state and four times in the waking state, and the order of testing was counterbalanced. Williams (1930) reported that performance in the trance state was not superior to that in the waking state.

The effect of hypnosis on running distances of 100 and 1000 m was evaluated by Simonson (1938). He found the time for both distances to be faster during hypnosis. Also, threads attached to electrical circuits were placed at 4-m intervals, allowing computation of within-run velocities. Typical patterns involved a rapid acceleration followed by a plateau and then a slowing down toward the end. In addition, it was noted that the greatest variability between runners occurred at the level portions of the curves.

The influence of hypnotic suggestions designed to enhance and decrease strength of grip has been reported by Crane (1940). Five male Ss were tested in the waking state, and their maximal strength of grip averaged 101 lb. Under conditions of hypnosis they were told that they were weak and feeble, and their average performance decreased to 69 lb. Of course, it is obvious that such a decrement could be evoked in any cooperative S under waking conditions. However, their performance averaged 140 lb following the suggestion that they were now powerful. In other words, a decrease of 30% and an increase of 40% in strength of grip was evoked following suggestion of decreased and increased strength, respectively.

A fundamental question that remains unanswered regarding Crane's (1940) report is whether these same changes could have been produced in the waking state. It is obvious that decreases could readily be produced in the cooperative S. However, the matter of evoking increments is far more complex. It is unlikely that the pretest mean of 101 lb represents a valid base line for these five soldiers. One would anticipate an average of about 125 lb. At any rate, the hypnotic condition demonstrated that the average performance of 101 lb was indeed a pseudo-base line. Since the order was not counterbalanced it is conceivable that the Ss consciously or unconsciously depressed their performances on the pretest. The importance of considering order effects is illustrated in the work of Evans and Orne (1965). At the same time, a score of 140 lb is well above expectations, and therefore it would appear that hypnotic suggestion of enhanced strength was effective. However, since it is generally accepted that most Ss are capable of performing above their normal levels in various circumstances, it is not at all clear that hypnosis per se evoked the observed increases; that is, state and suggestion were confounded.

Eysenck (1941)* tested one 50-year-old male S who was capable of

* Eysenck (1941) also tested a 25-year-old female, but he presented detailed results only for the male S.

entering a deep trance with complete posthypnotic amnesia. The *S* performed 24 successive maximal pulls on a grip dynamometer with 10-second rest periods between contractions. The trials were alternated between normal and hypnotized states with five trials for each, but suggestions of enhanced performance were not given under either condition. At no point did the fatigue curve in the normal state rise above the hypnotic curve. Also, the distance between the two curves grew greater and greater until finally the difference was approximately seven times as large as at the beginning. Eysenck commented that ". . . in the normal state the subject is nearing exhaustion, in the hypnotized state he goes on machine-like, without tiring (p. 312)." The *S* performed 24 successive maximal pulls and Eysenck simply interpreted the beginning of the curve as representing strength and the latter portion endurance. He interpreted his findings as indicating that fatigue levels differed for the two states but grip strength did not. Since the *S* was clearly performing an endurance task this conclusion seems questionable regarding grip strength. In other words, the *S* was not tested for strength of grip alone in the two states. This investigation supports the view that hypnosis per se facilitates muscular performance. Also, Eysenck (1941) found that variability was less under the hypnosis condition.

The effect of hypnosis on the physical performance of 11 female *S*s was evaluated by Mead and Roush (1949). One hundred volunteers were screened, and the 11 *S*s selected were all capable of achieving amnesic somnambulism. Strength of grip, elbow flexion strength, and an endurance test that consisted of gripping an overhead bar and hanging for as long as possible served as dependent variables. The *S*s received stereotyped suggestions designed to enhance performance in both the hypnotic and control states. Suggestions in the hypnotic state resulted in a significant increment in performance for the test of elbow flexion strength. Significant changes were not observed, however, for the bar hang or the grip dynamometer test. This study is important for at least three reasons. First, treatment (hypnosis versus control) was not confounded with suggestion; that is, the same stereotyped suggestion was employed under both conditions. Second, the number of *S*s employed in this study was greater than that reported in previous investigations. Third, these are the first investigators to discuss the reliability of their test instruments. By today's standards their test–retest reliabilities for muscular endurance would not be acceptable. In addition, the investigation raises a question regarding task specificity; that is, hypnotic suggestion was demonstrated to enhance performance on the elbow flexion strength test but not for the tests of endurance or strength of grip.

Therefore, even with the same group of Ss the matter of task specificity is quite important.

Roush (1951) replicated this investigation with fifteen females and five males who were all capable of achieving amnesic somnambulism. These Ss were screened from 250 volunteers by means of hypnoinductive techniques, and therefore it is reasonable to assume that Roush was employing Ss who were responsive to hypnotic suggestion. The results of two experiments are presented in her discussion. Eleven female and five male Ss participated in the first series and ten female Ss took part in the second series. Six of the Ss in the second experiment had also participated in the first series of tests. In the first experiment stereotyped suggestions designed to enhance performance on a strength of grip, elbow flexion, and a bar-hanging task were administered in both the waking and trance states. Performance in the hypnotic state was significantly superior to that in the waking state for elbow flexion strength. Significant differences were not observed, however, for the test of grip strength and bar-hanging tasks. This finding was in agreement with the earlier report of Mead and Roush (1949). Similar stereotyped suggestions were employed, but they were changed slightly to minimize the experience of pain. The Ss were tested in the waking, hypnotic, and posthypnotic states with the same suggestions used in all states. Elbow flexion strength in the hypnotic and posthypnotic states was significantly higher than that in the waking state, but performances in the hypnotic and posthypnotic states did not differ from each other. Also, strength of grip was significantly greater in the hypnotic and posthypnotic states when compared with waking performance. Endurance as measured by the bar-hanging task differed significantly between the hypnotic and control states. Roush (1951) concluded that ". . . when given instructions to disregard pain, subjects showed an increased performance in all three tests in the hypnotic state. There are indications that this increased performance probably results from removal of inhibitory influences during the hypnotic state" (p. 410).

It will be recalled that Mead and Roush (1949) earlier reported that, while hypnotic suggestions facilitated elbow flexion strength, the same suggestions did not enhance grip strength or bar-hanging endurance. This was again observed in the first phase of Roush's (1951) later work. However, in the second phase, elbow flexion strength, grip strength, and bar-hanging endurance were all facilitated in the hypnotic state. It should be emphasized that the latter study also incorporated suggestions designed to minimize pain. It is difficult to accept the view that enhanced performance resulted from instructions to disregard pain since the same instructions were apparently employed in the control state as well. One interesting observation in the Mead and Roush (1949) study was not emphasized by the authors. They reported that the test–retest reliability for elbow flexion strength was $r = 0.66$ in the waking state and $r = 0.94$ in the trance state. Since the reliability of this test was considerably higher in the trance state, it might be possible that differences between the two states are simply related to relative levels of measurement precision. Such a proposal is entirely speculative and should be tested systematically. At any rate, the reports of Mead and Roush (1949) and Roush (1951) support the view that hypnotic suggestion can facilitate muscular performance.

Mierke (1956) reported that hypnotized Ss ceased to work on an ergograph task sooner than Ss in the waking state. However, the hypnotized Ss increased their effort when they were told that they were in a competitive situation. This observation emphasizes the important role played by the type of suggestion used. Also, it relates to the matter of social facilitation discussed in Chapter 9.

Hottinger (1958) tested 12 Ss in the waking state on hand, back, and leg dynamometer strength, as well as on a jump and reach task. Six of these Ss were considered "good" hypnotic Ss (highly suggestible) and assigned to the experimental or hypnotic group, while the remaining six Ss were regarded as "poor" hypnotic Ss (low suggestibility) and assigned to the control group. Both the hypnotic and control Ss were retested following suggestions of enhanced performance. Back and leg strength were increased significantly in the hypnotic Ss, but the hand dynamometer and jump and reach tasks were not influenced. The control group did not increase significantly for any of the tests. Unfortunately, there is no way of knowing whether the "good" hypnotic Ss (highly suggestible Ss) would have also increased their performance with similar suggestions in the waking state; that is, suggestion and state were confounded.

Nine Ss* were tested by Orne (1959) on a muscular endurance task consisting of holding a kilogram weight at arm's length. The Ss were first tested in the hypnotic state with suggestions that the right arm would not experience pain or fatigue, and these Ss were instructed to hallucinate a table supporting the extended arm. Suggestions were also administered throughout performance of the task to the effect that the S's arm would not get tired and that he would continue to see the table. After completion of the task, care was taken to insure that the S was in deep trance,

* Orne implies that these Ss were male and Barber (1966), in his review, states that "Orne (1959) tested nine selected 'hypnotizable' male subjects" (p. 46). Orne (1959), however, indicates elsewhere that at least one of the Ss was a female (see footnote c, Table 4, in Orne's article).

and then posthypnotic amnesia was induced. The S was retested in the waking state within 30 minutes of the first test, and various task-motivating instructions were administered. For example, the S was told that females could hold the weight a certain length of time, which was actually the length of time the S held the weight in the hypnotic state (see footnote, p. 204). The S was also told that he would receive a monetary reward if he surpassed specific goals. In the task-motivating situation seven of the nine Ss surpassed their trance performances. The other two Ss also improved when given a second chance and additional task-motivating instructions.

It should be emphasized that the treatments were not counterbalanced; that is, trance performance preceded waking performance by approximately 30 minutes. In a later report Evans and Orne (1965) demonstrated that muscular endurance scores obtained under hypnosis in a waking–hypnosis order are superior to those for a hypnosis–waking order. Also, exercise physiologists might suggest that enhanced performance in Orne's (1959) study might simply reflect an effect due to warm-up. This point is pursued in Chapter 6. It is also possible that trance performance resulted in learning or a realization of performance potential. It is quite common for Ss to score higher on subsequently administered trials for a wide variety of physical tasks. A number of reviewers have interpreted Orne's findings to mean that performance in the motivated waking state can be equal or superior to performance in the hypnotic state. Such an interpretation is not justified for the portion of his article just reviewed. An alternative explanation might be that the "maximal" performance elicited in the hypnotic state resulted in a sort of "psychological breakthrough" that persisted into the waking-state setting. Such a view is plausible when one considers the case of the professional football player discussed by Johnson and Kramer (1961).

An experiment dealing with the effects of posthypnotic suggestions on an all-out effort of short duration was reported by Johnson *et al.* (1960). The Ss performed an all-out "dash" of 100 revolutions on a bicycle ergometer that was loaded at 26.8 lb. The average performance time was approximately 40 seconds. Hypnotic suggestions designed to enhance performance were not facilitative. These investigators pointed out, however, that the Ss invariably reported feeling better after the ride when the posthypnotic suggestions were given, even though they presumably were not aware that suggestions had been given to them at all. It should also be emphasized that all of the Ss in this investigation had high levels of physical fitness and were former athletes who had previously experienced "all-out" efforts on many occasions. Therefore, it is quite conceivable that the waking base-line performance represented not only operational but functional levels as well. This, of course, is fine if one intends to infer such findings to a population of highly fit former athletes. On the other hand, if one intends to generalize about the effect of hypnosis on muscular performance in the general population, then such a sample would obviously be inadequate.

Johnson and Kramer (1960) also evaluated the effect of different types of hypnotic and posthypnotic suggestions on muscular endurance. The endurance task consisted of pressing a 47-lb barbell to exhaustion. It was found that moderate "pep talk" type of suggestions tended to get better results than more quietly reasoned suggestions or suggestions intended to take effect posthypnotically, but this trend was not statistically significant. At the same time, suggestions designed to impair performance were always successful. As a matter of fact, the investigators reported that the Ss were so upset that their efforts failed to equal customary performance levels. Also, the Ss rationalized their failure in various ways such as suggesting that the weight was actually heavier under such conditions.

In a related investigation Johnson and Kramer (1961) compared the effects of nonhypnotic, hypnotic, and posthypnotic stereotyped suggestion on strength, power, and endurance. Ten male Ss were tested under conditions of (a) no hypnosis, (b) in a trance, (c) in a deep trance, and (d) out of trance, before performance of the three tests. The tests included a grip dynamometer task (strength), the jump and reach task (power), and supine press of a 47-lb barbell to exhaustion (endurance). The testing extended over a 4-day period. The only statistically significant improvements found were in endurance when two of the hypnotic conditions were compared with the no-hypnosis treatment, and none of the hypnotic conditions was found to be consistently superior. However, it should be pointed out that one S in this study experienced what might be regarded as disinhibition of inhibitory phenomena. This case will be discussed in detail because of its unusual nature.

The S was a professional football player who bench pressed the 47-lb barbell 130 times in the first testing session where suggestions were given but hypnosis was not utilized. Hypnosis was then introduced and on the next three testings his scores were 180 (when he was stopped by the investigator), 230, and 233, respectively. In contrast, the next-strongest athlete began the study at 57 presses and eventually reached a maximum of 75 repetitions. Since our own research has revealed that a performance of 100 repetitions is exceptionally high, it is reasonable to regard this S's hypnotic performance as a superhuman feat. To determine whether the professional football player was dependent on hypnosis to perform in this way, he was later retested without hypnosis and was stopped by the investigator at 350 presses!

There are several points of interest regarding this case. First, it is inconceivable that this weight-trained, mesomorphic, professional football player could almost double his initial performance in the hypnotic state since such Ss are generally thought to perform at or near their maximums when tested in the waking state. Also, Johnson and Kramer (1961) have pointed out that this S recovered quickly from each bout, and he did not report soreness at any time. Age regression was employed with this S several months following the experiment and the S was led to relive the first test in the trance state. The S gave the impression that he had accepted the suggestions as vivid reality and his performance became a matter of life and death. Under age regression he also reported that he would give up in complete fatigue and then watch in amazement as his arms seemingly lifted the weight by themselves. This case is an example of the type of performance cited to support the view that man is capable of performing far above his "maximal" capacity under certain conditions.

A recurring problem in exercise physiology has been the extent to which physical warm-up facilitates muscular performance. One of the inherent difficulties associated with the study of such a problem relates to the S's past experience with warm-up and his attitude toward its value. Indeed, as pointed out in Chapter 6, one's attitude toward the value of warm-up influences performance under warm-up and no-warm-up conditions. In order to control for this particular variable, Massey *et al.* (1961) conducted a study in which the Ss presumably did not know whether they had warmed up prior to performing the criterion task, which consisted of pedaling a bicycle ergometer 100 revolutions at a resistance of 26 lb. The 15 male Ss first performed active physical warm-up or rested quietly in the hypnotic state under the two conditions. The ergometer rides were performed in the posthypnotic state that followed. Warm-up had no influence on physical performance, and there was no indication that lack of warm-up resulted in muscle injury or soreness. While this investigation does not answer the question of whether hypnotic suggestion can facilitate muscular performance, it does illustrate one of the many possible applications of hypnosis to the study of human performance.

Nine male Ss and one female S were tested under hypnotic and waking conditions on a test of elbow flexion strength by Ikai and Steinhaus (1961). The Ss exerted maximal forearm flexion once a minute for 30 minutes. This procedure resulted in an overall decrement of about 10%

for the 30-minute period, and it should be emphasized that suggestion was not employed. Of the ten Ss tested under control conditions seven were capable of entering a trance. Trance criterion consisted of responsiveness to suggestions of rigidity and limpness of the arms and legs, and the S was not tested until his arm could be held so rigidly that neither investigator could bend it. The Ss were then tested (a) in the trance state with suggestions of enhanced strength, (b) in the posthypnotic state with suggestions of weakness, (c) in the posthypnotic state with suggestions of enhanced strength, and (d) in the waking state after hypnosis. Suggestions of enhanced strength resulted in significant increments in performance during the trance and posthypnotic states as compared to the waking control state. Also, this increase persisted in the waking state after hypnosis as compared with the control waking state. Negative suggestions resulted in significant decrements in the posthypnotic state. These investigators indicated that six of the hypnotic Ss demonstrated identical response patterns. The seventh S was an experienced weight lifter, and he was skeptical of hypnosis. His control performances exceeded the hypnotic, posthypnotic, and waking-state performances. The posthypnotic suggestion of weakness, however, was very effective for this S. The authors suggested that this S's superefforts in the control state were related to his skepticism of hypnosis and his desire to disprove its efficacy. They stated, "We interpret the findings in this subject to indicate that he was able, probably because of long training, to approximate his physiologic limit in the waking state and therefore suggestion could lower but not further his performance." (Ikai and Steinhaus, 1961, p. 160). Such an interpretation seems reasonable, but it will be recalled that Johnson and Kramer (1961) have discussed the performance of a weight-trained, mesomorphic, professional athlete who exhibited outstanding efforts in the waking control state and then went on to experience significant increments following hypnotic suggestion.

Several points must be emphasized regarding the report of Ikai and Steinhaus (1961). First, suggestions of enhanced and decreased performance were given in the hypnotic but not the control state; that is, there was experimental contamination due to confounding of treatment and suggestion. Therefore, the suggestions employed with hypnosis might have produced comparable effects under control waking conditions. Second, there was no discussion of the test–retest reliability of the strength test. Third, the control and hypnotic states were not counterbalanced. Fourth, only the six Ss who had identical response patterns were included in the analysis. It will be recalled that the seventh S scored much better in the control state. The authors did not offer any justification for excluding this S from their analysis and, more importantly, they failed to relate the effect of deleting his scores. It is quite possible that inclusion of this S in the analysis would modify their results appreciably.

The "human plank" feat is commonly employed by stage hypnotists to dramatize the power of hypnotic suggestion. The S is normally suspended between two supports which are placed beneath the ankle in the region of the Achilles tendon and between the occipital protuberance and fifth cervical vertebra. The effect of hypnotic suggestion on performance of the "human plank" feat was evaluated by Collins (1961). The task criteria consisted of endurance time and body sway. Sway was measured by attaching a nylon line in the region of the umbilicus and passing it over a pulley and then to a paper recorder. In other words, the amount of time taken for the S to collapse was defined as muscular endurance. The onset of fatigue and ability to recover during work were also measured. Forty-eight Ss were classified as being (a) insusceptible, (b) medium, or (c) somnambule Ss. Eight of each classification were placed in the experimental group ($n = 24$) and eight of each classification were assigned to the control group ($n = 24$). The Ss in the experimental group were given trance induction and suggestions of catalepsy followed by suggestions that they were "stiff and rigid," "stiffer and stiffer," "unable to bend," etc., every 5 seconds. The control Ss were given the average scores for men (6–6½ minutes) and women (5–5½ minutes) prior to the test. In addition, they were advised at the end of every 5-second block as to how they were doing in order that they might compare their efforts to the previously cited norms. Also, as the S began to fall the investigator appealed to his will, ego, and cajoled him to do better. Collins (1961) concluded that the suggested cataleptic state of the hypnotic Ss was not superior to the motivated waking state of the control Ss for increasing muscular endurance. Also, there was no significant difference in the muscular performance of Ss scoring high, medium, or low on hypnotizability. This paper tends to lend support to the "skeptical view" of hypnotic phenomena. It is unfortunate that the suggestions to the hypnotic and control Ss differed. Indeed, one might argue that hypnotic suggestions of "stiff and rigid," "stiffer and stiffer," and "unable to bend" might in fact hasten the onset of fatigue rather than enhance performance.

London and Fuhrer (1961) assessed weight-holding endurance, strength of grip, and performance on a tremor task in 32 female Ss. Sixteen of the Ss were rated as highly susceptible to hypnosis and the remaining 16 Ss were regarded as possessing low susceptibility. All Ss were retested following suggestions designed to enhance performance. The posttesting was performed under both hypnotic and waking conditions, and the order was balanced. The unsusceptible Ss performed better than the susceptible Ss throughout the study. Also, hypnosis without suggestion had no effect on muscular performance. Furthermore, motivational instructions were just as effective in the waking as the hypnotic state.

In a related investigation Rosenhan and London (1963) evaluated grip strength and weight-holding endurance in 78 male undergraduate students without their knowledge that the experiment dealt with hypnosis. They were then asked to volunteer for a hypnosis experiment, and 68 of the original Ss volunteered. Of the 68 volunteers it was found that 16 were susceptible to hypnosis and 16 were relatively unsusceptible. The Ss were administered the same physical performance tests in the waking and hypnotic states. The conditions were not balanced, and motivational instructions were not employed. It was found that strength of grip did not differ under the three conditions for either group. Also, both groups performed better on the endurance task prior to learning that the experiment dealt with hypnosis. This suggests that hypnosis per se reduced performance since serial testing of this nature would normally be characterized by slight to moderate increases as a function of trials and then eventually level off. Certainly it would not be expected that lower performances would result unless there were interactive effects due to behavioral artifacts such as experimenter expectancies. On the other hand, it is also conceivable that the nature of the hypnotic induction was such that a lethargic state was created.

The investigations of London and Fuhrer (1961) and Rosenhan and London (1963) were replicated by Evans and Orne (1965) and amplified to include a third group consisting of Ss classified as possessing "medium" hypnotizability, as well as Ss scoring "high" and "low" in susceptibility. Each group consisted of 12 males and 8 females. The tasks consisted of strength of grip,* weight-holding endurance, hand tremor, and rote learning. The order of testing was counterbalanced with half of the Ss tested under hypnosis first and the other half under the waking condition first. The mean strength and endurance scores were lower under hypnosis for both susceptible and unsusceptible Ss, but these differences were not

* Mean performance for the strength of grip task ranged from 76 to 200 lb under the various conditions. The mean waking performance was 175 lb. Since college males and females would be expected (Kellor *et al.*, 1971) to score approximately 125 and 65 lb, respectively, the mean waking performances reported by Evans and Orne (1965) are at least 3 SD above the population mean. Therefore, it would not be reasonable to expect increases under hypnosis. Of course, the unusually high strength scores reported by Evans and Orne (1965) may reflect differences in instrumentation or testing procedures, and therefore comparisons to norms may not be appropriate.

significant. An important finding related to the influence of testing order, is that base-level measures of muscular endurance were significantly higher when the waking base-level performance preceded the hypnosis performance. Furthermore, the only difference between base-level and hypnosis trials occurred when the endurance test was first administered in the waking state. A similar trend was also observed for the strength of grip test; that is, the waking–hypnosis order was superior. It will be recalled that 36 males and 24 females participated in this investigation. It is important to note that sex did not serve as an independent variable since actual effects may have been masked due to grouping males and females.

Strength of grip and weight-holding endurance of 60 female Ss were evaluated by Barber and Calverley (1964). Fifteen Ss were then randomly assigned to each of the following groups: (a) task-motivating instructions, (b) hypnotic induction procedure, (c) hypnotic induction procedure plus task-motivating instructions, and (d) control. None of the experimental treatments affected strength of grip significantly. The hypnotic induction procedure per se depressed weight-holding endurance. Significant increments in endurance followed task-motivating suggestions in both the hypnotic and waking states, which implies that suggestion, not hypnosis, may be the ergogenic aid. At any rate, Barber's views represent a decade of systematic inquiry, and his work has been summarized in a recent book (Barber, 1970).

Barber (1970) and his associates have generally found that suggestions administered in the motivated waking state produce effects comparable to those resulting from the same suggestions in the hypnotic state. Of course, in the case of experimentation with student nurses there are obvious restrictions with respect to external validity. For example, such Ss would not be expected to be at or near their muscular performance *Endkrafts,* and consequently they would not be expected to possess an appreciation of their true performance potentials. In other words, generalization of such results to the highly trained male S would have to be made with caution. These latter comments are not intended to imply that Barber and Calverley's (1964) findings are not relevent. On the other hand, Hilgard (1971) has also studied hypnotic behavior for many years, and he has arrived at an entirely different interpretation of hypnotic phenomena. Hilgards' (1971) recent article places the "credulous" versus "skeptical" view of hypnosis in historical perspective.

Levitt and Brady (1964) also evaluated muscular endurance in the hynotic and motivated waking states. The Ss consisted of eight student nurses, and the endurance task was performed by holding a 2-lb sand bag in the open palm with the arm extended at a 90° angle to the body.

Performance was assessed (a) under hypnosis, (b) under hypnosis with the upper arm and shoulder anesthetized hypnotically, and (c) in the waking state with motivation. Motivation was provided by means of verbal exhortation and monetary payment. There were no significant differences among the conditions, which is in disagreement with the report of Barber and Calverley (1964), who reported that hypnotic induction depressed weight-holding endurance.

The influence of instructions on hypnotic and nonhypnotic performance in high- and low-susceptible Ss was evaluated by Slotnick and London (1965). The Ss consisted of 50 females, and they were assigned to one of three experimental groups or two control groups. One of the control groups always performed in the waking state, while the remaining groups performed under both hypnosis and waking conditions. The physical tasks consisted of a tremor test, grip dynamometer test, and an endurance test in which the S held her hand in the outstretched position with a 2½-kg weight on the back of her hand. Comparisons were made between various instructions involving exhortative and analgesic suggestions. It was found that special instructions improved performance in the hypnotic but not the waking state. Also, exhortative instructions were more effective than analgesic instructions.

Slotnick *et al.* (1965) evaluated the effect of exhortation and exhortation plus "involving instructions" on muscular endurance. Twelve female students served as Ss and all were in the upper 20% of hypnotic susceptibility as measured by the Stanford Hypnotic Susceptibility Scale. The task consisted of supporting a 2½-kg weight attached to the outstretched hand (palm down) by means of a strap. Each S performed the weight-holding task following exhortative instructions in the hypnotic state. On the basis of performance in this test the Ss were placed into two matched groups. In the next session Group 1 received the "involving instructions"* in addition to exhortation in the hypnotic state. Group 2 received the same instructions but performed the weight-holding task in the waking state. Since other investigators (Barber and Calverley, 1964) have reported that task-motivating instructions in the waking state are just as effective as the same instructions in the hypnotic state, the present design permitted an assessment of the interaction between hypnosis and instructions. It was found that the second session, which included the "involving instructions" in addition to the exhortations, resulted in significant increments for both the hypnotic and waking Ss. However, the performance

* The exhortations were essentially those reported by London and Fuhrer (1961). The "involving instructions" were designed to elicit S commitment and involvement in the production of enhanced performance, and the S was required to verbalize her desire to do well.

of the hypnotic group increased significantly more than that of the waking group. The investigators interpreted this finding to demonstrate the ". . . differential efficacy of various instructions" (Slotnick *et al.*, 1965, p. 44). This study provides insight into much of the contradictory hypnotic literature. Furthermore, one cannot expect true replications across laboratories until some agreement can be reached regarding optimal instructions.

It seems appropriate at this point to consider the external validity or generalizability of results with respect to many of the studies discussed thus far. Hilgard (1965) has demonstrated that hypnotizability is distributed in a bimodal fashion which imposes statistical limitations, as well as restrictions on external validity. Also, most of the hypnotic studies reported in the literature are concerned primarily with the responsivity of Ss scoring high on hypnotic suggestibility. In those studies that have employed Ss scoring in the extremes of suggestibility, the high-suggestible Ss have generally performed better than the low-suggestible Ss. In addition, most of the recent hypnotic experimentation concerned with muscular performance has employed female Ss. Since a basic premise involved in hypothesis testing relates to statistical inference from the sample to its population, these methodological factors become very important. It seems reasonable to suggest that much of the recent research concerning hypnosis and muscular performance must limit generalizations to physically untrained, hypnotizable female Ss. Such a restriction, of course, limits the application of such findings to human-performance settings.

The above considerations prompted Morgan and Coyne (1965) to conduct an investigation dealing with stereotyped suggestion and muscular performance in the motivated waking state. Their Ss consisted of 18 male students enrolled in a physical education weight-training class. The Ss were trained on various exercises directed toward progressively overloading the major muscle groups of the body. The Ss attended 40-minute exercise sessions twice weekly for 2 months in an attempt to minimize pseudo-base lines during the experimental session that was to follow. The authors reported their belief that the Ss were functioning at or near their theoretical *Endkraft* when the actual experiment was conducted. Therefore, the Ss consisted of males who were not selected on the basis of high suggestibility, and each S had recently participated in a weight-training program designed to acquaint him with his maximal physical capabilities. In short, these Ss were presumably performing at their actual maximums under conditions of base-line testing.

All Ss were then administered a test of grip strength and a weight-holding task. Strength of grip was measured by means of a Naragansett grip dynamometer, and weight-holding endurance was assessed by having the Ss abduct their arms in the lateral plane with a 9-lb dumbbell in each hand. The length of time the S held the weights parallel to the floor was defined as muscular endurance. The 18 Ss were then assigned to one of the following groups: (a) control group ($n = 6$), (b) stereotyped-suggestion group ($n = 6$), or (c) placebo group ($n = 6$). The stereotyped suggestion was similar to that employed previously by London and Fuhrer (1961). The placebo control was employed for purposes of evaluating the Hawthorne effect, and the Ss in this group were given a placebo (sodium bicarbonate) with the suggestion that it was a pep pill that might improve muscular performance. The control Ss reported to the environmental room and rested quietly for the same length of time the other two groups received the respective treatments. While the suggestion group had a mean increase of 15 seconds for the weight-holding task this increment was not statistically significant. None of the groups experienced significant increases in weight-holding endurance or strength of grip, which contradicts the view that task-motivating instructions in the waking state facilitate muscular performance. Of course, had highly suggestible Ss who had not undergone physical training been employed, it is reasonable to assume that confirmation would have been obtained.

One serendipitous finding emerged, however. The Ss in the placebo group had a significant decrease in both muscular strength and endurance. Since Luoto (1964) had earlier reported that placebo responsivity was related to personality type, Morgan and Coyne (1965) requested the six placebo Ss to complete a battery of psychological tests, which were administered by a clinical psychologist not acquainted with the study. He reported that all six Ss were significantly more extroverted than normal, and five of the six were significantly more neurotic than normal. The sixth S, while not significantly more neurotic than normal, did score in the same direction as the other Ss. This observation agrees with Luoto's report (1964), namely that neurotic extroverts are negative placebo reactors. Subsequently, Morgan *et al.* (1967) conducted a double-blind study that dealt with strength of grip and weight-holding endurance following a double-blind placebo administration to extroverts and introverts. Their findings again were in general agreement with those of Luoto (1964). Probably the most significant lesson to be learned here relates to the danger of using intact classes for experimental purposes. Is it possible that students with given personality traits gravitate toward certain physical activities when confronted with an elective program of course work? There, of course, is evidence to suggest that this does occur.

The work of Slater (1967) adds another dimension to the study of hypnotically induced changes in muscular performance. He studied the influence of expectancy on strength of grip. The muscular strength of 72 male Ss was tested and then they were asked their expectation (yes, no, or undecided) as to whether hypnosis would enhance dynamometer performance. Hypnotic and nonhypnotic groups were then formed by random assignment of Ss differing in expectancy, and they were retested following the administration of task-motivating instructions. While neither hypnosis nor expectancy per se influenced performance, there was a significant interaction effect for the two variables. In other words, hypnosis was effective when expectancy favored hypnosis.

In a yet to be published report dealing with motivation and hypnosis, Evans (1971, personal communication) discusses the replication and extension of earlier work by him and his associates. This research reveals that deeply hypnotized Ss who report (nod of head) that they have successfully experienced the suggestion of enhanced muscular strength exhibit a greater relative increase in strength of grip than do insusceptible Ss who fail to experience the suggestion. In some respects, this finding is similar to the earlier observation of Slotnick *et al.* (1965), who reported that "involving suggestions" were more efficacious than standard suggestions. However, Evans (1971, personal communication) has stated that susceptible Ss ". . . appear to depress waking performance rather than increase hypnotic performance, presumably to 'protect' the integrity of their own hypnotic experiences" (p. 40). This observation implies that randomized-group designs might be superior to a repeated measures schedule in hypnotic experimentation involving attempts to enhance muscular performance.

Summary

The studies reviewed in this section have dealt with the effect of hypnosis on muscular strength and endurance. The tasks have involved tests such as strength of grip, elbow flexion strength, weight-holding endurance, bench pressing, vertical jumping, the bar hang, and bicycle ergometry. Certain of the investigations reviewed have been concerned with the influence of hypnosis per se on muscular performance, whereas other studies have concentrated on the effect of various hypnotic, posthypnotic, and waking suggestions. Hypnosis per se has been found in some cases to have no influence on muscular performance and, in others, to provoke increases and decreases; that is, the literature is clearly equivocal on this point. While a number of investigators have reported that hypnotic suggestions designed to facilitate muscular strength and endurance are effective, an equal number of studies have not found this to be the case. Also, there is some evidence that task-motivating instructions in the waking state are just as effective as the same suggestions in the hypnotic state. On the other hand, there is limited evidence that suggestions of an "involving" nature are superior in the hypnotic state. However, there is also evidence that Ss depress waking performance in order to insure facilitated efforts under hypnosis conditions. The only point on which widespread agreement exists is that negative suggestions designed to impair muscular strength and endurance are usually effective. Hull stated in 1933 that the literature in this area was contradictory, and unfortunately the present review suggests that 40 years of research have failed to provide clarification. However, it is clear that much of the confusion can be explained at a methodological level and this point will be pursued further at the conclusion of the present chapter. While hypnotic suggestions of enhanced muscular strength and endurance are sometimes effective, they cannot be counted upon to consistently facilitate performance. On the other hand, decrements in functional capacity can be routinely evoked under hypnotic conditions. However, even the most credulous operators would admit that the latter would be possible in the waking state as well.

C. Metabolic Effects of Suggested Work

A number of investigators have attempted to manipulate metabolic responses in hypnotic Ss at rest by presenting suggestions of imagined work. Heart rate, oxygen consumption, carbon dioxide production, respiration rate, total ventilation, and cardiac output have been examined, and these investigations are reviewed in the present section.

It was reported by Bier (1932) that hypnotic suggestions of rest produced a decrease in pulse rate, while suggestions of happiness and excitement produced an increase. Also, the suggestions of excitement caused a rise in the P and R peaks of the ECG. In a related study, Whitehorn *et al.* (1930) demonstrated that hypnotically induced anxiety increases the metabolic rate about 22%, while suggested moods of elation, irritability, and depression have little influence on metabolism (e.g., 1.3, 2.5 and 0.9%, respectively). This view has been corroborated by Hepps and Brady (1967), who observed a mean increase of 15.9 beats/minute (from 75.8 to 91.7) in 13 hypnotic Ss following the production of anxiety, and such anticipatory heart rates presumably reflect elevated state anxiety. In our own research preexercise heart rates as high as 160 beats/minute have been observed.

Ventilation and oxygen uptake increase as the beginning of hypnosis approaches (Fulde, 1939). However, values for these variables are about the same as those under normal waking conditions in a quiet hypnotic state (Fulde, 1937). Since metabolic changes are associated with the initial induction procedure, it is necessary that continuous monitoring be performed in order to make meaningful comparisons. Also, Fulde (1937) has reported that "suggested excitations" cause increases in ventilation, oxygen uptake, and carbon dioxide production. Therefore, the type of trance employed is another variable to be considered.

The hypnotic suggestion of light exercise was found to increase the resting ventilation of four Ss from 4.35 to 11.27 liters and oxygen uptake from 177 to 320 ml by Nemtzova and Shatenstein (1939). Furthermore, hypnotic suggestion of heavy exercise resulted in increases to 14.5 liters and 409 ml/minute in ventilation and oxygen uptake, respectively. These changes reflect three- and twofold increases over resting values.

Total ventilation, oxygen uptake, and heart rate following hypnotic suggestion of work in resting Ss were evaluated by Levin and Egolinsky (1936). Ventilation, oxygen uptake, and heart rate averaged 5.7 liters, 239 ml, and 75 beats/minute at rest under hypnosis, and these values were elevated to 14.5 liters, 331 ml, and 88 beats/minute following the suggestion of work. The cost of hyperventilation, which is under voluntary control in the normal S, could account for the increased oxygen uptake and cardiac frequency.

Berman *et al.* (1954) evaluated the electrocardiographic effects of hypnotically suggested anxiety and exercise in 14 healthy students. Also, four of these Ss completed a 10-minute treadmill walk at 3 mph and 5% grade in order to compare the effects of actual and suggested work. The suggestion of anxiety produced a mean increase of 26.4 beats/minute and the suggestion of exercise evoked a similar response of 24.1 beats/minute. This latter increment was considerably lower than that observed for actual exercise, which was 42 beats/minute. Also, 50% of these normal Ss experienced various changes in the ECG T wave, and depression of the ST segment was observed in one S following hypnotic suggestion.

Most investigators have instructed their Ss to imagine that they are performing a specific form of exercise. Such an approach has the advantage of presumably creating a standard stimulus. At the same time such an approach conceivably might inhibit physiological responsivity in certain Ss. This would be especially true in the S who lacked the appropriate background experience required for interpretation of the suggestion. In this context, the report of Dudlye *et al.* (1964) represents an exception. These investigators chose to employ hypnotic suggestion in which the Ss were ". . . asked to relive a type of physical exercise in which they had actively participated" (p. 51). Postexperimental debriefings revealed that Ss had imagined various forms of exercise including mild calisthenics, running a race, playing tennis, and mountain climbing. The total ventilation and oxygen uptake of the 11 Ss were found to increase from 4.3 to 12.7 liters/minute and from 271 to 377 ml/minute, respectively, under these conditions. Also, suggestions of anxiety- or anger-provoking situations and pain elevated ventilation and oxygen consumption, while the suggestion of depression had no influence on the same variables. This observation is in agreement with the earlier report of Whitehorn *et al.* (1930).

Agosti and Camerota (1965) evaluated the influence of hypnotic suggestions of imagined work on respiratory frequency, total ventilation, oxygen uptake, and heart rate. The imagined work resulted in an increase for total ventilation but none of the remaining variables differed significantly. For example, the mean heart rates for the control period and conditions of imagined work were identical (84 beats/minute). These investigators concluded that suggestions of imagined work ". . . have their primary effect on the rate and depth of breathing" (Agosti and Camerota, 1965, p. 155).

The hypnotic suggestion of heavy leg exercise was found to increase cardiac output to a level consonant with expectations for actual exercise by Bevegård *et al.* (1968). Under such conditions the oxygen consumption reached 1100 ml/minute, which is approximately the requirement for working at 600 kpm on a bicycle ergometer. Furthermore, the increased cardiac output resulted from increases in both heart rate and stroke volume, which averaged 19 and 30%, respectively. These investigators interpreted this finding to reflect a centrally induced general vasodilatation in muscles since forearm blood flow increased with hypnotic suggestion of leg exercise.

Cobb *et al.* (1967) evaluated the influence of hypnotically suggested exercise on heart rate, respiration, blood pressure, and free fatty acid mobilization. The six Ss were first given hypnotic suggestions of tranquility for 10 minutes, and this was followed by suggestion that exercise was being performed on a bicycle ergometer. The exercise simulation gradually progressed to maximum over a 20-minute period, and arterial blood was collected at 5-minute intervals for purposes of measuring free fatty acid levels. Also, three of the Ss were retested following the administration of a beta adrenergic blocking drug. Two of the Ss had no changes in any of the variables measured, while the other four Ss developed significant elevations (55–190%) in free fatty acid levels with suggestion of exercise. The increase in heart rate ranged from 19 to 40 beats/minute, but consistent changes were not observed for blood pressure. Beta adrenergic blockade prevented catecholamine-induced lipolysis, but it did not have a consistent effect on free fatty acid response during hypnosis. This indicates that the initial responses were evoked by factors other than catechols, and these investigators concluded that ". . . experimental stimuli of this study effected a rather nonspecific arousal of the nervous system" (Cobb *et al.*, 1967, p. 197).

Two unpublished reports from the Laboratory of Hypnosis Research at Stanford University suggest that bradycardia as well as tachycardia may accompany hallucinated exercise. In the first investigation (Hilgard and Boucher, 1967) hallucinated exercise was associated with a slight decrease in cardiac frequency. However, the investigators reported that resting heart rate values averaged about 8 beats/minute higher when hypnosis was to follow. In the second investigation (Marshall, 1970) hallucinated exercise resulted in an elevation of heart rate, which failed to corroborate the earlier report, but the findings regarding a higher anticipatory heart rate for the hallucinated exercise condition were confirmed. Also, while Marshall (1970) observed an increase in heart rate with hallucinated exercise, this increase did not equal the cardiac frequency for actual exercise.

In Section II,D a number of paradoxical metabolic shifts will be described for hypnotic conditions involving the suggestion that actual work is becoming easier.

Summary

A series of investigations over the past 40 years has revealed that hypnotic hallucination of exercise tends to increase heart rate, and such increases are usually commensurate with the level of work suggested. Also, increases in respiration, total ventilation, and oxygen consumption have been reported by a number of investigators. In addition, cardiac output has been found to increase under such conditions, and it is felt that such increments reflect a centrally induced general vasodilatation in muscles. The question of whether metabolic decreases and increases can be evoked in the exercising S will be examined in the following section.

D. Metabolic Changes during Work

A number of investigators have evaluated the influence of hypnotic suggestion on the metabolism of exercising Ss. Tasks such as the rhythmical lifting of weights and bicycle ergometry have been employed, and the dependent variables have consisted of heart rate, oxygen consumption, oxygen debt, carbon dioxide production, respiratory quotient, ventilation, and rectal temperature. These investigations will be reviewed in the present section.

Levin and Egolinsky (1936) examined the effect of various hypnotic suggestions on pulse rate, oxygen consumption, and ventilation in three subjects. The subjects were 12, 14, and 17 years of age, and the work task consisted of pedaling a bicycle ergometer for 3 minutes at a rate that would result in 1500 m distance. Assessments were made (a) at rest, (b) during hypnosis at rest, (c) during work, (d) during work in the hypnotic state, (e) at rest during hypnosis with suggestions of work, and (f) at work during hypnosis with suggestions of rest. Repeated measurements were performed and the averages are presented in Table I.

The mean responses for heart rate, oxygen consumption, and ventilation were all higher when the *Ss* exercised in the hypnotic state. This suggests that hypnosis per se evokes a metabolic increase in the exercising *S*, and it probably reflects a sympathoadrenomedullary response. While cardiac frequency was the same in both states at rest, ventilation and oxygen consumption were lower at rest for the hypnotic condition. Also, when suggestions of work were administered to these *Ss* at rest, ventilation increased 9 liters, oxygen uptake 92 ml, and heart rate 13 beats/minute. In other words, the suggestion of work resulted in metabolic gains that equalled those for actual work, with the exception of oxygen uptake. This suggests that heart rate and ventilation are under conscious control, but oxygen uptake is probably regulated by tissue need. Also, the observed increase in oxygen utilization can be attributed to the cost of hyperventilation.

The effect of hypnotic and posthypnotic suggestion on ventilation and

TABLE I

EFFECT OF HYPNOTIC SUGGESTION ON EXERCISE METABOLISM[a]

	Variable		
Condition	Ventilation (liters/minute)	O_2 uptake (ml/minute)	Pulse rate (beats/minute)
Waking			
Control	6.2	262	75
Exercise	15.7	735	92
Hypnosis			
Control	5.7	239	75
Exercise	19.1	867	100
Suggestion of work	14.5	331	88
Suggestion of rest	17.0	824	106

[a] From Levin and Egolinsky (1936).

oxygen consumption of exercising Ss was evaluated by Nemtzova and Shatenstein (1939). Two male and two female Ss lifted weights at a rate of 20 repetitions/minute, and the distance of each excursion was 0.5 m. Three of the Ss lifted 15.5-kg weights and the fourth a 10-kg weight. The work resulted in ventilations ranging from 13.69 to 22.88 liters, and the oxygen consumption ranged from 610 to 929 ml/minute. The Ss were then given suggestions of light work (300-gm weights) and heavy work (30 kg). The suggestions of light work resulted in a decrease in ventilation and oxygen consumption that ranged from 20 to 30%, while suggestions of heavy work evoked increases of about 50%. The resting ventilation and oxygen consumption averaged 4.35 liters and 177 ml, respectively, and the suggestion of light work during rest resulted in increases to 11.27 liters in ventilation and 320 ml/minute in oxygen uptake. Furthermore, suggestions of heavy work administered during rest evoked a mean ventilation of 14.5 liters and an oxygen consumption of 409 ml/minute. Therefore, while such suggestions resulted in ventilation rates equal to actual work, the oxygen uptake remained well below the requirements for actual work. Also, it is difficult to attribute these changes to hypnotic suggestion since there was not a waking control condition.

Morgan (1970) conducted an experiment in which two male Ss exercised under hypnotic conditions and their performances were compared to those of two male Ss who simulated (faked) hypnosis. On the first day of the experiment the Ss lifted 9-lb dumbbells for 5 minutes at a rate of 25 excursions/minute for each arm. Oxygen consumption was measured throughout exercise, as well as prior to and following the task. On the second and third days of the investigation the Ss received either heavy- or light-work suggestions (counterbalanced order) prior to performing the same task. The suggestions were designed to distort the S's percept of the work task in such a way that the weights would appear considerably heavier or lighter on the 2 days. However, it should be noted that 9-lb weights were used on all 3 days. The amount of oxygen consumed during exercise was not altered under either experimental condition for any of the Ss. However, hypnotic and simulatory Ss did seem to differ on oxygen debt. The simulatory Ss had an increase in oxygen debt following the suggestion of heavy work and a reduction following suggestion of light work, whereas the hypnotic Ss had a decreased debt following suggestions of heavy work and an increment following suggestions of light work. Morgan (1970) interpreted the paradoxical effects observed for the hypnotic Ss within the context of "trance logic." It will be recalled that Levin and Egolinsky (1936) also observed a similar paradox under related circumstances; that is, administration of suggestions of rest to Ss who were exercising resulted in slight increases in ventilation, oxygen uptake, and heart rate.

The influence of various hypnotic suggestions on perceptual and metabolic responsivity to a standard bicycle ergometer task has been evaluated by Morgan *et al.* (1973). Five male Ss pedaled a bicycle ergometer at a work load of 600 kpm and a rate of 50 rpm for 5 minutes. However, the S was told that he would exercise at a light, moderate, and heavy load under hypnotic conditions A, B, and C, respectively. Responses under these conditions, as well as suggestions of moderate work in the waking state, were compared. The dependent variables were perceived exertion, heart rate, oxygen uptake, oxygen debt, respiratory exchange ratio, excess carbon dioxide production, ventilatory minute volume, ventilatory efficiency, and rectal temperature. While several investigators have attempted to distort the S's perception of work in similar studies, they have not employed objective psychophysical assessments to corroborate the attempted perturbation. For this reason the S was asked to rate the level of perceived exertion on a psychophysical scale (Borg and Linderholm, 1967) following each treatment. The ratings of perceived exertion were consonant with the suggestions administered, and these findings are illustrated in Fig. 1.

It will also be noted in Fig. 2 that manipulation of perceived exertion was accompanied by certain physiological changes. For example, cardiac frequency following the suggestion of heavy work was significantly higher than that following the light-work suggestion. It will be recalled that the work load was always the same. The major finding regarding oxygen uptake was that at no time during heavy-work suggestions was a steady-state condition obtained. Also, a steady-state condition was not achieved following hypnotic suggestions of either light or moderate work until the final minutes of exercise. By comparison, the Ss had achieved a steady state following 1 minute of exercise in the waking state. This investigation demonstrates that man's perception of work, as well as his physiological response to work, is governed in part by psychic phenomena.

Summary

In the previous section it was reported that the hypnotic hallucination of exercise in the resting S can induce tachycardia, increase cardiac output, alter respiration rates and total ventilation, and increase oxygen uptake. The present review demonstrates that metabolic changes can be provoked in the exercising S as well under hypnotic conditions, but such changes have not been entirely consistent. Also, hypnosis per se

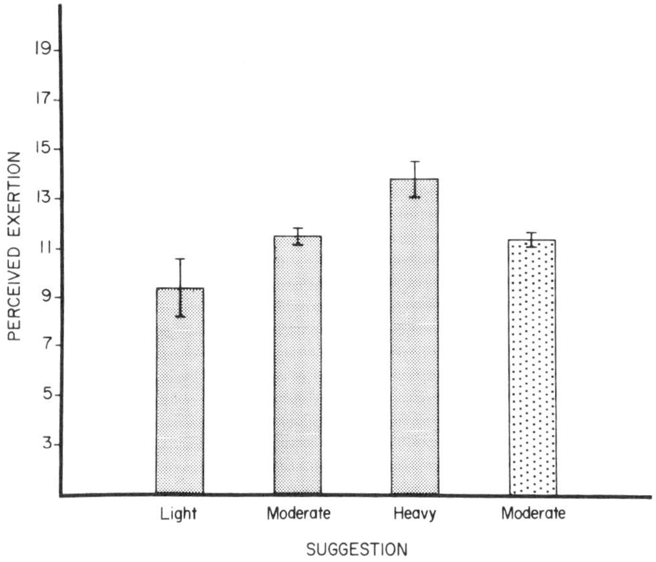

Fig. 1. Means and standard errors of the means for the perceived exertion ratings following 5 minutes of exercise at 600 kpm and 50 rpm. Densely stippled bars represent hypnotic condition and lightly stippled bar represents waking condition. (Reprinted from Morgan *et al.*, 1973.) Perceptual and metabolic responsivity to standard bicycle ergometry following various hypnotic suggestions. *Int. J. Clin. Exp. Hypnosis* **21** (in press). Reprinted from the *International Journal of Clinical and Experimental Hypnosis* 1973.

seems to increase the energy cost of standard work. A major shortcoming of most of the investigations reviewed has been the general failure to compare hypnotically altered metabolic rates with changes induced following the same suggestions in the waking state.

E. Psychomotor Behavior

The preceding review section dealing with muscular strength and endurance actually represents performance, which relates to the psychomotor domain. The decision to present a separate section entitled psychomotor behavior is largely a matter of convenience. The reports reviewed in this section deal primarily with the influence of hypnotic suggestion on reaction time and motor learning.

The effects of hypnosis and motivational instructions on kinesthetic learning have been evaluated by Edmonston and Marks (1967). Twenty-four male Ss participated in an experiment in which equal numbers received either (a) hypnotically administered task-motivating instruc-

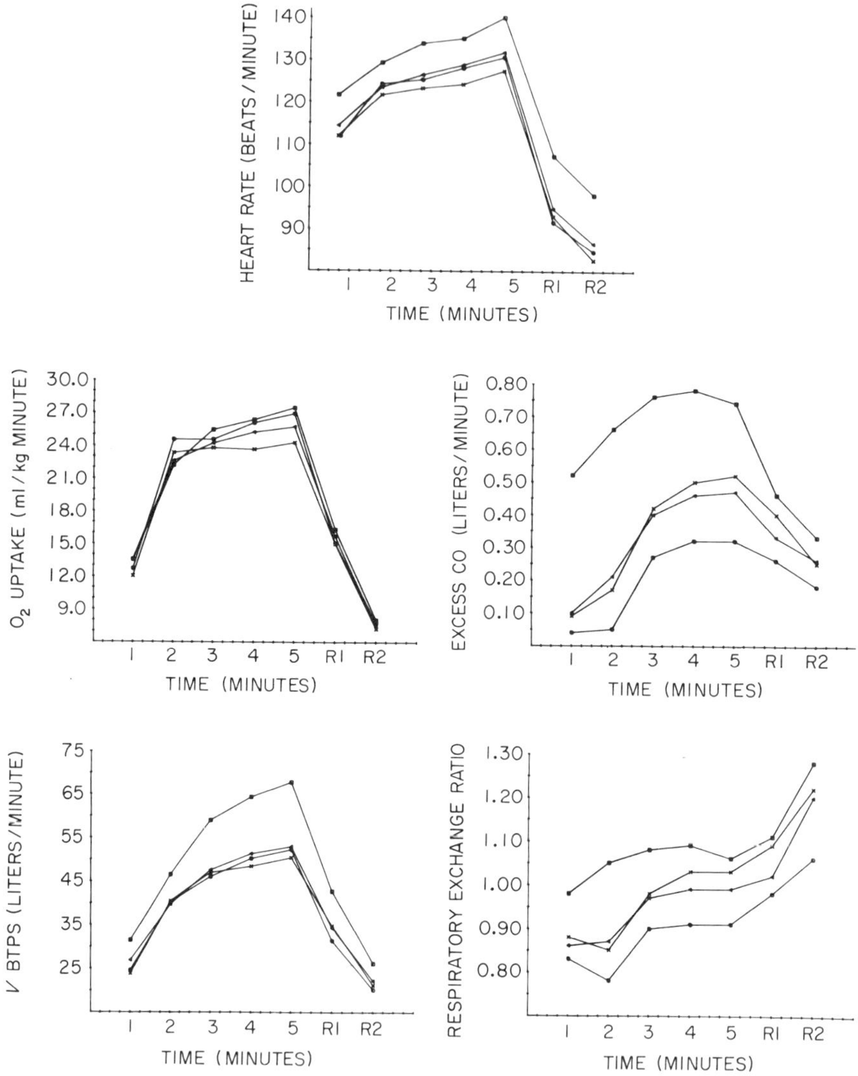

Fig. 2. Mean responses during exercise for heart rate, oxygen uptake, ventilatory minute volume, excess carbon dioxide production, and respiratory exchange ratio. Suggestion, hypnosis condition: ○, of light work; ▲, of moderate work; □, of heavy work. Suggestion, waking condition: ■, of moderate work. (Reprinted from Morgan *et al.*, 1973.) Perceptual and metabolic responsivity to standard bicycle ergometry following various hypnotic suggestions. *Int. J. Clin. Exp. Hypnosis* **21** (in press). Reprinted from the *International Journal of Clinical and Experimental Hypnosis* 1973.

tions, (b) the same treatment as the first group plus deepening instructions, (c) task-motivating instructions and a short story, or (d) a control treatment. The criterion variable was a kinesthetic learning task consisting of a 10-choice-point stylus maze. Performance on this task was unaffected by the various treatments, and these investigators concluded that neither hypnosis nor motivational instructions enhance kinesthetic learning. Also, Edmonston and Marks (1967) interpreted their findings as being at variance with much of the literature dealing with the influence of motivating instructions on strength and endurance. Furthermore, they have provided an explanation of this apparent contradiction largely based on task specificity and the imbalance between cortical excitation and inhibition in the respective tasks. A more fundamental distinction would seem to be that the investigation of Edmonston and Marks (1967) was concerned with learning, whereas the muscular strength and endurance literature has been concerned with performance.

Graham *et al.* (1968) evaluated the influence of hypnotically induced fatigue on the reaction time of 10 male Ss. Reaction time was assessed (a) under a hypnotic or control condition, (b) under hypnosis, (c) under hypnosis with the suggestion of fatigue, and (d) under a posthypnotic condition. Hypnosis per se was found to retard reaction time by 21%, the hypnotically suggested fatigue state evoked a performance decrement of 57%, and posthypnotic performance was comparable to prehypnotic. It is not surprising, of course, that reaction time was increased following hypnotic suggestion of fatigue. The same phenomenon could readily be demonstrated under waking conditions in cooperative Ss. The increased reaction time under hypnosis without suggestion is important, however. This observation suggests that hypnosis per se produces psychomotor retardation. While the potential role of hypnosis in the study of motor learning and motor performance is quite clear, this latter observation suggests potential methodological contamination in such paradigms. Alternative procedures such as "alerting" inductions might be appropriate in such circumstances.

The effect of posthypnotic suggestion on reaction time has been studied by Eskridge (1969). Seven female Ss were administered repeated measures of a simple visual reaction-time test on four different occasions in the waking state. These responses were taken to represent the Ss baseline reaction time. The Ss were then tested (a) following posthypnotic suggestion of improved reaction time and (b) 3 weeks later without any further hypnosis, practice, or instruction. Performance under the posthypnotic condition was increased. Since the waking prehypnotic condition always preceded the hypnotic condition, it is not at all clear that the hypnotic suggestion was responsible for the enhanced performance. For example, it is conceivable that these Ss suppressed their performances in the waking state in order to make possible the observed gains under subsequent hypnotic conditions. This view was supported by the observation that the enhanced performance persisted for 3 weeks in the absence of further hypnosis, practice, or suggestion. The investigator might have intentionally or unintentionally communicated desired outcomes to the Ss. Such possibilities are discussed in detail in the first chapter of this volume. While this investigation suggests that posthypnotic suggestion is capable of facilitating simple reaction time, there are several alternative explanations for the observed outcomes.

Ham and Edmonston (1971) compared the effect of an "alert" hypnotic induction, relaxation hypnotic induction, and a relaxation control treatment on the simple visual reaction time of 30 male Ss. The Ss in the control group received relaxation instructions, those in the standard hypnotic induction received a traditional induction, and those in the "alert" induction group received a hypnotic induction patterned after that of Liebert *et al.* (1965). The mean reaction time for the alert induction group was significantly lower than that for either of the other groups. However, the waking relaxation and traditional hypnotic induction groups did not differ. This report is in disagreement with the observations of Graham *et al.* (1968), who reported that hypnosis per se retarded reaction time. Ham and Edmonston (1971) emphasized that investigators concerned with facilitation of motor performance should employ alerting instructions, in contrast to the relaxation–drowsiness type of suggestions used effectively in the reduction of pain and anxiety.

Repeated one-choice reaction-time trials were compared for one female S under three motive–incentive conditions by Blum and Wohl (1971). The S received performance feedback following each trial, and the feedback related to (a) levels of predetermined monetary rewards, (b) posthypnotically cued pleasure or anxiety, and (c) an intrinsic incentive condition having no additional value. The monetary, affective, and intrinsic incentives did not evoke different levels of response. This report demonstrates an imaginative application of hypnosis to the study of motor performance. At the same time, its uniqueness prohibits comparison with the earlier reports, since direct hypnotic suggestions designed to influence performance were not employed. Also, it is conceivable that all three incentive conditions may have been superior to base-line measures of reaction time.

The effects of hypnosis on the learning of two selected motor skills were studied by Arnold (1971). He reported that 45 highly "tranceable" Ss and 15 "nontranceable" Ss were tested following various suggestions on motor learning tasks involving mirror tracing and ball bouncing.

Arnold (1971) apparently uses the term "tranceable" as a synonym for suggestible or susceptible, since this state was defined as performance on the Stanford Hypnotic Susceptibility Scale. This may not be an accurate assumption, however, since the criterion employed for high suggestibility was not consonant with contemporary views. The effects of positive posthypnotic suggestions were compared with the effects of similar suggestions in the waking state, as well as with a no-suggestion waking condition, and none of the conditions was found to be superior. However, it is difficult to comment on the findings of this investigation because of numerous statistical and design inelegancies.

Summary

In many respects the findings of investigations dealing with reaction time parallel those of the muscular strength and endurance studies reviewed earlier. That is, hypnotic suggestions of increased (slower) reaction time are effective, and suggestions of decreased (faster) reaction time may do so, but not consistently. Also, the type of hypnotic suggestion seems to be an important variable in that alerting suggestions are more likely to facilitate performance than are traditional hypnotic induction procedures. Generalizations regarding motor learning variables, in contrast to performance variables, are not possible at this time.

F. Athletic Performance

There have been countless reports in the popular literature pertaining to the use of hypnotic suggestion in the facilitation of athletic performance. Unfortunately, the authenticity of such reports is difficult to substantiate for a wide variety of reasons. However, there have been a few systematic studies dealing with the application of hypnosis to sport problems and these will be reviewed in the present section. These reports relate to complex movement behaviors in contrast to the simple motor behaviors reviewed in the preceding section.

Johnson (1961b) reported on a case study involving body movement awareness in the nonhypnotic and hypnotic states. The *S* was a baseball player who was having problems with his batting performance. The player had requested help in solving his batting problem, but he was completely unable to explain what was wrong with his batting. However, following various approaches in deep hypnosis the *S* presented a detailed analysis of his swing, citing distinct errors throughout the analysis. When asked whether he desired total recall of this analysis or to simply have the information "just come to him" gradually, he preferred to have it return in time rather than immediately. The player's performance improved immediately, and he went on to complete the season with an outstanding .400 average. The player thanked the hypnotist at the close of the season for providing him with such an excellent analysis of his batting problem! He would not believe that he had actually performed the analysis himself until the hypnotist advised him that he had never seen him play, and therefore would not have been able to diagnose and present a psychomotor prescription.

Johnson (1961b) has interpreted this case report within the context of Henry's (1960) "memory drum" theory of neuromotor reaction in the sense that he postulated, ". . . it is suggestive of an extensive body movement awareness which is apparently not ordinarily accessible to conscious verbal representation" (Johnson, 1961b, p. 263). This case study, like most, suffers from the lack of methodological controls; however, it illustrates an interesting clinical approach to the interpretation of complex motor behavior.

Another application of hypnosis to sport has been reported by Ryde (1964), who employs hypnosis in his practice of sports medicine. While he does not apparently attempt to facilitate performance as such, he does make participation possible for athletes disabled by a wide variety of injuries. Ryde's (1964) report contains a discussion of 35 cases consisting mainly of minor trauma resulting from athletic competition, as well as similar injuries sustained in nonathletic settings. He reports on the successful hypnotic treatment of conditions such as tennis elbow, shin splints, chronic Achilles tendon sprain, bruised heels, arch sprains, as well as other common ailments of uncertain minor pathology. As a matter of fact, his hypnotherapeutic achievements have been so good that he now offers ". . . to treat these disabilities initially by hypnosis and only proceed with conventional methods, should hypnosis fail or be refused" (Ryde, 1964, p. 244). Many sports injuries are disabling and the ailments frequently have uncertain minor pathology. To the extent that hypnotherapy is successful in mobilizing the disabled athlete, it would appear that hypnosis can, in fact, facilitate muscular performance. Sports medicine practitioners will find that Ryde's (1964) report provides various insights into the understanding of sports trauma.

Johnson (1965) has discussed a series of case studies dealing with the role played by sex and aggression conflicts in athletic competition. Resolution of the conflicts was possible through the application of hypnosis, and the cases represented a variety of sports. He has approached aggression in sport from the standpoint that, like sex, ". . . it is perceived as being simultaneously good and bad" (Johnson, 1965, p. 189). The cases cited by Johnson (1965) illustrate the situations in which athletes attempt to deal with aggression conflicts in competition. Hypnotherapists concerned with the treatment of problems in athletes will find Johnson's (1965) paper of interest.

Another application of hypnosis in sport has been reported by Naruse (1965), who has been concerned with the treatment of "stage fright" in champion athletes. Precompetition anxiety is probably present in some form in all athletes at every level of competition. Anxiety in such settings can be so mild as to have little influence on performance or so disabling that the athlete is completely incapacitated and unable to compete. Naruse (1965) has likened such anxiety attacks to "war neurosis" and he has labeled the state as "stage fright." His Ss consisted of champion Japanese athletes who had participated in the 1960 Olympic Games in Rome. He discusses the use of direct hypnotic suggestion, posthypnotically produced autohypnosis, and self-hypnosis in conjunction with autogenic training and progressive relaxation in the treatment of athletes for "stage fright." The actual method employed for a given athlete was determined on an individual basis and governed by factors such as the athlete's personality, as well as the unique nature of his "stage fright." Naruse (1965) discusses a series of cases, and the hypnotherapist will find his techniques of value in treating psychodynamic problems arising in athletes.

Summary

This section has considered the role of hypnosis in the clinical treatment of numerous problems arising in the competitive athlete. While the reports that have been reviewed are not characterized by the type of methodological control called for in Chapter 1, they do illustrate the approaches employed by practicing hypnotherapists from various parts of the world.

III. Summary

Investigations dealing with the influence of hypnosis per se and hypnotic suggestion on muscular performance have been reviewed in this chapter. The review has been categorical, with emphasis on muscular strength and endurance, metabolism at rest, metabolism during work, psychomotor behavior, and athletic performance.

An examination of earlier reviews pertaining to the enhancement of muscular performance by means of hypnotic suggestion reveals the literature to be equivocal. The purpose of the present chapter has been to update these earlier reviews as well as examine the methodological adequacy of both the earlier and current research. It seems reasonably certain that much of the disagreement in this research area reflects statistical and design inelegancies to a great extent, and this point has been emphasized throughout.

Hypnosis per se has been reported by several investigators to have no influence on muscular strength and endurance, but an equal number of investigators have reported that simply being in a trance can evoke both increments and decrements in performance. The literature on this point is clearly equivocal. On the other hand, there is widespread agreement that hypnotic suggestions designed to decrease muscular strength and endurance are almost always effective. Unfortunately, investigators have failed to evaluate whether the same suggestions would be effective in the waking state. However, one would intuitively expect negative suggestions to be effective in the cooperative waking S. The influence of hypnotic suggestions designed to enhance muscular strength and endurance is less certain. It is difficult to advance generalizations at this time without citing numerous qualifications relating to task specificity, S characteristics, and type of suggestion. In other words, in certain circumstances hypnotic suggestion facilitates muscular strength and endurance, but there are a number of factors that govern such response. For example, Ss who are not normally accustomed to performing at their maximal levels experience gains in strength and endurance following the administration of "involving instructions" in the hypnotic state. Therefore, prior to advancing generalizations on this point it is imperative that systematic investigations be conducted that take into account the many variables interacting in this human-performance domain.

Additional psychomotor variables such as simple reaction time have been evaluated under hypnotic conditions, and the findings of this research parallel those cited in the strength and endurance literature. For example, hypnotic suggestions of increased (slower) reaction time are usually effective in much the same way that suggestions designed to decrease strength and endurance are effective. Of course, there is little reason to believe that the same effects could not be produced in the cooperative waking S. Attempts to produce lower (faster) reaction time by means of hypnotic suggestion are sometimes effective but not consistently so. Also, there is limited evidence suggesting that the type of suggestion employed may hold the key to facilitation of reaction time.

Facilitation of complex motor behavior, characteristic of sport competition, has been reported by a number of investigators. These reports have been based on clinical case studies involving psychodynamic analysis followed by hypnotic resolution of complex motor problems. For example, precompetition anxiety states have been managed through hypnosis, and pain minimized, in order to improve performance.

Hypnosis has also been employed in an attempt to alter metabolic responsivity to hallucinated exercise, as well as in studies of the metabolic dynamics of exercise. This research has revealed that hypnotically suggested exercise tends to increase heart rate, respiration, total ventilation, oxygen consumption, and cardiac output. These findings have obvious implications for the human-performance investigator concerned with the definition of base-line metabolic rates. It has also been observed that a tendency exists for metabolism to be slightly elevated in the S exercising in the hypnotic state. While metabolic changes have been evoked in the exercising S by means of hypnotic suggestion, these alterations have not been consistent.

In summary, it can be said that attempts to decrease muscular performance by means of hypnotic suggestion are almost always effective. Intuitively, however, one would anticipate similar success in cooperative Ss tested in the waking state. Attempts to facilitate muscular performance by means of hypnotic suggestion have been successful where hypnotherapists have attempted to correct psychomotor problems, reduce pain, resolve aggression conflicts, and control anxiety states in the competitive athlete. However, the experimental literature on this topic at first appears to be equivocal. Further examination reveals that this apparent equivocality can be explained on the basis of numerous methodological considerations. For example, the S characteristics, criterion task, induction procedure, and type of suggestion are interactive variables in hypnosis research. Therefore, it seems reasonable to suggest that Ss scoring high on hypnotizability and low on physical performance will experience increases on performance tasks in which "alerting" hypnotic inductions and "involving" instructions are employed. While there are numerous exceptions to these qualifications in the clinical literature, these interpretative restrictions seem appropriate for the experimental literature. It is hoped that citation of these qualifications will be heuristic rather than frustrating or confusing. A great deal of systematic research involving rigorous methodological controls must be conducted before the influence of hypnosis per se and hypnotic suggestion on muscular performance is understood.

References

Agosti, E., and Camerota, G. (1965). *Int. J. Clin. Exp. Hypn.* **13,** 149.
Arnold, J. (1971). *Res. Quart.* **42,** 1.

Barber, T. X. (1966). *Brit. J. Soc. Clin. Psychol.* **5**, 42.
Barber, T. X. (1970). "Hypnosis: A Scientific Perspective." Van Nostrand-Reinhold, Princeton, New Jersey.
Barber, T. X., and Calverley, D. S. (1964). *Can. J. Psychol.* **18**, 156.
Berman, R., Simonson, E., and Heron, W. (1954). *J. Appl. Physiol.* **7**, 89.
Bevegård, S., Arvidsson, T., Åström, H., and Jonsson, B. (1968). *Proc. Int. Union Physiol. Sci.* **7**, 42.
Bier, W. (1932). *Psychol. Abstr.* **6**, 586.
Blum, G. S., and Wohl, B. M. (1971). *Psychonom. Sci.* **22**, 69.
Borg, G., and Linderholm, H. (1967). *Acta Med. Scand.* **472**, 194.
Charcot, J. M. (1889). "Lectures on Diseases of the Nervous System" (translated by T. Savill). New Sydenham Soc., London.
Cobb, L. A., Ripley, H. S., and Jones, J. W. (1967). *In* "Physical Activity and the Heart" (M. J. Karvonen and A. J. Barry, eds.), pp. 192–199. Thomas, Springfield, Illinois.
Collins, J. K. (1961). "Muscular Endurance in Normal and Hypnotic States: A Study of Suggested Catalepsy." Honors thesis, Univ. of Sydney, Sydney, Australia.
Crane, C. W. (1940). "Psychology Applied." Northwestern Univ. Press, Evanston, Illinois.
Dudlye, D. L., Holmes, T. H., Martin, C. J., and Ripley, H. S. (1964). *Psychosom. Med.* **26**, 46.
Edmonston, W. E., Jr., and Marks, H. E. (1967). *Amer. J. Clin. Hypn.* **9**, 252.
Eskridge, V. L. (1969). "The Effects of Limited Training in Hypnosis upon Reaction Time." Master's thesis, Western Kentucky Univ., Bowling Green.
Evans, F. J. (1968). *Behav. Sci.* **13**, 477.
Evans, F. J., and Orne, M. T. (1965). *Int. J. Clin. Exp. Hypn.* **13**, 103.
Eysenck, H. J. (1941). *Brit. J. Med. Psychol.* **18**, 304.
Fulde, E. (1939). *Psychol. Abstr.* **13**, 368.
Gorton, B. E. (1959). *In* "Hypnosis in Modern Medicine" (J. M. Schneck, ed.), pp. 246–280. Thomas, Springfield, Illinois.
Graham, C., Olsen, R. A., Parrish, M., and Leibowitz, A. (1968). *Psychonom. Sci.* **10**, 223.
Hadfield, J. A. (1924). "The Psychology of Power." Macmillan, New York.
Ham, M. W., and Edmonston, W. E., Jr. (1971). *J. Abnorm. Psychol.* **77**, 329.
Henry, F. M. (1960). *Res. Quart.* **31**, 448.
Hepps, R. B., and Brady, J. P. (1967). *J. Nerv. Ment. Dis.* **145**, 131.
Hilgard, E. R. (1965). "Hypnotic Susceptibility." Harcourt, New York.
Hilgard, E. R. (1971). *Amer. Sci.* **59**, 567.
Hilgard, E. R., and Boucher, R. G. (1967). Hypnosis Research Memorandum 59, Department of Psychology, Stanford Univ., Stanford, California.
Hottinger, W. L. (1958). "Effect of Waking and Hypnotic Suggestion on Strength." Master's thesis, Univ. of Illinois, Urbana.
Hull, C. L. (1933). "Hypnosis and Suggestibility." Appleton, New York.
Ikai, M., and Steinhaus, A. H. (1961). *J. Appl. Physiol.* **16**, 157.
Johnson, W. R. (1961a). *J. Sports Med.* **1**, 71.
Johnson, W. R. (1961b). *Res. Quart.* **32**, 263.
Johnson, W. R. (1965). *In* "Proceedings, 1st International Congress of Sport Psychology" (F. Antonelli, ed.), pp. 187–189. F.M.S.I., Rome.
Johnson, W. R., and Kramer, G. F. (1960). *Res. Quart.* **31**, 469.
Johnson, W. R., and Kramer, G. F. (1961). *Res. Quart.* **32**, 522.

Johnson, W. R., Massey, B. H., and Kramer, G. F. (1960). *Res. Quart.* **31**, 142.

Kellor, M., Frost, J., Silberberg, N., Iversen, I., and Cummings, R. (1971). *Amer. J. Occup. Ther.* **25**, 77.

Levin, S. L., and Egolinsky, I. A. (1936). *Psychol. Abstr.* **10**, 421.

Levitt, E. E., and Brady, J. P. (1964). *Int. J. Clin. Exp. Hypn.* **12**, 21.

Liebert, R. M., Rubin, N., and Hilgard, E. R. (1965). *J. Pers.* **33**, 605.

London, P., and Fuhrer, M. (1961). *J. Pers.* **29**, 321.

Luoto, K. (1964). *J. Abnorm. Soc. Psychol.* **68**, 54.

Manzer, C. W. (1934). *Psychol. Clin.* **22**, 248.

Marshall, G. D. (1970). Hypnosis Research Memorandum 113, Department of Psychology, Stanford Univ., Stanford, California.

Massey, B. H., Johnson, W. R., and Kramer, G. F. (1961). *Res. Quart.* **32**, 63.

Mead, S., and Roush, E. S. (1949). *Arch. Phys. Med.* **30**, 700.

Mierke, K. (1956). *Psychol. Abstr.* **30**, 356.

Moll, A. (1913). "Hypnotism" (translated by A. F. Hopkirk). Scribner's, New York.

Morgan, W. P. (1970). *In* "Contemporary Psychology of Sport" (G. S. Kenyon, ed.), pp. 283–286. Athletic Institute, Chicago, Illinois.

Morgan, W. P., and Coyne, L. L. (1965). Paper read before 43rd annual session, Amer. Congress of Physical Medicine and Rehabilitation, Philadelphia, Pennsylvania.

Morgan, W. P., Cooper, J., and Goeckerman, R. (1967). Paper read before annual meeting, Amer. College of Sports Medicine, Las Vegas, Nevada.

Morgan, W. P., Raven, P. B., Drinkwater, B. L., and Horvath, S. M. (1973). *Int. J. Clin. Exp. Hypn.* In press.

Naruse, G. (1965). *Int. J. Clin. Exp. Hypn.* **13**, 63.

Nemtzova, O. L., and Shatenstein, D. I. (1939). *Psychol. Abstr.* **13**, 422.

Nevski, I., and Sryashchich, K. (1930). *Psychol. Abstr.* **4**, 494.

Nicholson, N. C. (1920). *Bull. Johns Hopkins Hosp.* **31**, 89.

Orne, M. T. (1959). *J. Abnorm. Soc. Psychol.* **58**, 277.

Orne, M. T. (1970). *Nav. Res. Rev.* **23**, 1.

Rieger, C. (1884). "Der Hypnotismus." Gustav Fisher. Cited by Hull (1933). pp. 226–227.

Rosenhan, D., and London, P. (1963). *J. Abnorm. Soc. Psychol.* **66**, 77.

Roush, E. S. (1951). *J. Appl. Physiol.* **3**, 404.

Ryde, D. (1964). *J. Sports Med.* **4**, 241.

Simonson, E. (1938). *Psychol. Abstr.* **12**, 21.

Slater, C. (1967). "Expectancy and Hypnotic Performance." Dissertation, Washington State Univ., Pullman.

Slotnick, R., and London, P. (1965). *J. Abnorm. Psychol.* **70**, 38.

Slotnick, R. S., Liebert, R. M., and Hilgard, E. R. (1965). *J. Pers.* **33**, 37.

Toews, J. V. (1964). *Arch. Phys. Med. Rehabil.* **45**, 413.

Weitzenhoffer, A. M. (1963). "Hypnotism: An Objective Study in Suggestibility." Wiley, New York.

Wells, F. L. (1928). *J. Abnorm. Soc. Psychol.* **24**, 264.

Whitehorn, J. C., Lundholm, H., Gardner, G. E. (1930). *Amer. J. Psychiat.* **9**, 661.

Williams, G. W. (1929). *J. Abnorm. Soc. Psychol.* **24**, 318.

Williams, G. W. (1930). *Amer. J. Psychol.* **42**, 83.

Young, P. C. (1925). *Amer. J. Psychol.* **36**, 214.

Chapter 8

Music

*Luigi F. Lucaccini and Leonard H. Kreit**

I. Introduction

If one accepts the premise that psychological truisms are reflected in the myths, proverbs, anecdotes, and literary creations of man, the folklore of music is well worth considering. Although this chapter is largely confined to the effects of music on work and muscular performance, a cursory examination of the folklore of music may lend perspective to the scientific review that comprises the major portion of this chapter.

A comparison of musical folklore with scientific studies of the effects of music reveals an interesting discrepancy. According to tradition, the effects of music on the human psyche are powerful indeed, and sometimes little short of miraculous; on the other hand, while some scientific

* The views expressed in this chapter are solely the responsibility of the authors and reflect in no way the official position of the Division of Dental Health, B.H.M.E., N.I.H.

investigators have found music to affect man's behavior, the impact is flat and weak by comparison.

Let us briefly consider a few of the many myths and beliefs that have been held regarding the power of music. In her book "Music Therapy," Alvin (1966) notes that Apollo was the god of both medicine and music. The implication is that music possesses healing powers, and, in fact, music was an integral part of the armamentarium of primitive medicine men. But not any song would do. "In a number of magic healing rites, the medicine man tried to discover the sound to which the sick man, or the spirit inhabiting him, would respond" (Alvin, 1966, p. 16).

Alvin cites several legends illustrating the power of music. In the biblical story of David and Saul, David's harp playing enabled King Saul to overcome his depression. In a similar vein, the legend of Farinelli and the Spanish King is described as follows. "Philip was suffering from acute melancholia. The King had for many weeks refused to take part in the affairs of state, and this put the whole country in a critical situation. . . . When the King first heard him the singer was out of sight in an adjoining room. It was the impact of his music alone that shook the patient out of his state of despondency and was responsible for his first reaction" (p. 63).

Of course, any magic as powerful as music would have to contain negative elements in addition to positive aspects. There is "Odysseus telling of the songs of the sirens which cast a spell on the sailors who could not resist their appeal and were wrecked on the rocks" (p. 19). Similarly, there is the familiar legend of the Pied Piper, who entranced the town's children with his beautiful music and led them off, never to be seen again.

Again, it is noted that the vivid accounts of the effects of music, whether positive or negative, contrast with the findings from studies reviewed in this chapter. One possible reason for the discrepancy is the methodological difficulty of doing well-controlled research on music as an ergogenic aid. Another reason may be that the myths and literary passages deal with the effects of music on mental and physical health, while studies reviewed in this chapter focus upon its effects on work and athletic performance, covering lightly the other areas mentioned. Lest this explanation be prematurely convincing it should be noted that workers have historically benefited from music. Farnsworth (1969), for example, recalls "that Negro stevedores and laborers the world over have typically synchronized their work speeds to the tempos of music and have derived much benefit therefrom. Their morale has been lifted and their work movements have been made smoother and more efficient by the directing force of group singing" (p. 217). Thus, historical evidence suggests that, in its absence, workers spontaneously create music to alleviate their toil.

This chapter reviews recent work dealing with the effectiveness of music as an ergogenic aid. The emphasis is primarily on published scientific studies and unpublished dissertations of the last two decades; however, several citations date from the 1940's or earlier. The intention is to provide a balanced, comprehensive summary of the current "state of the art," rather than an exhaustive, historical review. Reference sources that were surveyed in selecting materials for inclusion were "Completed Research in Health, Physical Education and Recreation," "Masters Theses in Education," "Psychological Abstracts," and "The Education Index."

Several topics are covered in the remainder of this chapter. First, an overview of music in terms of its stimulus properties and its physiological and psychological effects is presented. Next, research studies of the ergogenic effects of music are reviewed which fall into three performance situations: athletic and related tasks, industrial production, and vigilance performance. Following the review of research findings, common methodological problems in measuring the ergogenic effects of music are discussed. The reader who wishes additional background is referred to Farnsworth's (1969) text and to reviews by Kirkpatrick (1942, 1943) and Uhrbrock (1961).

II. Music as an Independent Variable

To attempt a rigorous definition of the term "music" would involve controversial issues including theories of aesthetics and philosophy and would do little to elucidate the subject matter of this chapter. Suffice it to say that sound is the raw material of music.

Every musical instrument has in common the fact that it produces regular or periodic acoustic vibrations which are perceived by the listener as sound. The frequency of these vibrations determines the "pitch" of the sound. The intensity of vibration determines the volume of the sound, and the duration of the vibration determines how long the sound will be heard.

Each musical instrument has its own characteristic sound, sometimes denoted as "tone." Tone results from the fact that each musical instrument, in addition to producing a fundamental frequency, produces certain overtones or harmonics of the fundamental frequency. These harmonics fuse with the fundamental frequency in the listener's hearing to create one unitary auditory impression, the tone which characterizes that instrument.

Melodies are organized series of notes sometimes identified in the layman's mind with songs or tunes but which, strictly speaking, encompass any succession of notes, short or long, from a musical composition. "Tempo" refers to the speed at which a particular musical selection is played, while "rhythm" deals with such temporal organization factors as beat, accent, grouping of notes, and the like.

The large range of values that the musical variables cited above can assume and the combinations of these variables that vary among and within musical compositions make it appear to be an impossible task to develop a taxonomic system for classifying music and its effects. Nevertheless, some classification schemes, although far from perfect, have been developed. In the following section, one such classification system is briefly described, and the relationship between values of musical variables and their effects on mood and physiological responses is discussed.

III. Effects of Music on Mood and Physiology

A commonplace yet little-understood psychological phenomenon is the impact music has on the mood or emotional feeling of the listener. Some might hold that the changes in mood which accompany music are paralleled by corresponding changes in the underlying physiological state of the listener.

Everyday experience indicates that music exerts a psychological impact on the individual which cannot be denied. The case for corresponding variations in the traditional physiological measures of emotional response (e.g., heart rate and galvanic skin response) is not as compelling.

Before turning to the physiological evidence, one might ask how music achieves its effect on mood. One position is that the elements of music, described in the preceding section, affect the listener's mood in a precisely determined fashion. For example, Diserens and Fine (1939), as cited by Soibelman (1948, p. 74), state, "We believe that the compilation of a sufficient number of mood-change charts taken from all kinds of listeners to the Edison phonograph would result in a body of statistics indicating the probability of the appearance of any specific kind of emotion, in connection with various musical selections."

Although the simplistic approach of Diserens and Fine is not satisfying, it does contain a grain of truth. Certain songs, certain sounds appear to elicit characteristic emotional responses on the part of the listener.

Farnsworth (1969, p. 83) cites the work of Hevner (1935), who produced a system for classifying musical mood in accordance with the elements of the composition. Hevner's system includes six musical elements: mode, tempo, pitch, rhythm, harmony, and melody. Each element can assume one of two possible values, e.g., slow or fast for tempo, flowing or firm for rhythm, and ascending or descending for melody. Each of the values is assigned a numerical weight and a pattern is formed and named in much the same fashion as a factor in factor analytic procedures. The result of this system is a set of numerically defined patterns against which musical selections can be compared and hence classified. Names of patterns include dignified–solemn, sad–heavy, and graceful–sparkling, among others.

A problem with the foregoing approach is that it makes no allowances for individual differences. As Farnsworth (1969) states: "Although musical compositions can quite properly be placed into mood categories, they will not invariably arouse the moods in terms of which they have been described. We are thus forced to conclude that music can be reported as a language of mood and emotions in a very limited sense only" (p. 80).

One's cultural milieu, personal experiences, situational factors, and perhaps even genetic factors may all help to shape the mood that characterizes an individual's immediate response to a particular musical selection. For instance, learning theory may explain in part how music affects one's mood through past associations of music with happy, sad, or other emotionally toned events. The reappearance of music can act as a conditioned stimulus eliciting a conditioned emotional response. "So is the slowly acquired response to the tone of the organ associated with church and religious feelings" (Alvin, 1966, p. 88).

Although complete specification of resultant mood cannot be made in terms of the stimulus elements of the music played, what general statements are possible? Hevner (1937) concluded that tempo is the most important musical element that affects mood, followed by modality and pitch level. Washburn and Dickinson (1927), cited by Soibelman (1948), observed that subjects ranked the elements of music as contributing to enjoyment in the following order: melody, rhythm, harmony, design, and tone color. More work is needed to clarify the relationship of the basic stimulus elements of music to mood. Refinement and adoption of systems such as Hevner's (1935) would make possible more valid comparisons between studies and would reduce the confusion and inconsistencies apparent to those who seek to synthesize and interpret findings from diverse studies.

A somewhat heightened level of physiological arousal has been found to accompany music. Ellis and Brighouse (1952) found that respiration rate increased 5–10% during classical music, and Zimny and Weidenfeller (1963) reported that music judged to be exciting resulted in a significantly higher level of galvanic skin response (GSR) than music judged to be calming or neutral. On the negative side, Coutts (1965), Ellis and Brighouse (1952), and Zimny and Weidenfeller (1963) all failed to find significant changes in heart rate with the playing of a variety of selections.

The relationship between mood and physiology is neither consistent across measures nor strong. For example, Ries (1969) correlated respiration rate and GSR with subjects' affective reactions to a wide range of musical selections. Although GSR level was increased by music, the correlation of GSR and subjects' preference for specific selections was nonsignificant. The relationship ($r = 0.48$) between modal breathing amplitude and affective response was significant, however, indicating that the more a subject liked a selection the deeper his breathing was.

With respect to physiological measures of emotion, Ellis and Brighouse (1952) state that "the evidence indicates that the magnitude of an individual's reaction to music is fairly specific to the music employed. Evidently, there is no general trait of reactivity to music, and thus it would be hazardous to predict an individual's reaction to different musical selections on the basis of his reaction to one or two" (p. 46). Farnsworth (1969) points out that physiological responsiveness to music varies with the musical training of the listener, the personal "meaning" of the music played, and the particular selection played. Regardless of these factors, it appears that the physiological effects of music are neither striking nor closely related to mood.

IV. Athletic and Skilled Performance

One of the most interesting studies of the effects of music on athletic performance was reported in 1911 by Ayres of the Russell Sage Foundation. During a 6-day bicycle race held in New York City, Ayres recorded the average time per mile during periods when the band was playing and during periods in which no music was being played. The data included time recordings of 46 miles made over a period of three evenings. "The average time per mile while the band was playing was three minutes and four seconds or at the rate of 19.6 miles per hour. When the band was not playing the average time was three minutes and twenty-one seconds or at the rate of only 17.9 miles per hour. In other words, the miles ridden with music averaged 17 seconds faster than those ridden without" (p. 321).

Ayres' study raises two questions that cannot be answered by the data he reports. Was the increase in speed that occurred with music accompanied by a corresponding decrease in speed during the nonmusic period? If so, then the music did not really increase the overall performance of the bicycle riders, but simply caused it to be more variable. Unfortunately, there is no way to tell what overall performance might have been without music. A second question is whether the music by itself increased speed or whether the accompanying noise of the crowd caused the superior performance of the athletes. Ayres himself reports, "It often seemed as though the resulting faster riding came rather because the music stimulated the spectators and their shouts encouraged the riders than because it affected the riders directly" (p. 323).

A master's thesis by Olson (1960) tends to support the interpretation that crowd noise may have been a factor which influenced the results of Ayres' study. Olson studied the effects of music, recorded crowd noise, and quiet on high school athletes and nonathletes in a series of five tests of athletic performance: the Bass Tests of Static and Dynamic Balance, the penny cup test, the McCloy Blocks Test, and the basketball free-throw test. For nonathletes, performance was best during the quiet period or the music period; in four out of five comparisons, nonathletes were handicapped by noise to a statistically significant degree. In contrast, noise conditions aided the athletes; in four of the five comparisons they performed best with noise, while in the fifth comparison there was no statistically significant difference among performances in the noise, music, and quiet conditions.

Four recent studies concern the effects of music on performance on a bicycle ergometer. Nelson and Finch (1962) measured all-out performance on a 60-second bicycle ergometer ride under the following four conditions: fast march music, slow music, white sound with a mambo background, and no sound. Nelson (1963) measured all-out performance on a 90-second ride in a series of three experiments. The first experiment included the conditions described above, the second experiment compared rhythmically varying pure tones of constant intensity to no sound, and the third experiment compared variations in sound intensity of a musical selection to no sound. Hart (1965) compared the effects of march music with silence in an all-out ride on a bicycle ergometer in which subjects were required to maintain a preset work rate as long as possible. Coutts (1965) studied the effects of music on an all-out ride on a bicycle ergometer; experimental conditions included fast music, slow music, and silence. Coutts' study differed from the preceding ones in that the various auditory conditions were introduced and terminated prior to the test performance on the ergometer. In all four studies no statistically significant differences were found.

One may speculate as to why Ayres' study showed music (or at least music and crowd noises) to facilitate athletic performance on a bicycle, in contrast to the other studies cited above. It may be that motivation is at a peak during a task that requires only 60 or 90 seconds of all-out performance, so that music, noise, or any other ergogenic aid could not be expected to assist performance markedly. On the other hand, during a long and grueling 6-day bicycle race fatigue would be high and motivation low, and therefore athletes might be receptive to music, noise, or other ergogenic aids, at least temporarily. A second factor is that in a long race athletes deliberately pace themselves and thus have some reserve to call on when motivated, in contrast to subjects who are presumably already at peak performance levels in an all-out test.

If music facilitates athletic performance, a question that naturally follows is whether music can facilitate the learning of athletic skills. Some physical education teachers feel that, because the proficient execution of complex athletic skills such as swimming involves smooth rhythmic movements, music, with its element of rhythm, can be exploited as a teaching aid. Dillon (1952) states that "swimming to the accompaniment of music or with music as a background is not something new. In recent years many college swimming clubs have been using music as an accompaniment for their swimming. Some teachers interested in this type of swimming have used music with instructional swimming classes and have found that students, as a general rule, enjoy this type of instruction. Many coaches, instructors, and aquatic officials believe rhythm is important in both speed swimming and form swimming" (p. 1).

Dillon (1952) conducted a 3-year study to demonstrate the effects of music on the learning of swimming. This study included 240 intermediate swimmers divided into a nonmusic (control) group and a music (experimental) group. Performance measures were speed and form on the crawl and breaststroke. For the music group, the tempo of the music was used as a teaching aid when specific skills were practiced. It was found that the group taught by music improved significantly more than the control group in crawl and breaststroke form; the music group also improved more in speed, but the difference between the two groups was not significant.

Beisman (1967) carried out a study in which the rhythmic element of music was used to teach elementary school students such skills as throwing, catching, climbing, balancing, jumping, leaping, dodging, bouncing, and striking. Elementary school students in grades 1–6 participated in the study, which involved 10 weeks of practice sessions ranging from 10 to 20 minutes in duration. Experimental groups received instruction similar to that of control groups but in addition heard music during practice sessions. There was an overwhelmingly consistent difference in favor of the experimental treatment for all of the skills. In 57 of the 66 comparisons, the experimental groups showed significant improvement as contrasted to the control groups. In the remaining nine analyses, although significant differences were not found, the results favored the experimental treatment.

In contrast to the studies of Beisman (1967) and Dillon (1952), which showed that music can facilitate the teaching of athletic skills, several master's theses in physical education have reported negative findings. For example, Grocki (1967) found march music to produce no beneficial effects on push-ups and sit-ups, and to produce significant detrimental effects on teaching squat jumps. Similarly, Chipman (1966) reported that march music did not increase endurance significantly in the performance of sit-ups. McLellan (1964) likewise found that music did not help in the teaching of badminton. McLellan's study was limited to 41 subjects and included a waltz rhythm that may not have been in harmony with the rhythmic movements required in badminton. Bowers (1966) concluded that music tended to improve boys' but not girls' rope-jumping skills. It should be noted that Bowers and Grocki used intact classes instead of assigning subjects to groups at random.

Finally, Mikol and Denny (1955) compared the effects of synchronous and asynchronous rhythmic stimuli on performance in a pursuit rotor task under five conditions: metronome synchronous with rotor, metronome asynchronous with rotor, music synchronous with rotor, music asynchronous with rotor, and silence. Although the synchronized rhythm of the metronome did result in enhanced performance, synchronous (and asynchronous) music did not improve performance over that with silence. Rhythm was apparently effective as a teaching aid in this situation but synchronous music, or at least the specific selection employed, was not the proper vehicle to emphasize the rhythmical aspects of performance in the task.

The evidence for the utility of music as an aid in teaching athletic skills is fairly evenly divided. In such sports as swimming, properly chosen music may sometimes be effective because it paces the swimmer and reinforces desired rhythmical motor patterns. In activities such as conditioning exercises, in which endurance is more important than rhythm, music may be ineffective because it serves mainly as a motivator, in a situation in which motivation is already high. As noted previously, this would also appear to be the case with all-out performance on the bicycle ergometer. Pursuing this point, Beisman's (1967) overwhelmingly positive results appear to be more readily explained in terms of the motivating effects of music than through any possible contributions to the rhythmic aspects of performance. Given the diversity of skills taught and the fact that Beisman's subjects were elementary school children, it appears reasonable to hypothesize that music served to increase the enthusiasm and attention of her students rather than to reinforce any particular aspects of the skills practiced. These interpretations must be considered speculative, however, in view of the paucity of detail provided by most investigators regarding both the particular musical selections employed and the manner in which music was used in the teaching situation.

Since driving may be considered, with some justice, to be a national sport, it is perhaps fitting that the effects of music on driver behavior be mentioned in this section. In view of the importance of traffic safety and the fact that radios and tapes are played by many drivers, it is surprising how few scientific studies on the subject have been conducted.

Brown (1965) studied the effects of music on driving in light and in heavy traffic. Ballroom dance music was compared with a program of speech and with a quiet condition. Only eight subjects participated in the study. In light traffic, music reduced the use of the accelerator, brake, clutch, and steering wheel and increased driving speed as compared to driving with silence. The first two differences (i.e., the reduction in use of the accelerator and brake) were statistically significant. In heavy traffic, the effect was the opposite; control movements were more numerous with slow music than with quiet, and speed was reduced. Only the reduction in speed was significant. For both light and heavy traffic, driving performance with the speech program was intermediate to performance with music and with quiet.

Konz and McDougal (1968) measured control activity and speed changes for 24 subjects driving on a test circuit with light traffic. Each subject drove under three conditions: slow music, Tijuana Brass music, and silence. The slow-music condition resembled the condition of ballroom dance music in Brown's (1965) study and resulted in driving behaviors similar to those found by Brown in the light-traffic situation. Control activity with slow music was reduced and speed was increased in comparison to driving with silence; however, only the increase in speed was significant. Other findings of the study indicated that drivers were generally more active with Tijuana Brass music than when driving in silence; both speed and accelerator use increased significantly.

Unfortunately, it is not completely clear in these two studies whether the changes in behavior introduced by slow music were beneficial since no operational definition of optimal driver behavior was made in terms of speed and control activity. Konz and McDougal (1968), in a secondary analysis of their data, report that regardless of auditory background, subjects used the car controls less and took less time to cover the test circuit as they grew more familiar with the car and route. Presumably these learning effects are in the direction of more efficient and relaxed performance, suggesting that the similar changes noted in both studies with slow music in light traffic were beneficial. By the same token, Tijuana Brass music, which tended to increase control activity, would be judged detrimental.

V. Industrial Production

The economic advantages of a measure that can increase industrial output or reduce production errors even by a small margin are obvious. For this reason, music has been employed in many manufacturing situations with the expectation that enhanced production would result. Although it is difficult to demonstrate unequivocally the effects of a single factor such as music in a complex industrial setting, several studies have attempted to document the possible benefits to be derived. Table I summarizes 12 such studies involving a diversity of routine tasks. These studies focused on direct measures of productivity, although such auxiliary measures as absenteeism, accidents, and workers' attitudes were occasionally reported.

Some evidence exists to support the claim that industrial music can increase production significantly. Smith (1947) reported increases of 7 and 17%, respectively, on two radio equipment assembly shifts of 21 workers each when from 1 to 5 hours of music was presented daily. Similarly, Kalanevich (1950) found the output of five industrial clothes pressors to be increased by 8% when 2 hours of daily music programming was provided.

Twelve other experiments or subexperiments failed to support the results of Smith (1947) and Kalanevich (1950). Kerr (1945) found that 2–2½ hours of music daily in three studies of electronics assembly tasks resulted in statistically nonsignificant increases in quantity of production. A fourth study by Kerr (1945) failed to show any significant differences between "more-music" days (6 hours of programming) and "less-music" days (1 hour of programming). McGehee and Gardner (1949) reported that 80 minutes of music daily had almost no discernible effect on the production of rug loom setters as compared to working without music.

TABLE I

STUDIES OF INDUSTRIAL PRODUCTIVITY

Subjects	Music variables	Production measures	Effects on production[a]	Investigators
88 female radio tube assemblers	Four music conditions (64 minutes of slow, fast, mixture of slow and fast, or randomly chosen music) compared to no music; total playing time (64 or 96 minutes) was varied in slow, fast conditions	Scrappage over five 3-week periods; one period for each music condition	Scrappage was significantly lower with slow and fast music than in other conditions; no effect of total playing time was shown; Humes attributed results to confounding with extraneous variables	Humes (1941)
64 female electronics workers	Variety-music days (2 hours of music) alternated with no-music days in 2-day cycles	Quantity, scrappage, net good yield over 40-day period	No statistically significant differences	Kerr (1945)
53 female electronics workers	Music days ($2\frac{1}{2}$ hours of either variety, sweet, or peppy music daily) alternated with no-music days in 3-day cycles	Quantity, scrappage, net good yield over 107-day period	No statistically significant differences among types of music or between presence and absence of music	Kerr (1945)
520 female radio tube assemblers	"More-music" days (6 hours daily of either popular music, waltzes and Hawaiian music, or marches and polkas) alternated with "less-music" days (1 hour of requests and special programming) on a ratio of 3:1	Quantity and scrappage over 54-day period	No statistically significant differences	Kerr (1945)

53 female electronics workers	High- and low-quality-record days ($2\frac{1}{2}$ hours of music) alternated with no-music days in 3-day cycles	Quantity, scrappage, net good yield over 60-day segment of 107-day study	No statistically significant differences between recording qualities or between presence and absence of music	Kerr (1945)
42 female radio equipment assemblers in two shifts of 21 each	0, 1, 2, 3, 4, or 5 hours of music daily	Quantity (adjusted for overall production trends) over 8-week period	Production was significantly higher for 1, 2 hours music on day shift; production was significantly higher for 2, 3, 4, 5 hours music on night shift; on an overall basis, music resulted in 7% increase on day shift, 17% on night shift, both significant	Smith (1947)
142 female rug loom setters	Four unspecified music conditions (80 minutes daily) alternated with no music in 4:1 ratio within each week	Quantity over 5-week period	No statistically significant differences among types of program or between presence and absence of music; no statistically significant differences between overall production during study period and 5-week base-line periods without music before and after study period	McGehee and Gardner (1949)
Three male and two female clothes pressers	0 or 2 hours of music daily	Quantity (based on cleaning cost) over 4-week period	8% production increase with music was statistically significant	Kalanevich (1950)

TABLE I (*Continued*)

Subjects	Music variables	Production measures	Effects on production[a]	Investigators
22 female keypunch operators	0 or 2 hours of music daily	Quantity and errors over 4-week period	No statistically significant differences between music and no music or between overall production measures during study period and 4-week base-line periods without music before and after study period	Smith (1961)
20 female temporary employees	0 or 1 hour of music in 3-hour task sessions	Quantity and errors over 2- or 3-day periods in addition, anagram, manual assembly, and mark-sense coding tasks	No statistically significant differences	Konz (1964)
26 male and female mechanical assembly workers in a skateboard factory	Four music conditions (folk, dance, show, and popular music; 4 hours daily) alternated with no music on 4:1 ratio within each week	Quantity and percentage of rejects	No statistically significant differences	Newman *et al.* (1966)
31 male and female telecommunications operators	Show tunes and light classical selections for 24 minutes out of every half hour	Quantity over 12-week period	No statistically significant difference between production during study period and 4-week base-line periods without music before and after study period	Devereux (1969)

[a] References to significance or statistical significance are based on interpretations of statistical tests as reported in the references cited.

Smith (1961) found a nonsignificant increase in the production of 22 keypunch operators with the introduction of 2 hours of music daily. Konz (1964) compared the effects of 1 hour's programming within 3-hour work periods with a nonmusic condition. Four tasks were used: manual assembly, mark-sense coding, addition problems, and anagram solution. No differences in favor of music were found. Newman *et al.* (1966) reported that 4 hours of music daily had no effect on the productivity of assembly workers in a skateboard factory. Finally, Devereux (1969) found a nonsignificant increase in the output of 31 telecommunications operators with music presented during 80% of the work shift.

Taken together, these results do not provide a strong case for the ergogenic effect of music on industrial production. Given the diversity of tasks studied and music conditions employed, some disagreement in results would be expected; however, Smith's (1947) positive findings are not supported by allied studies involving assembly tasks, namely those of Kerr (1945), Konz (1964), and Newman *et al.* (1966).

There is little evidence that industrial music reduces production errors. No reduction in errors was noted with background music in a keypunch task (Smith, 1961), in the performance of mark-sense and addition tasks (Konz, 1964), in the mechanical assembly of skateboards (Newman *et al.*, 1966), or in four studies involving electronic assembly tasks (Kerr, 1945).

Humes (1941) reported statistically significant reductions in scrappage in three radio tube assembly tasks when four different music programs were employed. Of the four, a slow-tempo program and a fast-tempo program were the most effective in reducing scrappage rates in comparison with production without music. In view of the fact that the results were based on the manufacture of about 900,000 radio tubes by a work group of 88 employees over a 4-month period, Humes' (1941) caution in interpreting his results is surprising. He states that "while there are certain statistical indications of advantage in the use of music in general . . . the experimental observations were not recorded over a sufficiently long period to justify definite conclusions" (p. 585). Further, "Inconsistencies in the statistical results indicate that factors other than music, although none was observed, operated to produce some and possibly all of the differentiating effects noted" (p. 586).

When Humes' (1941) interpretation of his own results is taken into account, the evidence is uniformly negative. This is perhaps not suprising since industrial error rates may not be under the control of the worker. Environmental factors such as lighting, heat, humidity, and noise and task factors such as the quality of the raw materials themselves, the pace of activity imposed in assembly tasks, and the motor skill requirements of the work may overshadow possible internal effects resulting from background music.

Secondary measures were collected in some of the production studies reviewed in order to shed additional light on the relationship between music and industrial production. Smith (1947) attempted to show a relationship between the presence of background music and accident rates. Although he found that accidents decreased on two shifts with music, a large increase was noted on a third shift. Thus, on an overall basis, accident rate did not vary with the presence or absence of music. Smith (1961) included absenteeism as a secondary measure in a study of keypunch operators but noted only a slight, nonsignificant decrease in absenteeism with music. Others (e.g., Kalanevich, 1950; Konz, 1964) treated absenteeism as a methodological problem rather than as secondary experimental data and noted absentee rates only insofar as was necessary to correct experimental data.

The most common secondary measure in the studies reviewed was attitudes. Workers in many studies expressed a clear preference for background music (Devereux, 1969; Humes, 1941; McGehee and Gardner, 1949; Newman *et al.*, 1966; Smith, 1947; Smith, 1961). It is interesting to note, however, that worker impressions and preferences do not necessarily reflect performance changes on the job. Devereux (1969), McGehee and Gardner (1949), Newman *et al.* (1966), and Smith (1961) report that from 35 to 73% of the personnel in the work groups studied felt that background music raised performance or helped them to "work better." In none of these studies was a significant improvement in performance demonstrated.

That industrial employees generally prefer to work in an environment containing background music cannot be disputed. One instance has been reported in which employees went so far as to present a petition to management to restore music when it had been removed for experimental purposes (Humes, 1941). Whether industrial music improves production is questionable in light of the evidence at hand. At best, it appears that background music which otherwise might act to increase production is cancelled out by confounding variables inherent in most industrial settings.

VI. Vigilance Performance

Vigilance research is the study of human detection performance in prolonged, monotonous tasks in which stimuli that are infrequent, near threshold, and unpredictable in time and location must be detected. Military monitoring tasks and industrial inspection work often involve detection functions that can be classified as vigilance performance.

Engineering psychologists have been engaged in the study of human vigilance performance since World War II, when it was discovered that the detection efficiency of personnel who monitored radar screens was far from ideal. Operational and laboratory studies by Mackworth (1950) and others have shown that, although detection performance is high at the start of a task session, subsequent performance declines rapidly to a lower, relatively constant level of performance.

A critical feature of vigilance tasks appears to be the lack of stimulation confronting the monitor. Since the monitor spends the bulk of his time waiting for the occurrence of a signal, vigilance tasks have been aptly termed "do-nothing" tasks (Dunlap, 1961). Background music has been employed in some vigilance studies in an attempt to maintain a high level of performance by enriching the sensory environment of the human monitor. These studies, conducted in the well-controlled though artificial setting of the psychological laboratory, have yielded positive results.

Experimental research on vigilance generally supports the notion that music serves as an ergogenic aid at least in the laboratory setting (see Table II). Two experiments by Lucaccini (1968) and studies by McGrath (1963), Tarriere and Wisner (1962), Ware *et al.* (1964), and Wokoun (1963) all indicate that overall target detection performance is significantly higher when monitoring with background music than with noise or silence. Exceptions to these positive results are found in a third study by Lucaccini (1968) and one by Poock and Wiener (1966).

Several studies reporting positive results employed a music condition that included some form of stimulus variation in addition to music itself. Lucaccini (1968) interspersed short breaks between recorded selections on a tape recording. In McGrath's (1963) study, music formed only one part of the audio variety tape played during monitoring sessions; noises and audio portions of television programs were also presented in short segments throughout. Ware *et al.* (1964) employed local radio music programming, which presumably included announcements and commercial messages. Other studies that produced positive results employed relatively heterogeneous musical selections. Tarriere and Wisner (1962) presented a series of classical music selections which at first glance appear to be homogeneous. The authors note, however, that the selections, which span two centuries in composition and style, are distinguished for their rhythmic dynamism and instrumental richness. Wokoun (1963) employed a background music tape recording that had been specially

TABLE II

STUDIES OF VIGILANCE PERFORMANCE

Subjects	Music variables	Performance measures	Effects on performance[a]	Investigators
35 automobile factory employees	Continuous program of classical music versus silence, motor noise, and speech	Detection of small light spots on driving film during four 90-minute sessions	Detection performance with music showed a decrement from first to second half hour, but was significantly higher than performance without music throughout the task	Tarriere and Wisner (1962)
28 naval enlisted men	Variety audio tape including music, noise, speech versus white noise	Detection of brightness increments of intermittent light source during eight 1-hour sessions	Detection performance with variety audio declined over first half hour as did performance without music; over last half-hour, performance improved and was significantly higher than with noise	McGrath (1963)
14 government workers	Continuous program of commercial background music versus noise	Reaction times to colored lights during 1-hour task	Reaction time appeared to be lower for subjects performing on first session with music than with noise; on second session, in which conditions were reversed, no differences were found (overall significance tests were not performed)	Wokoun (1963)

112 army trainees	Radio music (either continuous or contingent on detections) versus no music	Detection of interruptions in pilot light during three 3-hour periods	Continuous radio music and no music both resulted in performance decrement over first hour; average detection level was significantly higher in both music conditions than with no music	Ware *et al.* (1964)
75 male college students	Preferred and nonpreferred music versus white noise	Detection of 30° needle deflections on voltmeter during 75-minute period	No statistically significant differences	Poock and Wiener (1966)
63 army enlisted men	Three continuous programs of commercial background music arranged with stimulation value selected to be in either ascending, descending, or increasingly variable order	Reaction time to change in size of opening displayed in "magic eye" electronic tube during 1-hour task	Reaction times were significantly lower with the ascending and variable sequences than with the descending sequence	Wokoun (1968a)
41 adult males	Wide frequency range and narrow frequency range filtering was applied alternately to selections in a 1-hour continuous program of commercial background music	Reaction time to change in size of opening displayed in "magic eye" electronic tube during 1-hour task	Reaction times were significantly lower with wide-range selections	Wokoun (1968b)

TABLE II (*Continued*)

Subjects	Music variables	Performance measures	Effects on performance[a]	Investigators
40 male college students	Instrumental music separated by short breaks (5–15 seconds) versus white noise	Detection of light flashes in pilot light during 40-minute task	A significant performance decrement occurred with noise but not with music; overall performance was significantly better with music	Lucaccini (1968)
40 male college students	Instrumental music separated by short breaks (5–15 seconds) versus white noise	Detection of target stimulus in complex visual search problems during 40-minute task	Performance was significantly better with music than with noise during second half of task	Lucaccini (1968)
20 male college students	Instrumental music separated by short breaks (5–15 seconds) versus white noise	Replications of both of the tasks (pilot light and complex visual search) described immediately above extended to 1 hour in duration	Performance decrements occurred with music and noise; no significant difference in overall performance between music and noise conditions	Lucaccini (1968)

[a] References to significance or statistical significance are based on interpretations of statistical tests as reported in the references cited.

prepared by a commercial background music firm to include selections differing in stimulation value.

The failure of Poock and Wiener (1966) to show an effect of background music may be attributable to the homogeneity of the conditions employed. In their "preferred" music condition, they used a popular tape recording of uninterrupted piano tunes made from a set of three record albums by the same artists. In the "nonpreferred" music condition, uninterrupted music from three albums by one musical combo judged to be unpopular with their students was presented. Both music conditions appear to be much less varied than those used in the studies reporting positive results. It should be noted that Poock and Wiener (1966) did find that presenting a more varied though nonmusical source of stimulation (pilot–control tower conversations from the local airport) resulted in significantly improved performance. The failure of the third experiment by Lucaccini (1968) to show an effect of music is more difficult to explain since it repeated music conditions from two preceding successful experiments.

The importance of a varied music program is supported by two studies comparing the relative effectiveness of specially designed music programs. In the first study (Wokoun, 1968a), a series of 23 selections was ranked according to "stimulation value" determined according to criteria (e.g., tempo, rhythm, instrumentation) developed by a commercial background music firm (O'Neill, 1966). Three sequences were constituted: ascending stimulation values, increasingly variable values, and decreasing values. Each sequence contained the same 23 selections. The ascending and the increasingly variable sequences resulted in significantly better vigilance performance than the descending sequence. The second study (Wokoun, 1968b) compared the effects of selections of wide frequency range and narrow (filtered) frequency range. Vigilance performance was superior with the wide-range selections, indicating the value of the greater range of auditory stimulation provided in the higher-fidelity recordings.

The studies reviewed here document the importance of background music in vigilance tasks. This contrasts with industrial production research in which the contribution of background music to productivity is questionable. Some differences between the two situations should be mentioned. First, the vigilance task presents an impoverished stimulus environment to the operator while the industrial situation, although often monotonous, is rarely as low in stimulation as the vigilance task. Second, the vigilance research reported does not span work periods comparable to those of the industrial production studies reviewed. Third, both independent and dependent variables are controlled and measured much more precisely in the laboratory vigilance study than in the operational production study.

It appears reasonable to conclude that background music, if it includes some element of variety, can be used to improve overall vigilance performance in the psychological laboratory. Whether it has the same effect in the operational military or industrial setting is less clear since its effect on vigilance performance is yet to be tested in those surroundings.

VII. Methodological and Theoretical Considerations

At least three arguments can be advanced for hypothesizing that music aids work and athletic performance. As noted in the introductory section, tradition and everyday experience indicate that music can affect man's behavior in striking fashion. Second is the nearly universal preference of workers for music on the job. And third are the well-controlled laboratory studies of vigilance which show that music functions as an ergogenic aid.

Why, then, do most researchers find that music has little if any impact on work and athletic performance? Concerning the former, it has previously been noted that many elements of the work situation may preclude marked increases in productivity that might follow the introduction of music. Concerning the latter, too little may be known about how to exploit music in such a way as to greatly improve athletic performance. The lack of experimental control characterizing most studies may constitute the most important reason for the inconsistent, largely negative findings reported in this review. Positive findings, too, are suspect since they may have been elicited by experimenter hopes and expectations or by the simultaneous introduction of other improvements along with music.

Perhaps the most important decision facing the experimenter intent on assessing the ergogenic effects of music is that of selecting a specific music program for his study. Unfortunately, many of the studies reviewed not only fail to justify the music program used in terms of some aspect of the musical elements it contains but also fail even to specify what selections were included and how they were used. Studies such as those by Beisman (1967) and Dillon (1952) do not meet minimal scientific standards of reporting in that the reader is given virtually no description of the way in which the music was used, thereby making it impossible to evaluate the results or employ them in some practical fashion.

A second weakness in the studies reviewed is the choice of subjects. The validity of generalizing from a sample to some population of interest depends on the relevance of the sample chosen to that population. When the results reviewed earlier are considered in light of the appropriateness of the samples employed, in many cases the reader's confidence in their generalizability is shaken. For example, with respect to sex of subjects, it is a curious fact that most of the industrial production studies were limited to female workers while, conversely, almost all of the vigilance research dealt with male subjects. We know, therefore, little about the effects of music on the productivity of male factory workers or on the vigilance performance of women.

The importance, at least in industrial productivity research, of employing experienced subjects is pointed out by Uhrbrock (1961). He states that "the test of the effectiveness of music as a work incentive comes when applied to skilled employees whose production has leveled off" (p. 33). Konz (1964), for example, introduced into his study two confounding variables, learning and motivation, by using naïve subjects. The effects of both of these factors may have overshadowed those of music and could have been avoided by choosing a group of subjects more experienced in the tasks. Even if Konz had demonstrated an ergogenic effect of music, it is not clear that the same results would have been obtained with experienced subjects.

A final point worth mentioning in the context of subjects is random sampling. An unfortunate characteristic of the majority of the industrial production studies reviewed is the use of intact groups of subjects. Although this may be the only practical approach if one is to study the effects of music on experienced workers in realistic settings, it violates the assumption of randomization that underlies statistical tests of inference. Results based on intact groups must be interpreted, therefore, with caution if they are to be accepted at all.

Good experimental control is difficult to achieve in studies that take place in an industrial setting. Humes (1941), for example, attributed his favorable results to unspecified extraneous factors which he could not control in his design. Similarly, Smith (1947) noted that changes in engineering techniques, supervision, and the incentive system accompanied the introduction of music in the work environment. These factors make his positive findings suspect. Finally, as previously noted, Konz (1964) introduced unwanted learning and motivation effects by using naïve rather than experienced subjects. All of these studies failed through inadequate experimental design to isolate the effects of the variable of interest, namely, music.

A related problem has to do with expectations on the part of the experimenter and subjects which may alter the effects of music. The "experimenter effect" has gained recognition as a potential source of bias in psychological research (Rosenthal, 1966). In studies in which the experimenter himself, rather than an associate who has no knowledge of the anticipated outcome of the study, deals with subjects, there is a possibility that subtle cues may be transmitted to the subjects which may influence task performance. Almost none of the studies reviewed eliminated this source of bias by employing someone other than the experimenter to work directly with subjects.

Experimenter effects notwithstanding, subjects may independently realize the purpose of a study in which music is presented only on alternate hours or days or in which radically different programs are alternated. Admittedly, it is difficult to manipulate music conditions in an unobtrusive fashion unless the changes are mild deviations from the normal conditions. Marked changes in the auditory environment are likely to attract the attention of subjects. Regardless of the "official" explanation advanced, some subjects may suspect the true purpose of the introduction of music. Wokoun (1963) reported that some subjects in his study "admitted that they had guessed the experimenter's hypothesis and had then tried harder to show that they could do the task equally well under either condition" (p. 17). In certain cases, the background of the subjects may be such that it is difficult for them not to guess the purpose of the study. Brown (1965), for instance, used as subjects members of the scientific and technical staff who could be expected to be familiar with his work and the goals of his study.

One solution is the use of a double-blind design in which both the person directly administering the study and the subjects are unaware of the purpose of the study and its anticipated outcomes. While this design may be difficult or impossible to implement in some situations, given the nature of music as a variable, it represents the level of control that must be sought if subject and experimenter effects are to be ruled out.

Another design problem is related to the time period over which music is assumed to act. Wokoun (1968b), for example, employed a music condition in which the quality of recording alternated between high fidelity and low fidelity every few minutes. In order to accept his conclusions about vigilance performance under these two closely intermeshed music conditions, one must make the unlikely assumption that the subjects' internal states alternated rapidly in correspondence with the frequent, regular changes in recording quality.

An implicit assumption in several studies is that music has an intermediate term effect which does not carry over from one day to the next. For example, Newman *et al.* (1966) and Smith (1947) employed designs in which workers experienced music on some days but not on others. Interpretation of the results of these studies is based on the validity of the assumption that the effects of the program presented on a particular day do not transfer to other days on which a different program or no music is presented. The point to bear in mind is that the experimenter should make explicit his assumptions about temporal effect when choosing a design, if he is to obtain an adequate test of his hypothesis. If not, he may be in the position of Smith (1961), who attempted to demonstrate a distraction effect of music in a keypunching task but played music only during nonwork periods. Unless Smith made the questionable assumption that music played before the task could interfere with performance during the task, his design would seem entirely inappropriate to the hypothesis he was testing.

The studies reviewed in this chapter, by and large, are lacking in theoretical perspective. The emphasis has been all too often placed on determining whether music is an effective aid in a given situation instead of clarifying how it achieves its effects or why it fails to achieve any effects. The absence of a guiding theoretical interest in these studies may be responsible in part for inattention to such experimental design factors as choice of appropriate subjects, selection of a music program, and the question of the time period over which music acts.

To the extent that music serves as an ergogenic aid, it is not clear that it enhances performance by the same mechanism in athletic, industrial, and vigilance task situations. In the vigilance task, music may increase physiological arousal which, in turn, causes increased alertness of the observer. Several versions of arousal theory exist which emphasize different aspects of the stimulus situation in increasing or maintaining the level of arousal (e.g., Fiske and Maddi, 1961; McGrath, 1963). Considerable attention has been focused on one aspect, variety of stimulation, as being of particular importance in maintaining a high level of arousal or alertness (Scott, 1957). Variety, although lacking a clear-cut definition, might be interpreted as the inclusion of some element of change in stimulation, as suggested in Section VI.

Industrial production may benefit from the introduction of music in several ways. One already discussed is that of increased arousal. Another might be the masking of noises that distract or annoy the worker. A third possibility is that of providing relief from the monotony of the routine work situation, as suggested by Ghiselli and Brown (1948) and implied by Smith (1966).

In the athletic performance situation, there are indications that music may act as a teaching aid and, with children, also as a motivator. Some writers suggest that it is the rhythmic element of music that accounts for its utility as a teaching aid, but this hypothesis is neither supportable nor refutable on the basis of research evidence reviewed in this chapter.

The intent of most of the studies reviewed has been a pragmatic one. Does music enhance performance in a particular task? If so, is program

X better than program Y? If one could rest assured that music was an unequivocal asset in the performance setting, it might not be necessary to deal with theoretical models or issues. The fact that music has not generally been shown to possess ergogenic effects suggests that attention to the theoretical issues mentioned above may help elucidate those situations and conditions in which music does function as an ergogenic aid.

VIII. Conclusions

The widespread use of music in athletic and industrial settings reflects the commonly held belief that music facilitates human performance. Is this belief realistic? Is music really an ergogenic aid, or is its use wholly without effect? No conclusive answers to these questions can be derived from the research reviewed in this chapter. Music does not appear to function as a powerful ergogenic aid over a wide range of settings. Nevertheless, in certain limited circumstances, music does facilitate some behavior.

Subjective reports indicate that music can affect one's mood and can improve workers' attitudes. Experimental studies show music to have a mild effect on one's physiological reactions. It seems reasonable to assume that physiological and/or psychological reactions to music are a necessary though not sufficient condition for music to function as an ergogenic aid. Therefore, the studies of the effects of music on mood and physiology do not contradict the hypothesis that music is an ergogenic aid.

This chapter reviewed the effects of music in three settings: vigilance performance in the laboratory, athletic performance, and worker production in industrial settings. Laboratory research on vigilance shows that music aids the monitor, probably because of the variety it introduces in an otherwise dull, monotonous task. Although one study (Ayres, 1911) suggests that music improves athletic performance, the preponderance of the evidence is negative; however, music does seem to facilitate the learning of athletic skills. Concerning the productivity of workers in an industrial setting, the few studies that report modest but positive increments as a result of music are more than outweighed by the negative findings.

In surveying the field, one encounters a lack of methodological rigor, which renders many of the findings suspect. Add to this the fact that most of the studies were done from an atheoretical frame of reference and it becomes justifiable to characterize this field of inquiry as confused and ill-defined.

The evidence appears too weak to support tradition and commonly held beliefs regarding the efficacy of music, although a few studies report findings that do support these beliefs. A systematic program of research, conducted within a theoretical frame of reference and in accordance with sound principles of experimental design, is needed if a satisfactory answer is to be provided to the general question of whether music functions as an ergogenic aid. Considering current trends, it will be a long time before a satisfactory answer is forthcoming.

References

Alvin, J. (1966). "Music Therapy." Baker, London.

Ayres, L. P. (1911). *Amer. Phys. Educ. Rev.* **16**, 321.

Beisman, G. L. (1967). *Res. Quart.* **38**, 172.

Bowers, I. W. (1966). "The Effectiveness of Instruction and the Use of Music as an Aid in Teaching Rope Jumping Skills to First Grade Children." Unpublished master's thesis, State Univ. of Iowa, Iowa City.

Brown, I. D. (1965). *Ergonomics* **8**, 475.

Chipman, L. (1966). "The Effects of Selected Music on Endurance." Unpublished master's thesis, Springfield College, Springfield, Massachusetts.

Coutts, C. A. (1965). *Res. Quart.* **36**, 17.

Devereux, G. A. (1969). *Personnel Pract. Bull. (Melbourne)* **25**, 24.

Dillon, E. K. (1952). *Res. Quart.* **23**, 1.

Diserens, C. M., and Fine, M. A. (1939). "A Psychology of Music." College of Music, Cincinnati, Ohio.

Dunlap, J. W. (1961). *Electro-Technol. (New York)* **67**, 128.

Ellis, D. S., and Brighouse, G. (1952). *Amer. J. Psychol.* **65**, 39.

Farnsworth, P. R. (1969). "The Social Psychology of Music." 2nd ed. Iowa State Univ. Press, Ames.

Fiske, D. W., and Maddi, S. R. (1961). "Functions of Varied Experience." Dorsey, Homewood, Illinois.

Ghiselli, E. E., and Brown, C. W. (1948). "Personnel and Industrial Psychology." McGraw-Hill, New York.

Grocki, J. M. (1967). "Music and its Effect on the Performance Level of Selected Physical Activities." Unpublished master's thesis, Springfield College, Springfield, Massachusetts.

Hart, K. (1965). "The Effect of Anxiety, Music, and Heart Rate on All-Out Performance of College Women." Unpublished master's thesis, Univ. of Illinois, Urbana.

Hevner, K. (1935). *Psychol. Rev.* **47**, 186.

Hevner, K. (1937). *Amer. J. Psychol.* **49**, 621.

Humes, J. F. (1941). *J. Appl. Psychol.* **25**, 573.

Kalanevich, E. M. (1950). "The Effects of Music on the Output of Clothing Pressers in a Dry Cleaning Establishment." Unpublished master's thesis, Pennsylvania State Univ., University Park.

Kerr, W. A. (1945). *Appl. Psychol. Monogr.* No. 5.

Kirkpatrick, F. H. (1942). *Psychol. Rec.* **5**, 197.

Kirkpatrick, F. H. (1943). *J. Appl. Psychol.* **27**, 268.
Konz, S. (1964). "The Effect of Background Music on Productivity of Four Tasks." Unpublished doctoral dissertation, Univ. of Illinois, Urbana.
Konz, S., and McDougal, D. (1968). *Hum. Factors* **10**, 233.
Lucaccini, L. F. (1968). "Vigilance and Irrelevant Stimulation: A Test of the Arousal Hypothesis." Unpublished doctoral dissertation, Univ. of California, Los Angeles.
McGehee, W., and Gardner, J. E. (1949). *Personnel Psychol.* **2**, 405.
McGrath, J. J. (1963). *In* "Vigilance: A Symposium" (D. N. Buckner and J. J. McGrath, eds.), pp. 3–19. McGraw-Hill, New York.
Mackworth, N. H. (1950). "Researches on the Measurement of Human Performance." Medical Research Council Special Report Series No. 268, London.
McLellan, M. I. (1964). "A Study of the Use of Music as an Aid in Teaching the Badminton Serve." Unpublished master's thesis, State Univ. of Iowa, Iowa City.
Mikol, B., and Denny, M. R. (1955). *Percept. Mot. Skills* **5**, 3.
Nelson, D. O. (1963). *Res. Quart.* **34**, 484.
Nelson, D. O., and Finch, L. W. (1962). *Res. Quart.* **33**, 588.
Newman, R. I., Jr., Hunt, D. L., and Rhodes, F. (1966). *J. Appl. Psychol.* **50**, 493.
Olson, R. S. (1960). "The Effect of Noise and Music on Performance in Tests of Mental and Physical Skills." Unpublished master's thesis, State Univ. of Iowa, Iowa City.
O'Neill, D. M. (1966). *Management Personnel Quart.* **5**, 17.
Poock, G. K., and Wiener, E. L. (1966). *J. Ind. Eng.* **17**, 318.
Ries, H. A. (1969). *Psychonom. Sci.* **14**, 62.
Rosenthal, R. (1966). "Experimenter Effects in Behavioral Research." Appleton, New York.
Scott, T. H. (1957). "Literature Review of the Intellectual Effects of Perceptual Isolation." Defense Research Board Report HR66, Canada.
Smith, H. C. (1947). *Appl. Psychol. Monogr.* No. 14.
Smith, R. L. (1966). "Monotony and Motivation: A Theory of Vigilance." Dunlap, Santa Monica, California.
Smith, W. A. S. (1961). *Psychol. Rep.* **8**, 159.
Soibelman, D. (1948). "Therapeutic and Industrial Uses of Music." Columbia Univ. Press, New York.
Tarriere, C., and Wisner, A. (1962). *Trav. Hum.* **25**, 1.
Uhrbrock, R. S. (1961). *Personnel Psychol.* **14**, 9.
Ware, J. R., Kowal, B., and Baker, R. A., Jr. (1964). *Hum. Factors* **6**, 111.
Washburn, W. F., and Dickinson, G. L. (1927). *In* "Effects of Music" (M. Schoen, ed.), pp. 121–130. Harcourt, New York.
Wokoun, W. (1963). "Vigilance with Background Music." U. S. Army Human Engineering Laboratories Technical Memorandum 16-63.
Wokoun, W. (1968a). "Effects of Music on Work Performance." U. S. Army Human Engineering Laboratories Technical Memorandum 1-68.
Wokoun, W. (1968b). "Work Performance with Music: Instrumentation and Frequency Response." U. S. Army Human Engineering Laboratories Technical Memorandum 9-68.
Zimny, G. H., and Weidenfeller, E. W. (1963). *Amer. J. Psychol.* **76**, 311.

Chapter 9

Social Facilitation

Robert N. Singer

I. Introduction

Although it is interesting and informative to examine the results of laboratory experiments dealing with behavioral modification and changes, the truth of the matter is that most of these efforts are at best suggestive of how an organism reacts in real life. Complaints registered about the artificiality of the laboratory task and experimenter effects on the performance of the subject are legitimate and recognized as sources of difficulty in generalizing experimental results beyond the laboratory testing. But what can be said of the testing procedures used in general? In almost all cases where learning and performance phenomena are investigated, the subjects are tested alone in cubicles or isolated chambers so as not to contaminate data. And rightfully so, since one can examine only a limited number of variables at any one time.

In reality, however, we live in a competitive–cooperative society. We learn to adjust to our environment, to behave in certain ways, and to acquire skills according to cooperative and competitive demands placed upon us and values instilled within us. Tasks may be learned and/or performed in front of other people. Thus, the solitary nature of the research laboratory conflicts with that of the social-oriented world in which man actually exists. It may be argued, on the other hand, that numerous behaviors and skills are acquired in part or full by an individual when not in the presence of others. Conceding the validity of this proposition, and not wishing to take issue with "typical" laboratory research, permit me to explore social influence and muscular performance.

In order to proceed in this manner, one must be able to compare "alone" performances with those involving the presence of others, either as passive or active spectators, as coactors, or as a part of a group with designated roles. In sociopsychological terminology, we shall examine the phenomenon entitled social facilitation. The question to be answered is, To what degree do other individuals affect one's performance? Do they facilitate or impede it?

Social facilitation, sad to say, has not been a well-researched area, as Zajonc (1965) in a well-read article has indicated. And, as is the case with almost all learning studies, motor skills have been employed on rare occasions. Fortunately, a renewed interest in the topic by Zajonc and other investigators (e.g., Martens, 1969a,b; Singer, 1965, 1970) is providing some direction for those concerned. In this chapter, social facilitation research on all sorts of learning matter and from various contrived situations will be reviewed. The obvious goal is to relate and apply research and theory to human muscular performance.

II. Cooperation and Competition

Of all the social situations related to behavioral effects investigated by researchers and discussed by educators, those involving cooperation and competition are most omnipresent. Early in life preschoolers demonstrate competitive tendencies for objects, favors, and rewards and must be taught how to sublimate these feelings in a cooperative manner. In school, competitive and cooperative situations are part of the present learning environment and in varying degrees are promoted by teachers who wish to elevate class motivation. Athletics represent the "real" world. Competition against rivals within a framework of agreed upon, stated, or implied rules and regulations, as well as ethically accepted standards, are displayed in sport and jobs. One must cooperate with fellow workers and supervisors, or teammates and coaches, or other students and teachers, while attempting to rise in status, win, or be best as compared to others. Thus, in order to achieve a number of personal goals that satisfy needs and desires, two different but not necessarily mutually exclusive forms of activity occur: competition and cooperation.

Competition may be personal or impersonal. The main goal in personal competition is to defeat an opponent, while a particular personal objective other than victory illustrates impersonal competition. Prestige or performing to acceptable self-determined standards represents the latter case. Voluntary and involuntary types of cooperation have been distinguished, the former exemplified by a personal willingness to strive for the common goals of the group, the latter by lack of choice and enforced conditions. Rather than becoming involved with the many ramifications of these sources of motivation, and in order to remain within the framework of this book, it might be advisable to look at these factors as they are deliberately deployed for incentive purposes, especially for increased physical performance. Coaches, trainers, or instructors can certainly contrive practice conditions that will encourage alone performance, competition, cooperation, or some combination of them. Unfortunately, it is not easy to answer the question as to which circumstance is best. In an early publication, May and Doob (1937), after summarizing conflicting research findings, suggested that ". . . it becomes all the more evident that so-called 'social facilitation' is not a product of the social situation, but of the situation as interpreted by a living personality who possesses psychological peculiarities of his own" (p. 33). But social incentive situations are defended and supported in industrial situations by Gagné and Fleishman (1959), in scholastic activities by Coleman (1961), and in athletic endeavors by Moore (1970). Research findings tend to bear these premises out.

Generally, the social facilitative effects of competition and cooperation on individual output are reasonably documented. Of course, individuals differ in their reactions to these situations. Disregarding learner personality variables and the many ways the setting of incentive situations can vary (which may lead to exceptions to the rule), competitive and cooperative activities produce better results than solitary practice and work conditions. In fact, most of the time, competitive opportunities are more successful in yielding favorable outcomes than working-together arrangements. Exceptions to this proposition may arise when certain objectives are specified, task-to-task distinctions are made, or in the considerations given to the arrangement of these situations. For example, the influence of competition on performance depends on such factors as the personality traits of the competitors, factors unique to the situation, and the nature of the task in the broad cultural context (Cratty, 1967). Nevertheless, it is apparently easier to derive beneficial effects from rivalry than from cooperation or solo undertakings.

However, when competition is included with a cooperative structure, most desirable effects may be noticed. Strong (1963) attempted to determine the effect of six motivating conditions on the performances of sixth grade children on seven physical fitness tests. The following testing circumstances were arranged.

1. A situation in which the subject was a member of a group that competed against another group
2. A situation in which the subject competed with a classmate of nearly equal ability
3. A situation in which the subject competed with a classmate of markedly different ability
4. A situation in which, to establish a class record, the subject competed with all his classmates
5. A situation in which the subject competed with himself
6. A situation in which the subject chose the level of performance he wished to attain

In this study, the team competition and the level of aspiration conditions were more effective motivators than the other competitive situations. Team competition produced greater gains in performance than did individual competition. In other studies, however, competition between groups led to lesser performance than did individual competition. Gagné and Fleishman (1959) conclude, "The reason seems to be that when responsibility is divided, the status needs of individuals are not as directly affected" (p. 81). Perhaps in Strong's investigation, how the person's status might contribute to group success was not considered. If individual incentives are raised within a group, and group and individual goals are similar, group competition can certainly be an effective measure in accomplishments. Additional evidence supporting the desirability of a group in a competitive situation was reported by Myers (1962). Subjects were divided into rifle teams; some were placed in competitive leagues while others were in noncompetitive leagues. The competitive teams demonstrated a significant increase in team esteem (positive attitudes toward the team); the others did not. When failure occurred in the competitive league, less deterioration of team esteem was noted than when failure happened in the noncompetitive league.

In a task requiring depressing the correct telegraph key in a gamelike situation, Bruning *et al.* (1966) found that the speed of a competitive group was considerably faster than that of the cooperative group. When Maller (1929) formed three groups of children and tested them in speed adding, individual competition was more effective than cooperation. Also, the no-incentive group was poorest. When competitive conditions are compared in their effect on performance with solo conditions, the former usually are shown to be more beneficial. Likewise, when cooperative and alone situations are examined, cooperation is often found to be more desirable.

Exceptions to these trends may be noted when such factors as the subject's personality are considered. Specifically, anxiety level evidently interacts with level of stress. (Competition may be regarded as a form of stress.) Highly anxious subjects perform significantly better in noncompetition, but low-anxious subjects are more effective under competitive conditions (Ryan and Lakie, 1965). It has been speculated (Spence and Spence, 1966; Zajonc, 1967) that, with increased practice and learning, the correct responses in the repertoire of possible responses become the dominant ones. Stress, motivation, or drive (e.g., caused by the presence of others, competition) tend to encourage general arousal and the emission of dominant responses, thereby facilitating performance in the case of the skilled individual. Conversely, it is theoretically proposed that in a newly introduced task incorrect responses are dominant. Anything in the environment that might stress the learner and heighten his drive level should facilitate the occurrence of the dominant responses (the incorrect ones).

Although Martens and Landers (1969) did not observe any differences in performance on a coincident-timing motor task of well-practiced subjects placed in competitive and noncompetitive circumstances, they did suggest that insufficient stress may have been produced by the nature of the competition employed in their experiment. In another study (Voor *et al.*, 1969), two groups of male subjects from collegiate intramural athletic teams undertook an isometric contraction endurance task. One group performed individually, while the other group competed for a prize in teams of three. The investigators concluded that "contrary to expectations, the factors of competition and team presence during the task did not significantly increase the mean endurance time . . ." (p. 217). Evidently, considerably more work will be needed to resolve the conflict between broad theory and research dealing with motor tasks and specific situations.

Turning to a related matter, let us consider competition in the framework of athletics and physical performance and a so-called "competitive ability." One may attempt to measure competitive ability in numerous ways. As a general technique, Kretch *et al.* (1969, p. 715) illustrate a rating scale with criteria for the measurement of the competitiveness trait on the following five-point scale, summarized below.

1. *Very competitive:* Extreme or hectic drive to surpass competitors; either will not play if he cannot win, or always picks inferior opponents, or cheats to win. Defeating his competitors is practically his only satisfaction in a play or work situation. Competitive drives dominate major part of his activities—a diffused set extending to many people and to all sorts of situations that to most individuals would not be competitive.
2. *Above average:* Enjoys surpassing competitors to the point of being upset when he loses; takes his failure to win very hard, or cannot restrain an overt expression of satisfaction when he wins. Not so extreme as 1 but characteristic and noticeable by anyone with whom he comes in contact. Either several fields in which competitive drive is very pronounced but not so extreme as 1 or one field in which it is terribly important to surpass others.
3. *Average:* Is stimulated by competitive situations and enjoys excelling but can accept defeat without much strain. Periodic competitive sprees but not persistent and pervasive nor extreme.
4. *Below average:* No real competitive relationship; enjoys games for the fun of playing them but relatively unimportant who wins.
5. *Very uncompetitive:* Sensitive to competitive situations but gets disorganized, is let down, unproductive, or flees from them. Resistive in negative way. Extremely discouraged about his abilities, or appears to seek defeat compulsively.

Presumably a person scoring high in ability should be expected to perform more successfully in competitive situations. Fitting the personality to the situation makes sense, all things being equal. Going a step further, Ryan (1958a) sent a questionnaire to track coaches throughout the country to ascertain the characteristics associated with the good competitor. He concluded that ". . . differences in competitive ability represent relative differences in freedom to achieve or to express aggression" (p. 122). In a follow-up report, Ryan (1958b) summarized the data and distinguished between good and bad competitors. For instance, the good competitor often exceeds practice performances; the bad competitor is variable and usually has lower performance in the actual contest than in practice. The two groups of competitors possess a different emotional ability to accept high-level athletic achievement. Ryan states that the good competitor is perhaps a temporary victim of overanxiety when he competes badly, whereas the poor competitor shows a ". . . feebleness of effort, almost a level of paralysis" (p. 125).

The good competitor demonstrates warm friendships with opponents, but not during competition. The poor competitor likes an atmosphere of friendliness; he does not get angry or bitter. He is self-condemning and constantly berates himself. He is fearful of error and takes a negative approach. Also, he seems to have an ". . . emotional inability to accept achievement" (p. 131). After competition, the poor competitor is in good spirits if he performs badly. The good competitor is difficult to live with. Thus, it can be seen that any discussion of the effect of competitive situations and social facilitation is insufficient if the personality of the individual is not considered.

Be that as it may, the importance and values of interscholastic athletic competition have so impressed Coleman (1961) that he recommends using forms of this kind of competition in scholastic matters, e.g., grades. Instead of the traditional frequent grading and evaluations, he prefers changing the system and structure to contests and games both within and among schools. Coleman wishes ". . . to change the structure of rewards in high schools—to shift from interpersonal competition, with its conflict-producing effects, to intergroup competition, in which group rewards reinforce achievement" (p. 322). This implies competition within a cooperative group venture. Let us now turn to coaction effects and examine cooperative behavior in more detail, especially as it contrasts with individual behavior.

III. Coaction Effect

Coaction activity includes the interaction of team members and the effects others have on one member's performance when all are actively and simultaneously involved in the same task or activity. Typically, subjects working together in groups are compared in their individual performances with those subjects working in isolated circumstances. In most of the published research, teams consist of two or three members, rarely exceeding four.

Teams may be found in many diverse places in society. As Blum and Naylor (1968) indicate, "References are frequently made to 'research teams,' 'management teams,' 'missile launch teams,' 'air defense teams,' etc." (p. 259). And, of course, there are always athletic teams. A team by definition is a small group of people attempting to realize a common goal. It is natural to ask whether members of the unit should be trained individually or as a team. Many sports are of a team nature and the coach is often uncertain how much time to allot to individual practice versus team practice. Since an athlete's skills are to be demonstrated in a team context, the coach must consider the best structure in which team tasks can be accomplished. Much of the recent research on the topic comes from military, aviational, and industrial situations, where increased concern has been displayed for team performance situations. An important concept in learning, feedback, can be individually or team initiated. A team can offer social reinforcers, information sharing, and motivation for the members. These factors must be weighed against the values of individual training, limitations due to the size and nature of the team, and the type of tasks (e.g., simple or complex, familiar or novel) to be learned.

A. Individual and Group Behavior Compared

In analyzing individual and team performance outcomes, we must determine whether the main concern is team behavior or individual proficiency. In other words, we might (a) seek to train people in a small group in order to stimulate the acquisition of individual skills and motivate behavior or (b) wish to train people as a unit because that is the way they will ultimately function in the "real" situation. Coaction effects can therefore be examined with at least a double purpose.

Abel (1938) found that a paper and pencil maze task was learned to a higher degree by boys and girls working in pairs than in isolation. In pursuit rotor performance, the value of group performance over individual performance was supported (Weyner and Zeaman, 1956). If we examine the behavior of lower forms of organisms, coactive effects become more apparent. From ant output in nest building (Chen, 1937) to amounts of the food consumed by chickens (Bayer, 1929) and rats

(Harlow, 1932), coaction situations stimulate greater activity than alone conditions. These tasks, it might be mentioned, require that some of the natural responses be emitted by the organisms. With unfamiliar and difficult learning tasks requiring attention, accompanied by few distractions and minimal stress, coactors may depress individual performance. This point will be elaborated on when the nature of the task is discussed (Section III,C), especially in the framework of Zajonc's (1965) theory. Staying with infrahuman behavior for examples of the negative effects of coaction, Gates and Allee (1933) observed such results in cockroaches learning a maze, as did Allee and Masure (1936) with parakeets learning a discrimination task.

In the learning of coordination skills involved in a simulated radar-controlled aerial intercept task, no difference in proficiency level was noted by Johnston (1966) between individually taught and team-taught subjects. However, this study employed activities requiring much more teamwork than those used in other studies. Also, the task was fairly difficult. Much of the research is in agreement on the social facilitative effect of team performance, especially when reciprocal information sharing and reinforcement are present. One possible exception will be noted when we consider the nature of the task as a variable. It should also be reemphasized that in most investigations the teams whose performance is being compared to solo performance are relatively small, e.g., dyads, trials, or quads. If teams become too large, other problems arise, possibly negating their value over individual performance conditions.

Social situations are certainly motivating. Working and learning in units provides a pooling of knowledge and mutual assistance. Feedback can be obtained immediately, thereby lending further support for the use of teams in learning situations. May and Doob (1937) considered the benefits not clear-cut, and they summarized the early literature by stating that "in general—with almost as many exceptions—it appears as though American students in psychology and social psychology courses do more or poorer work when they are brought together in a group than they do in isolation; and they tend to approach a greater degree of uniformity and conformity in respect to their activity and opinions" (p. 34).

Nevertheless, considering subsequent research findings and allowing for certain interfering variables, it can be said that a team process in learning is generally favored under appropriate conditions. The individuals working in a team situation can increase performance more readily when (a) their knowledge and abilities are positively related to the task, (b) they are a cohesive unit that can work together, (c) the size of the team is reasonable, (d) they are not passive but actively offer assistance, reinforcement, and feedback, or (e) they compete against each other within the group.

In the last situation, social competition should increase motivation more than individual performance. There are circumstances, however, in which the coactive effect might be disruptive to performance. When rivalry causes distraction and stress, it is better to practice separately. Even when the same subjects worked under both partitioned and social conditions, two different tasks yielded opposing outcomes in an experiment completed by Noble *et al.* (1958). With a discrimination reaction-time task, social competitive conditions stimulated greater increments in performance than did isolated practice. Behavior did not change, on the other hand, with a pursuit rotor task practiced under both social and nonsocial conditions. Perhaps unique task demands interacted with the experimental treatments to produce these results.

In the case where learners are ultimately to perform in a team context, it is preferable for them to experience group interactions as much as possible. A small proportion of the total variance on a group performance task can be predicted from individual performance on a similar kind of task (Comrey and Deskin, 1954a,b). Using the Purdue Pegboard Assembly Task, these investigators observed that individual skill alone cannot predict success in a group task. Additional variables must be considered. Other research (Kidd, 1961; Comrey, 1953) supports this concept. It was found in the latter experiment that less than half of the group performance variance could be predicted from a knowledge of an individual's performance. A logical question may well be, Why pair up people on the basis of individual ability if group performance is not dependent on individual scores?

Apparently, it is most desirable to practice under conditions most nearly like the actual situation. Wiest *et al.* (1961) concluded that team performance was less than the sum of individual performances. The greater the likeness of two members of the team in individual proficiency, the greater the probability for team success. At any rate, when transferring learned materials or skills to the actual situation, it is probably best to learn under conditions similar to those in which the application will be made.

B. Size of Group

In some cases, larger teams lead to more effective outcomes; in other cases, the opposite holds true. With small numbers, an increase in size is not only tolerable but perhaps desirable. When individual, dyad, and quad performance on a motor task was compared by Weyner and Zeaman (1956), it was found that the larger the team, the better the performance. But the mere increase in numbers on the team may not be the solution. With increases in the size of the group beyond four, decisions are more difficult to make, ingroups or cliques are formed, the atmosphere is less intimate, and the degree of satisfaction is reduced (Berelson and Steiner, 1964). For any given task there is probably an ideal number of members that should interact. A limited number of individuals provides an increased available resource input for the group, but too many restrict the means of communication.

C. Nature of the Task

Social facilitation is more likely to occur when the task at hand is familiar and reasonably well learned. Whether the social situation be that of an audience viewing an individual's behavior or a unit actively functioning, Zajonc's (1965) theory of the social facilitaton of the performance of well-learned responses and impairment of newly introduced responses appears plausible. Audience presence will be discussed later, so let us review coaction effects here.

A classic early study illustrates how the nature of the task interacts with solo and team performances. Allport (1920) introduced a variety of cognitive tasks to subjects, who attempted to solve them either alone or in groups. Loners performed more successfully than team members on a problem-solving test that required new responses. Team members were more effective with familiar tasks involving multiplication and word association. Perhaps novel tasks learned in a team context encourage the "pooling of ignorance," in addition to the stress (social presence and interaction) factor, which tends to elicit the dominant responses, the incorrect ones.

A team is function oriented and, as such, a high level of proficiency must be reached by the team in order to function capably. Thus, it pays to look at the functions of the group. Naylor and Briggs (1965) have suggested that tasks may be analyzed according to complexity and organization. Task complexity refers to memory demands placed on the learner, and task organization indicates the way the task components are interrelated. From the results of their data analysis, Naylor and Briggs concluded that highly organized tasks that require interaction and communication among members are best learned with team training. When the subtasks are hard, individual training is favored. Naylor and Briggs suggested that their task, a radar-controlled aerial intercept task, was of moderate or low organization and of medium or high complexity, favoring individual rather than team-cooperative activities. Briggs and Naylor (1965) have proposed that

> . . . the subject has a given capacity for information processing; if working independently, he can devote the entire capacity to the direct demands of the task; but if allowed, encouraged, or required to interact with another subject, he must divide this capacity between the task and the inter-person-interaction requirements, that is, interaction per se is a time- and capacity-consuming function which can detract from exclusively task-oriented behavior (p. 391).

Extending the argument, team performance is a function of task structure, work structure, and communication structure (Naylor and Dickinson, 1969). Teams must master task complexity (individual cue-criterion relationships) before they can handle task organization (complex subskill interaction relationships).

In summary, there are a number of tasks that are handled best when individual strengths are totaled, as in a unit. Activities that are not too complicated and unfamiliar, which by their very nature enable learners to produce better performance from knowledge sharing and social motivation and reinforcements, are examples. On the other hand, there are tasks that do not favor group participation over work in isolation. Jones and Gerard (1967, p. 640) warn:

> At least in some group contexts creativity may be stifled by certain fears of derision for deviance, and the group solution may reflect the lowest common denominator of talent. There are also tasks in which the component jobs are so interrelated that the failure of one person disrupts the performance of everyone else.

We would all welcome, as Jones and Gerard wistfully speculate, a detailed classification system with guidelines for the best combinations of social situations with learning tasks.

IV. Group Influences

A. Group-Task Motivation

The effectiveness of the individual in a group is obviously dependent on such variables as (a) cooperative striving, (b) satisfactory competitive–cooperative arrangements and outcomes, and (c) personal responsibility. The group can increase individual efforts, but only when the above-mentioned factors as well as the nature of the task are considered. A number of these problems have been reviewed in previous sections of this chapter. In any event, a well-defined, logical unit, formed in a meaningful way, can demonstrate social facilitative effects on the individuals in many activities. Motivation for productivity and learning, as well as reinforcement in a social context, occur in real-life situations as well as in contrived experimental settings. Cooperation among members of the group is advanced under a favorable and fair reward system for all. Personal goals as well as group goals, when perceived as being furthered, promote a more favorable work climate.

The group tends to influence individual behavior in the direction of conformity. Schonbar (1945) noticed that individual judgments in perceiving certain visual stimuli were modified to some degree in the group. The social norm is strongly influential in the way individuals establish personal standards and references. In other words, individuality is lost to a considerable extent within the context of group behavior. The consequences of such interactions should be weighed according to expectations placed on individuals and the group in any given situation.

B. Hawthorne Studies

The interesting results of a series of studies, begun in 1927 and terminated 12 years later (Roethlisberger and Dickson, 1939), have often been referred to by those concerned with various aspects of work production, management–worker relationships, environmental conditions surrounding performance, and experimental design. The effects of changes in illumination, temperature, rest periods, wage rates, and such on the productivity of workers were studied. The findings of this research have been summarized in Chapter 1. Essentially the data revealed the ironical finding that production increased regardless of the manipulation employed. Many interpretations were offered to explain the unusual results.

An acceptable analysis of the increased output lies in the social aspects of the situation. The subjects became closer and friendlier due to the prolonged experimentation. Their attitudes toward the company, their work, and their observer improved when they were being measured. They were apparently honored to be part of the study. The change in attitudes and increased cohesiveness of the group inspired greater work productivity. Hanson (1967) has demonstrated the "Hawthorne effect" in the performance of physical skills. A summarization of a series of three studies led to the following conclusions. (a) Subjects experiencing a group-centered approach displayed a greater improvement in endurance training than subjects experiencing an individualized-centered approach; (b) a placebo administered following a pretest and after no physical practice for 6 weeks resulted in a significant improvement in posttest endurance; and (c) bench-stepping endurance was increased due to the psychological effect of a placebo. The subject's attitude toward his "treatment" evidently has an impact on his performance, even though the treatment itself may be of no value. Social situations may facilitate group productivity when the individuals' perceptions are psychologically modified by the way working conditions are arranged.

C. Interpersonal Relationships

Groups have been described and analyzed according to various criteria, e.g., intimacy, homogeneity, hedonic tone, individual autonomy, stratification, permeability, goal orientation (polarization), cohesiveness, and participation (Gagné and Fleishman, 1959). According to the authors, social structure and group characteristics affect individual behavior. Space does not permit an appraisal of these factors and their influence on group behavior. Suffice it to mention them in passing and to realize that the way the group interacts and communicates is in part the function of the leader, instructor, or teacher. A homogeneous group, characterized by a common expression of unity, may exceed a group without cohesion in performance, although an exception to this belief has been reported by Cratty and Sage (1964). In learning a large maze task, a secondary group (no deliberate attempt at group cohesiveness) was superior to a primary group (presumably cohesive). The findings, however, may be unique to the conditions of this experiment and the methods employed by the respective groups to solve the problem of learning how to quickly transverse the maze pathway.

D. Morale

The spirit emanating from a desire to cooperate for a common goal and a feeling of togetherness express the meaning of morale. The presence of morale within a team or group indicates a social-motivating influence to achieve individually as well as for the good of the unit. Morale is constantly referred to in sports, the military, and industry and its importance stressed within the group structure. High morale results from the possible interaction of a number of variables, namely, group cohesiveness, payoffs, communication and interaction among group members and the leadership, effective leadership, and a common group goal. Surely the difficulty in describing and analyzing the precise nature of morale does not preclude the commonsense observation of its importance to group success.

E. Leadership

Depending on the structure of the group, leadership may not be pronounced or obvious, as, for example, in small units; it may be self-imposed, a natural outgrowth, or democratically determined; it may be autocratic in nature or democratic in approach. Without a doubt, a larger group requires some form of leadership and, in turn, as the size increases, the leadership role becomes more difficult and demanding and the leader is more isolated from the group. Leadership is task specific. Effective direction of a particular group under certain conditions is no assurance that similar success will prevail in other circumstances. Thus, effective leadership can be evaluated only within the restrictions of the given situation and the results derived. There is no one set of personal characteristics that best describes all leaders. But regardless of the conditions, the leader plays the role of a social facilitator; his presence and actions are meant to stimulate individual and group efforts.

V. Personal Factors

A. Social Class

Since a cohesive group is more apt to effectively fulfill its charges, it is important that we continue to examine those factors leading to group cooperation. Leadership, morale, motivation, interpersonal relationships, and common goals have previously been discussed. Now let us turn in the direction of social class or status. Evidence indicates that many functions are carried out within particular social strata. Although the trend is changing to more flexibility and less conformity, it will do well to keep in mind that Jenson and Kirchner (1955) found that 71% of the sons of fathers in occupations of a manual nature entered similar positions. With regard to nonmanual occupations, the father–son relationship was 63%. Furthermore, people tend to have characteristic attitudes, values, and identifications associated with certain social classes. Thus, the group social facilitative effect in individual physical performance may be lessened (at least at first) when there are representatives of social classes far apart. If interpersonal relationships are lowered and levels of aspiration widely divergent within the group due to class differences, group functioning is impaired. One solution is to attain group homogeneity in social status. Another solution is the recognition of intragroup problems that might exist when class heterogeneity is present, and to resolve conflicts.

B. Family

The Jenson and Kirchner study revealed mobility attitudes and possibilities related to family occupational status. In sports, Gedda *et al.* (1964) have shown that family members of Olympic athletes tend to engage in similar activities. Inheritance and the environmental conditions of the home influence attitudes toward various activities and possible success in them. Cratty (1960) has reported high relationships between father and son in physical performances when both were freshmen in college. If one were to analyze the backgrounds of champion oarsmen in England in the 19th century, he would notice the tendency for one family to dominate this event. The family exerts a powerful influence in shaping activity interests and individual drive for accomplishment. As such, it should be recognized for its role as a social mediator in its own way. Even family size and birth order are variables in determining pusuits of the individual members. For example, first born and secondborn children in the same family display different characteristics, even to the extent of sport interests (Nisbett, 1968).

C. Cultural Influences

Countries differ in the values they emphasize for their respective citizenry. This point is quite apparent in sport and physical training. Thus, popular sports vary from one country to another or even from one community to another. Respect for physical fitness and discipline can also be shown to vary according to the cultural influence. Members of a particular society tend to instill in other members an attitude to behave in a common way, in an accepted way. We are "shaped" by our culture in every way by the recognition of status symbols, reward systems, authority structure, child-rearing practices, and the like. The society and its structure encourage certain behaviors, discourage others. Although many of us like to think in terms of freedom of choice and independence, the fact is that it is quite difficult to conceive of any individual whose behavior has not been molded by social pressures, obvious or subtle.

D. Personality

One's characteristic way of behaving, often referred to as his personality, is related to his ability to influence or be influenced by group actions. Those concerned with social facilitation will want to go beyond generalizations concerning cooperative, competitive, and audience-presence effects. Vroom (1959) warned of the dangers in not considering the interaction between participation and personality when studying group behavior. Certainly individuals placed in competitive or cooperative situations will show the complex relationship between skill level, anxiety level, and induced stress. A person may feel the stress of the social situation surrounding the learning of a skill. Research findings suggest that facilitating or depressing effects depend on the proficiency level of the performer (the higher the skill, the more beneficial should be the stress induced from the social climate). High-anxiety people may be hurt more by the social circumstances, especially with complex acts, in the early stages of acquisition. Social facilitation does not operate independently of the participants' personalities, for the ability to cope wth stress, or indeed to be motivated to higher performance, is an individual matter.

VI. Audience Effect

The effects of coaction, whereby individuals actively participate in the same activity, and audience effects, as represented by a situation in which one performs in the presence of others, are the two major classifications in social facilitation research. The effect of spectators on human performance is a natural area of interest for those concerned with athletics and the performing arts. Verbal presentations in front of groups occur in many situations as well. Since one may perform in a different manner when alone as compared to when in the presence of others, it is of theoretical and practical concern to determine how and in what predictable ways behavior is altered under these contrasting conditions.

If one wishes to specify relationships even further, the nature of the audience, i.e., its size, gender arrangement, proximity to the subject, and degree of passivity, should be examined. Furthermore, the type of task, skill level, and personality of the performer might also be considered as they interact with audience effects. May and Doob (1937) warned that the different effects from social facilitation situations are dependent on whether others are "competitors, cooperators, on-lookers, 'rooters,' 'bystanders,' etc., or are physically present or psychologically present, or when they have certain predetermined attitudinal relations to the subjects of the experiments" (p. 34).

A. Passive Audience

The term "passive audience" connotes a group not directly participating in the activity with the subject and, even more, perhaps abstaining from motion or sound. In reality, spectators are vocal continuously at many athletic events. They are noticeably controlled except at appropriate times at gymnastic, dance, bowling, diving, and golf events. Experimental situations that afford the researcher the luxury of control and manipulation of subjects and events can thus be devised with active or completely passive spectators. Unfortunately, difficulty arises when a "realistic," active audience is desired in a particular study.

Such was the case in one study (Singer, 1965) in which athletes and nonathletes were to perform a gross motor task in front of a small group of spectators. Although an audience that would respond in a "natural" open way to each subject during his performance was intended, exploratory work revealed experimental weaknesses associated with such an approach. The six spectators responded too dissimilarly from subject to subject. Hence, this would probably facilitate performance in some subjects and impede performance in others. It was decided that a completely passive audience would yield the necessary control for the investigation. Other researchers, no doubt noticing similar problems, have resorted to the same type of audience control in their experimentation. Little wonder, then, that the majority of reports (and there are not many) dealing with audience effects on individual performance contain passive viewers.

In an early article, Travis (1925) produced data to confirm the hypothesis that an audience would help to improve an individual's performance. The motor task required tracking with a rotary pursuit apparatus. The subject first learned the task to some degree of proficiency while practicing alone. When the subjects were confronted with a small number of quiet spectators, their performance levels were raised. In addition, Abel (1938) used a simple maze test, Gurnee (1937) a large visual maze, and Dashiell (1930) such tasks as word association and simple multiplication, and all three reported improved performance as a result of the presence of others. Hollingsworth (1935) stated that working in front of an audience yields a greater output of work, especially if it involves muscular performance. With the purpose of determining the effect of different conditions of peer-group observation on physical performance tests, Chevrette (1968) administered a shuttle run, grip strength test, and vertical hang to fourth graders (a) unobserved, (b) in front of members of the same sex, (c) in front of members of the opposite sex, and (d) in front of a mixed group. The girls were unaffected by the experimental treatments. The peer motivating conditions were noticeable with the boys, but only with the shuttle run test. Perhaps motivation was optimally high for the subjects performing the tasks and the respective treatments generally could not elevate performance any further.

Some of the early research, on the other hand (e.g., Pessin and Husband, 1933; Pessin, 1933), indicates an inhibiting and disturbing effect of spectators on individual performance. Most of the early evidence, however, supports the notion of a positive effect of an audience, certainly when the task involves motor and muscular components. Zajonc (1965) has attempted to theoretically resolve conflicting findings in audience effects on performance, and his position will be discussed shortly. More recent experimentation has raised more questions and controversy, but these as well as Zajonc's theory in handling some of these discrepancies will also appear. First let us turn to evidence concerning active audiences.

B. Active Audience

As was pointed out, responsive spectators are typically not incorporated in the design of experiments. Sport situations reveal to us that, when examined on a subjective basis, emotional spectators tend to upset some performers, elevate the output of others, and apparently have no influence on still other athletes. The nature and magnitude of the audience reactions could also be a factor in performance. Why else do crowds yell in support of the home team and hysterically boo the opponent? Unfortunately, the predictable result of this interaction has not yet been determined through experimentation.

One attempt at utilizing a reacting audience was presented by Laird (1923). Four motor tests (tapping, the 3-Hole Test, and hand steadiness —standing and sitting) were administered by fraternity pledges. The first time the audience remained quiet; the second time they razzed each subject before he took the tests. Razzing impaired performance. When Gates (1924) tested the effect of an encouraging audience on the performance of tasks, only a slightly favorable difference was observed. Obviously, it is quite hazardous to extrapolate from these few investigations to predictable outcomes in similar situations in which physical performance occurs in competition in more realistic settings.

An audience can provide the necessary stress for motivating or worsening performances. It can also reinforce the actions of the individual. The effects on verbal behavior of positive reinforcement (praise, reward) versus negative reinforcement (criticism, punishment) have been studied by researchers for a long time. But, as Roberts and Martens (1970) observed, research dealing with these effects on complex motor behavior is almost nonexistent. They formed groups of college-aged subjects to receive one or four treatments in learning a motor task involving timing: positive social reinforcement; negative social reinforcement; nonreinforcement; and a control. All groups improved their performances with practice, but unexpectedly, no differences were found among the groups. One might assume from other research and theory that some form of reinforcement would be more effective than none at all and that positive reinforcement influences performance more than negative reinforcement. Certain experimental limitations, such as the lack of knowledge the subjects had of the respective reinforcement contingencies, may help to explain the findings of Roberts and Martens.

C. Cheerleaders

Nowhere is the belief in active verbal support for performers better represented than by cheerleaders in athletics. Presumably, their actions stimulate the crowd, which in turn positively influences the contestants. If "the bodily presence of another individual is a stimulus to the performer as an inspiration to greater effort" (Triplett, 1897, p. 516), then active encouragement by many people may be thought to help much more.

Continuing this conjecture, Herkimer (1967) has written of the importance of proper and appropriate cheers timed at different points of the contest. He believes that games have been won or lost due to the good or poor efforts of the cheerleaders. Unfortunately, Herkimer does not document that statement. Nor does he support the statement that "the players report that they many times give a better effort when the crowd is cheering for them" (p. 729). Nonetheless, it may be true, as he has written, that there is a psychological advantage for the players if spectators are cheering for them.

An early study by Ayres (1911) does support the use of an active band for stimulating spectators and athletic performance, at least in a bicycle race. Twenty-three miles (one-half of the 6-day bicycle race) were ridden while the band played. During this period, the miles ridden averaged 17 seconds faster than miles ridden without the band. Ayres observed the apparent effect the band music had on the spectators and speculated that their overt responses in turn encouraged the bicycle riders to higher levels of performance.

D. Skill Level

It would be wise at this point to examine the problem of audience effects on performance in more detail. One variable that must be reckoned with is the level of proficiency of the individual when he confronts an audience. It is conceivable that the effects are not the same on novice learners as on highly proficient performers. Zajonc (1965) supports the view that one might expect different outcomes depending on the learner's skill level.

When the dominant responses in the repertoire of responses are correct ones, as is the case with the skilled performer, the presence of an audience should be of benefit to the individual. Conversely, if the dominant responses are incorrect ones (exemplified early in learning), the audience effect should be detrimental. In other words, dominant responses tend to be activated and emitted under stress—the audience presence—thereby influencing the quality of the response. In practical terms one should expect the performance of outstanding athletes with spectator presence not to be impaired but probably enhanced. The learning process is negatively affected but performance, once high levels of proficiency are reached, is facilitated.

Does the research support these contentions? Marten's (1969a) data suggest that a well-learned motor task is performed better in the presence than in the absence of the audience. When the subjects were learning the task, the audience caused them to make more errors, to be less consistent, and to take more time to learn than subjects learning in isolation. These results were confirmed to some degree in another study by Martens (1969b). Other recent research in verbal learning situations tends to support such findings and Zajonc's theory.

Contrary to expectations, Singer's (1970) findings indicated that the presence or absence of spectators had no noticeable effect on early stages of learning as contrasted with later stages of performance. Four groups of college subjects were tested on a mirror-reversal star-tracing task on two occasions under the following conditions: spectators–no spectators,

spectators–spectators, no spectators–no spectators, no spectators–spectators. When conditions remained the same between the two test conditions, fewer errors were made. Speed was generally increased under altered task conditions. Although isolated studies like this one tend to refute Zajonc's predictions, the brunt of the evidence supports his proposal.

Taken at face value, then, the research might be interpreted in practical terms in the following simplified version. Learn a complex motor task under alone conditions and, when a reasonable level of achievement is attained, the individual is ready to stand the stress of an audience. He should not only bear it, but perform better as a result of it.

Are athletes, individuals who are accustomed to performing in front of spectators, better able than nonathletes to demonstrate a resistance to spectators when learning new tasks? In other words, can we expect athletes in general to react more effectively than nonathletes under stressful (audience-presence) conditions? Using 16 athletes and 16 nonathletes selected at Ohio State University, Singer (1965) had each subject receive 10 trials on the stabilometer (balance platform) in isolation. The next day, each subject was administered three more trials in which performances were recorded in front of a six-person audience. Unexpectedly, nonathletes performed at a greater level of skill in the presence of the audience than did athletes. Why did athletes fail to perform the motor task well in front of people even though they had successfully executed other motor (athletic) skills before crowds on many previous occasions? Possibly athletes are more sensitive than nonathletes to people watching them perform and feel uncomfortable demonstrating before a group a skill at which they are not extremely competent.

E. Anxiety Level

Performers react to a situation in accordance with their respective personalities. One aspect of personality that has been measured as it interacts with audience effects on performance is anxiety. Essentially, the question asked has been, Will highly anxious individuals perform differently than lower-anxious ones in front of an audience? Abel (1938) implied that the "more high-strung individuals are overstimulated with consequent decrease (in efficiency) in the group performance" (p. 379). If we can assume that the presence of others provides stress to the learner, its presence may also affect highly anxious and lowly anxious people in a differential manner, being more disruptive to anxious persons.

Confirmation of this hypothesis has come from Cox and Ganzer. Using a marble-dropping task, Cox (1966) determined the effect of mothers, teachers, peers, and strangers on the performance of primary grade children. Low-anxious boys displayed better performances during spectator presence, while the high-anxious boys were poorer in the presence of their mothers or teachers. With only the experimenter present, the low-anxious boys showed a response decrement; high-anxious boys improved. Ganzer (1968) found that spectator presence was detrimental to high-anxious female college students learning a list of nonsense syllables but not so for low-anxious subjects. Contradictory data by Martens (1969a) and Roberts and Martens (1970) suggest no interaction between anxiety level and performance in front of an audience. The performance of high-anxious subjects was superior to that of low-anxious subjects in both studies of coincident timing.

Several questions are therefore posed. Will different kinds of tasks, e.g., motor or verbal, difficult or simple, interact differently with anxiety level and audience presence? Does the sex and/or age of the performer make a difference? Finally, can anxiety be appropriately measured? Tests have been designed to measure general or specific states of anxiety, and researchers use different tests in their research depending on their preference. Problems like these create difficulties in interpreting research and making generalizations from findings.

F. Task Difficulty

When individuals are in a learning situation, task difficulty can be evaluated in terms of (a) its acknowledged complexity or simplicity to most subjects or (b) its meaningfulness and familiarity to the subjects. In either case, Zajonc's (1965) social facilitation theory provides an interesting framework to handle research findings that appear to conflict with each other on the effect of audience presence on performance. A complex task or a nonfamiliar, unusual one, represented by maze learning or nonsense-syllable learning, is apt to elicit from the performer many more wrong responses than right ones in the early stages of training as compared to a simple task or a familiar task. Zajonc has written that "audience enhances the emission of dominant responses" (p. 270). If the correct responses are dominant, spectators will benefit the performer, while social presence will harm the performance of an individual when incorrect responses are dominant.

G. Integrating the Variables

The situation appears quite confusing, for so many factors may influence social facilitation. An attempt will be made here to integrate the material presented and apply it to physical skill performance.

Simple tasks demanding physical energy, repetition, power, strength, or endurance are probably benefited by social presence. An audience motivates the person and stimulates his motor behavior. However, motor skills requiring complex coordination, finely executed movements, and intense concentration may easily be impaired by the presence of observers until they are well learned. The demonstration of any skill, once developed to a high degree of proficiency, should be favorably affected by an audience. Certainly, skilled behavior is not expected to be disrupted by the presence of spectators.

The more reactive audience adds to the possible effect on an individual's performance. Assuming its reinforcing and motivating properties, the audience should raise the drive level of the person. Dominant responses, right or wrong, probably tend to be emitted even more when an active audience, rather than a passive audience, is on the scene. Contrary to expectation, the best-skilled athletes in various sports are infrequently affected by crowd behavior. Their performances are relatively stable, consistent, and predictable. They have learned how to perform effectively under all kinds of favorable and nonfavorable conditions. That is why they are labeled "skilled."

For the average person, working in a motivated state is necessary for a reasonable performance yield. Every task requires that an ideal level of motivation be expressed by the learner. When the highest level of motivation is operating, audience presence can overstimulate and impair muscular coordination. The highly skilled athlete is able to control his emotions in front of spectators so that they work in a favorable way in his behavior. What of the athlete who does well in practice but cannot match his performance during the contest?

This problem was recognized by Triplett (1897). "It is a well known fact that some athletes, who in private can perform excellently, fail to distinguish themselves when the actual contest is run in the presence of the public. The weakening effect of nervous agitation has been ascribed as the cause" (p. 530). If skill is defined as the ability to execute proper spatially and temporally timed responses to appropriate cues under varying environmental conditions, the "practice athlete" is obviously not highly skilled. He must learn to perform in front of spectators. Experience and emotional adjustments are the necessary remediation.

Social presence may be distracting as well as motivating but inevitably produces some effect on behavior. We must not forget that the performer places himself in a position of evaluation and appraisal when he demonstrates in front of spectators (Jones and Gerard, 1967). The attitudes and anxieties of the performer to being critically observed indicate sensitivity to the situation. Familiar and friendly audiences tend to make the average individual more comfortable, while unknown and even unseen audiences can have a deleterious effect on performance (Wapner and Alper, 1952). If the subject is self-conscious, he is more likely to suffer under social-presence conditions. The gymnast who is concerned as to how he appears to the spectators viewing the contest is more likely to score more poorly than another gymnast who concentrates on his executions and form.

Zajonc (1965) simplified the research on social facilitation with a bit of wit in saying that "he would advise the student to study all alone, preferably in an isolated cubicle, and to arrange to take his examinations in the company of many other students, on stage, and in the presence of a large audience. The results of his examination would be beyond his wildest expectations, provided, of course, he had learned his material quite thoroughly" (p. 274). However, in fact, "a theoretical understanding of audience effects will ultimately require detailed analysis of the many varieties of tasks, performers, audiences, and observation settings that may be involved" (Jones and Gerard, 1967, p. 608).

H. Summary

The concept of social facilitation includes many and varied social parameters surrounding behavior. Competitive and cooperative ventures have been compared with each other and against solitary conditions, revealing their positive effects on performance. Further analysis of the cooperative situations indicates the positive effect of coactors on output. Research and theory suggest that the audience effect on performance is detrimental in the early going but facilitating when the individual is operating at a high level of skill. Beyond these general statements, consideration should be given to, and possible exceptions may arise from, the nature of the performer, e.g., his personality, the type of task, be it simple or complex, the skill level of the performer, and the characteristics of the group, coactors, or audience. Further investigations dealing with these and other variables will help to determine the general acceptance of social conditions as having facilitating effects on performance.

References

Abel, T. M. (1938). *Amer. J. Psychol.* **51**, 379.
Allee, W. C., and Masure, R. H. (1936). *Physiol. Zool.* **22**, 131.
Allport, F. H. (1920). *J. Exp. Psychol.* **3**, 159.
Ayres, L. P. (1911). *Amer. Phys. Educ. Rev.* **16**, 324.

Bayer, E. (1929). Z. *Psychol.* **112,** 1. Cited in Zajonc (1965).
Berelson, B., and Steiner, G. A. (1964). "Human Behavior: An Inventory of Scientific Findings." Harcourt, New York.
Blum, M., and Naylor, J. (1968). "Industrial Psychology." Harper, New York.
Briggs, G. E., and Naylor, J. C. (1965). *J. Appl. Psychol.* **49,** 387.
Bruning, J. L., Sommer, D. L., and Jones, W. R. (1966). *J. Soc. Psychol.* **68,** 369.
Chen, S. C. (1937). *Physiol. Zool.* **10,** 123.
Chevrette, J. M. (1968). *J. Psychol.* **70,** 113.
Coleman, J. S. (1961). "The Adolescent Society." Free Press, New York.
Comrey, A. L. (1953). *J. Appl. Psychol.* **37,** 207.
Comrey, A. L., and Deskin, G. (1954a). *J. Appl. Psychol.* **38,** 116.
Comrey, A. L., and Deskin, G. (1954b). *J. Appl. Psychol.* **38,** 178.
Cox, F. N. (1966). *J. Exp. Child Psychol.* **3,** 100.
Cratty, B. J. (1960). *Res. Quart.* **31,** 12.
Cratty, B. J. (1967). "Social Dimensions of Physical Activity." Prentice-Hall, Englewood Cliffs, New Jersey.
Cratty, B. J., and Sage, J. N. (1964). *Res. Quart.* **35,** 265.
Dashiell, J. F. (1930). *J. Abnorm. Soc. Psychol.* **25,** 190.
Gagné, R. M., and Fleishman, E. A. (1959). "Psychology and Human Performance." Holt, New York.
Ganzer, V. J. (1968). *J. Pers. Soc. Psychol.* **8,** 194.
Gates, G. (1924). *J. Abnorm. Soc. Psychol.* **18,** 334.
Gates, M. J., and Allee, W. C. (1933). *J. Comp. Psychol.* **15,** 331.
Gedda, L., Milani-Comparetti, M., and Brenei, G. (1964). *In* "International Research in Sport and Physical Education" (E. Jokl and E. Simon, eds.), pp. 693–698. Thomas, Springfield, Illinois.
Gurnee, H. (1937). *J. Psychol.* **3,** 437.
Hanson, D. (1967). *Res. Quart.* **38,** 723.
Harlow, H. F. (1932). *J. Genet. Psychol.* **43,** 211.
Herkimer, L. R. (1967). *In* "Motivation in Play, Sport and Games" (R. Slovenko and J. A. Knight, eds.), pp. 727–730. Thomas, Springfield, Illinois.
Hollingsworth, H. L. (1935). "The Psychology of the Audience." American, New York.
Jenson, P. G., and Kirchner, W. K. (1955). *J. Appl. Psychol.* **39,** 419.
Johnston, W. A. (1966). *J. Appl. Psychol.* **50,** 1966.
Jones, E. E., and Gerard, H. B. (1967). "Social Psychology." Wiley, New York.
Kidd, J. S. (1961). *J. Appl. Psychol.* **45,** 195.
Kretch, D., Crutchfield, R. S., and Livson, N. (1969). "Elements of Psychology." Knopf, New York.
Laird, D. A. (1923). *J. Exp. Psychol.* **6,** 236.
Maller, J. B. (1929). "Cooperation and Competition." Columbia Teachers College Contribution to Education, No. 384, New York.
Martens, R. (1969a). *J. Pers. Soc. Psychol.* **12,** 252.
Martens, R. (1969b). *Res. Quart.* **40,** 317.
Martens, R., and Landers, D. M. (1969). *J. Mot. Behav.* **1,** 1.
May, M. A., and Doob, L. W. (1937). "Competition and Cooperation." Social Science Research Council, New York.
Moore, J. W. (1970). "The Psychology of Athletic Coaching." Burgess, Minneapolis, Minnesota.
Myers, A. (1962). *J. Abnorm. Soc. Psychol.* **65,** 325.

Naylor, J. C., and Briggs, G. E. (1965). *J. Appl. Psychol.* **49,** 223.
Naylor, J. C., and Dickinson, T. L. (1969). *J. Appl. Psychol.* **53,** 167.
Nisbett, R. E. (1968). *J. Pers. Soc. Psychol.* **8,** 351.
Noble, C. E., Fuchs, J. E., Robel, D. P., and Chambers, R. W. (1958). *Percept. Mot. Skills* **8,** 131.
Pessin, J. (1933). *Amer. J. Psychol.* **45,** 263.
Pessin, J., and Husband, R. W. (1933). *J. Abnorm. Soc. Psychol.* **28,** 1933.
Roberts, G. C., and Martens, R. (1970). *Res. Quart.* **41,** 175.
Roethlisberger, F. J., and Dickson, W. J. (1939). "Management and the Worker." Harvard Univ. Press, Cambridge, Massachusetts.
Ryan, E. D., and Lakie, W. L. (1965). *J. Pers. Soc. Psychol.* **1,** 342.
Ryan, F. J. (1958a). *In* "Psychosocial Problems of College Men" (B. M. Wedge, ed.), pp. 113–122. Yale Univ. Press, New Haven, Connecticut.
Ryan, F. J. (1958b). *In* "Psychosocial Problems of College Men" (B. M. Wedge, ed.), pp. 123–139. Yale Univ. Press, New Haven, Connecticut.
Schonbar, R. A. (1945). *Arch. Psychol.* No. 299.
Singer, R. N. (1965). *Res. Quart.* **36,** 473.
Singer, R. N. (1970). *J. Mot. Behav.* **2,** 88.
Spence, J. A., and Spence, K. W. (1966). *In* "Anxiety and Behavior" (C. D. Spielberger, ed.), pp. 291–326. Academic Press, New York.
Strong, C. H. (1963). *Res. Quart.* **34,** 497.
Travis, L. E. (1925). *J. Abnorm. Soc. Psychol.* **20,** 142.
Triplett, N. (1897). *Amer. J. Psychol.* **9,** 507.
Voor, J. H., Lloyd, A. J., and Cole, R. J. (1969). *J. Mot. Behav.* **1,** 210.
Vroom, V. H. (1959). *J. Abnorm. Soc. Psychol.* **59,** 322.
Wapner, G., and Alper, T. G. (1952). *J. Abnorm. Soc. Psychol.* **47,** 222.
Weyner, N., and Zeaman, D. (1956). *J. Gen. Psychol.* **55,** 127.
Wiest, W. M., Porter, L. W., and Ghiselli, E. E. (1961). *J. Appl. Psychol.* **45,** 1961.
Zajonc, R. B. (1965). *Science* **149,** 269.
Zajonc, R. B. (1967). "Social Psychology: An Experimental Approach." Brooks-Cole, Belmont, California.

Part III

SUBSTANCES

Chapter 10

Water and Electrolytes

David L. Costill

I. Introduction

Water has seldom, if ever, been considered as an ergogenic aid to muscular performance. Despite the body of physiological information compiled on the subject of body fluids, athletic participants and industrial workers generally adhere to traditional habits in regulating both water and electrolyte (salt) intake. Recent commercial advertising has glamorized the role of fluid replacement and has hinted at the possible ergogenic value of ingesting an electrolyte solution. On the other hand, some athletic events seem to offer an advantage to participants who lose body weight by dehydration, thereby becoming eligible to compete against a smaller opponent. The purpose of the following discussion is to assess the ergogenic value of water and electrolyte administration and restriction. First, however, let us review the normal physiological responsibilities and regulatory mechanisms for water and electrolytes.

A. Physiological Importance of Water

Water is, by far, the most abundant component of the human body, constituting 45–75% of the body weight (Elkinton and Danowsky, 1955). This large fluid reservoir furnishes an environment that is essential to the survival of the body tissues. In addition to providing a medium to support the internal activities of the cell, body fluids play major roles in delivering nutrients from the external environment and eliminating metabolic by-products.

The outstanding functional divisions of body fluids are extracellular fluid and intracellular fluid, which are separated from one another by the aggregate of cell walls. Somewhat more than half of the total body water is contained inside the cells (intracellular fluids) and constitutes 30–40% of body weight (Pitts, 1963). In this state water supports the cell and many of its organelles (e.g., nucleus, mitochondria), contains dissolved organic and inorganic material (e.g., lipids, salts), and participates in hydrolysis.

Body fluids outside the cell are responsible for 20–25% of the total body weight (see Fig. 1). These extracellular fluids include blood plasma; interstitial fluid; transcellular fluid such as water in the gastrointestinal tract; small amounts of fluid in the serous cavity, joint spaces, and tendon sheaths; and cerebrospinal fluid. In terms of sustained muscular activity the water fraction of blood is responsible for transporting essential nutrients, metabolic heat, and muscle metabolites.

Unless affected by extraneous factors, the distribution and volume of intracellular and extracellular fluids remain surprisingly constant. However, such maintenance is not achieved without compensatory adjustments for body water increases and decreases. Water is constantly being lost from the body via urine, respiration, perspiration, and defecation. Under rest conditions, the normal urine volume varies from 30 to 60 ml/hour (Ladell, 1965; Robinson, 1954) but may decrease to 5 or 10 ml/hour during prolonged exertion and/or negative water balance (Costill *et al.*, 1970a, 1969). For a more detailed discussion of the kidney's role in water and electrolyte balance see Pitts (1963).

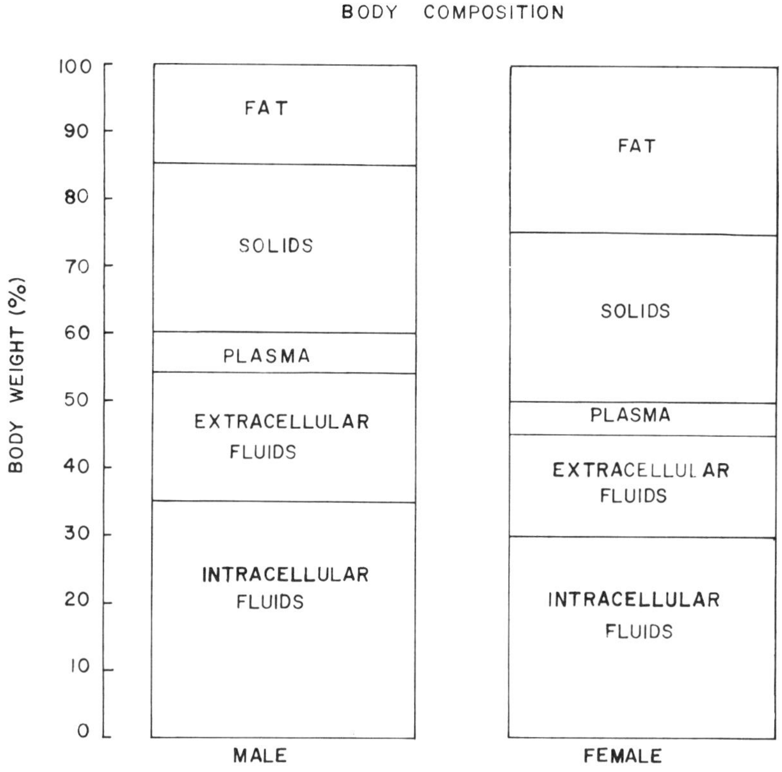

Fig. 1. Fractional components of body composition for men and women.

The average respiratory water loss, under normal conditions, is about 15 ml/hour and may exceed 130 ml/hour during heavy exercise (Pugh *et al.*, 1967). A distinction is commonly made between the body water evaporated from the respiratory tract and that from the skin. Furthermore, part of the cutaneous loss may not involve secretory activity of the sweat glands, since the epidermis itself is slightly permeable to water vapor. Human skin provides relatively poor protection against water loss in hot, dry environments. Adolph (1947) pointed out that even without the activity of the sweat glands men at rest may lose a liter of water by evaporation from respiratory and skin surfaces each day. With the greater thermal loads of muscular exertion and/or hot environments, the sweat glands are activated to facilitate body heat dissipation through evaporation. The sweat rate of heat-acclimatized men exercising under heat stress has been reported in excess of 1.8 liters/hour (Robinson, 1949; Pugh *et al.*, 1967) and may even exceed 10 kg (22 lb) in a 24-hour period.

Formed stools when the diet is normal account for about 100 ml of body fluid loss each day (Elkinton and Danowsky, 1955); when little water is consumed and the diet is dry, few feces are formed, with a total water loss of 10–20 gm every 2 or 3 days. In extreme water deprivation, as is often the case in "making weight" for wrestling, the bowels cease to work (McGee, 1906). On the other hand, water losses from the bowel may be great during diarrhea. Marriott (1950) has indicated that diarrhea water losses may reach 3 liters (6.6 lb) per day.

It is obvious from the foregoing discussion that the rate of water turnover is quite rapid in man. As demonstrated in Table I, body fluid losses are replaced by (a) metabolically produced water and (b) the intake of water, in both food and drink. Only small amounts of water are gained from chemically combusting endogenous fuels. In the moderately active individual, the total water produced in this manner probably does not exceed 300 gm/day. With the elevation of metabolism during exercise, water production has been estimated at 1.1 liters/hour among men who were metabolic exercising at 75% of their maximal oxygen uptake capacity (Kozlowski and Saltin, 1964).

The volume of ingested fluids and the frequency of ingestion are normally dictated by the sensation of thirst. Unlike some animals, man's thirst exhibits a time lag between fluid losses and the desire for replacement. When dehydrated by as much as 20.5 liters, the burro will ingest an equal volume of water in about 2.5 minutes (Schmidt-Nielsen, 1964; Dill, 1938; Bullard *et al.*, 1970). In contrast, Greenleaf and Sargent (1965) have reviewed the literature on voluntary dehydration and have concluded that man voluntarily maintains a water deficit of as much as 4% of his body weight for many hours after dehydration.

While body water losses are generally dictated by metabolic and environmental factors, under normally active conditions, water balance is effectively gauged by the sensation of thirst. Thirst, while slow in

TABLE I

NORMAL DAILY WATER EXCHANGE FOR MEN IN TEMPERATE CLIMATES

Water source	Water intake (ml)	Water release via:	Water output (ml)
Beverages	1200	Insensible perspiration	
Water of foods	1100	Lungs	700
Water of oxidation	300	Skin	300
		Sweat	100
		Feces	100
		Urine	1400
Total intake	2600	Total output	2600

responding to water deficits, is effective in maintaining man's total body water to within 1% of normal. Two theories have been advanced to explain the mechanism by which the thirst sensation is aroused. According to one view, thirst is due to the drying of the pharyngeal mucous membrane, the salivary glands being given a role in the regulation of the water balance of the body. When the water content of the body falls below a certain level, salivary secretion is depressed. The consequent drying of the mucous membrane of the throat then elicits the characteristic sensation. The second view suggests that thirst is a sensation resulting from changes in blood composition, probably due to a rise in its osmotic pressure, which stimulates the afferent nerve endings or perhaps acts on the central nervous system. Although the question of the thirst receptors is still under discussion, it is now generally agreed that there is a hypothalamic thirst center which controls the drive for water and is cholinergically controlled (Andersson, 1962; Stein and Seifter, 1962; Stein, 1963).

B. Physiological Importance of Electrolytes

By definition, electrolytes are substances that, when placed in water, dissociate into charged particles called ions. Those that are negatively charged are referred to as anions, while positively charged particles are cations. In each fluid compartment of the body, the total number of cations must always equal the number of anions. If this were not the case, the solution would be charged relative to its environment. During glandular secretion, muscular innervation, and the transmission of a nerve impulse, localized imbalances of ions may occur.

Simply because there are equal quantities of positively and negatively charged materials in a given biological fluid does not mean that all compartmental fluids have the same electrolyte compositions. To the contrary, intracellular (ICF) and extracellular (ECF) fluids are markedly different in terms of electrolyte content, as illustrated by Fig. 2. Sodium and chloride are the chief electrolytes of the ECF, while potassium is the main electrolyte constituent of the ICF. The predominant extracellular cation is the sodium ion, which makes up 90% of the total cations in the ECF. Because of its quantitative dominance and the fact that it is restricted from entering into the ICF, sodium plays a primary role in controlling the distribution of water throughout the body. The concentration of sodium in the serum is carefully controlled by nerve receptors in the hypothalamus that are sensitive to changes in tonicity (concentration) of the blood.

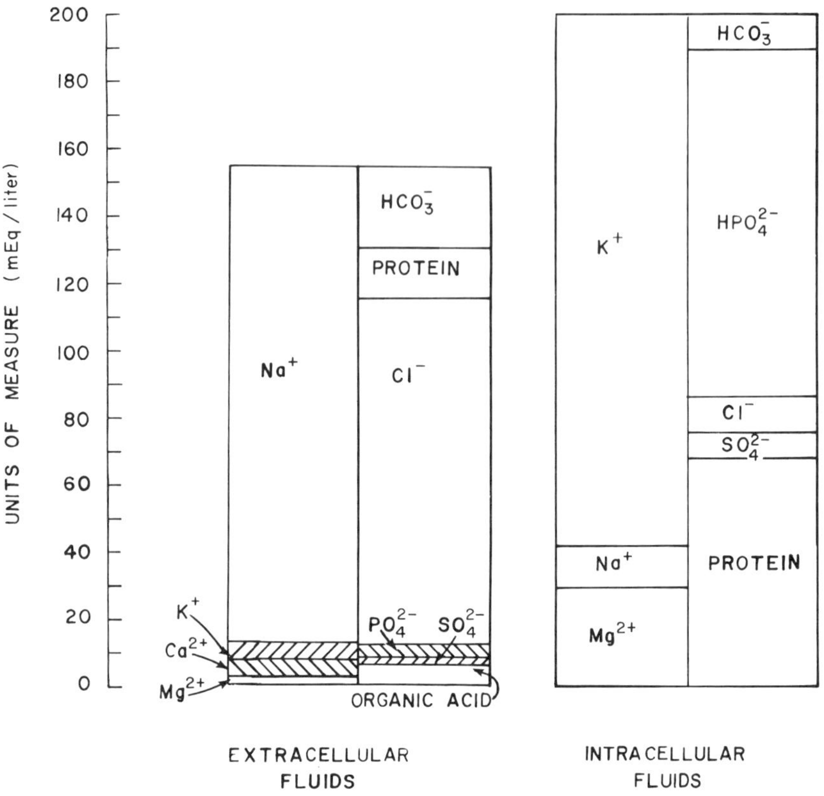

Fig. 2. Anion (negatively charged) and cation (positively charged) materials in extracellular and intracellular fluids.

Constancy of the concentration of the cations is important for three reasons. (a) The concentration of each cation, both individually and in relation to the others, has a marked influence on the activities of many vital tissues, including nerve conduction, neuromuscular irritability, energy metabolism, muscle contractility, cardiac conduction, bone growth, and the regulation of blood volume and renal function. (b) The sum of the concentrations of the cations determines the quantity of anions that can be kept in electrical neutrality at the pH of serum. (c) The sum of the cation concentrations is the determining factor in the total osmotic pressure of serum and interstitial fluids and, therefore, of intracellular fluids.

The differences in ionic concentrations across the cell membranes are derived from the active accumulation of certain ions within the cells and the active extrusion of others from the cells. Cells are, therefore, effectively but not actually impermeable to ions. The mechanism that extrudes sodium from cells and accumulates potassium within cells is called an "ion pump" (Pitts, 1963) and has been discussed in some detail by Guyton (1961).

Since the cell membrane is semipermeable, any imbalance in the nondiffusible molecules of the ECF or ICF elicits an osmotic pressure, causing water to pass through the membrane toward the side with the greater concentration. This phenomenon is called osmosis. As an example, if water is removed from the ECF, the remaining nondiffusible materials become more concentrated, thereby inducing an osmotic imbalance. As a result, osmosis of water begins immediately from the ICF to the ECF, diluting the ECF while concentrating the ICF. When the ECF becomes sufficiently diluted to equal the concentration of the ICF, further osmosis occurs so rapidly that any lack of osmostic equilibrium between the two fluid compartments is usually corrected within seconds and at most within a minute or more.

In order to balance the electrolytes lost with sweat, urine, and water from the gut, man normally ingests salt as a natural component of his food and partly from added seasoning. In normally active men, salt balance may be maintained with a daily salt intake of less than 17 mEq (Elkinton and Danowsky, 1955).

During prolonged exertion and exposure to hot environments sweating may account for a sizable loss of electrolytes. Unlike other body fluids, sweat contains relatively minor quantities of electrolytes. This means that, while large volumes of body water are lost, the body's total electrolyte content is reduced by a much smaller degree. It is not suprising, therefore, to observe elevated concentrations of serum electrolytes following severe dehyration, as a result of hemoconcentration.

The concentration of serum sodium is maintained relatively constant through the involvement of two hormones, aldosterone and the antidiuretic hormone (ADH), in the reabsorption and excretion of sodium and water from the renal tubules. A drop in blood volume is usually followed by increased adrenal secretion of aldosterone, which, by causing increased renal tubular reabsorption of sodium, promotes a restoration of the blood volume. Thus, the effect of ECF sodium on aldosterone is seen as an indirect effect by way of blood volume changes.

The ADH plays a very important role in the renal control of water loss. In a condition of dehydration, the osmolality of the blood is increased, the osmoreceptors in the hypothalamus are stimulated, ADH is released from the posterior pituitary, and water is reabsorbed by the collecting tubules of the kidney. Conversely, when a normally hydrated individual ingests a large volume of water,. the dilution of blood so produced reduces the release of ADH. Water reabsorption in the collecting tubules abates, and a more dilute urine is produced.

C. Water, Electrolytes, and Acid–Base Balance

So far in our discussion, we have considered the distribution of body water in its compartments and the forces involved in maintaining constant the volume and composition of these compartments. However, one of the major responsibilities of the body fluids during muscular effort must be the maintenance of an acid–base balance.

According to the Brønsted schema (Brønsted, 1923; Kaufman and Rosen, 1956) an acid is a molecular or ionic substance that yields protons or H^+, while a base is a substance or ion that combines readily with H^+. The plasma buffer anions HCO_3^- (bicarbonate) and protein ions are regarded as strong bases. Thus, when bicarbonates are exposed to the metabolically produced hydrogen ions (H^+) a weak acid is formed, H_2CO_3. The formation of HCO_3^- at the lungs and kidney plays a vital role in maintaining the pH of plasma at 7.4. At a pH of 7.4 the plasma has 1 part of CO_2 in free solution for 20 parts in the form of bicarbonate. Since the normal plasma bicarbonate concentration is about 27 mEq/liter, 1.35 mEq of CO_2 is in free solution for each liter of plasma. In order to maintain the pH of plasma at 7.4, the ratio between bicarbonate and free CO_2 must remain 20:1.

The bicarbonate buffer is the pivotal point for control of the acid–base balance of the plasma and interstitial fluids. With any accumulation of metabolic acids—through ingestion, overproduction or under-excretion by the kidney—the plasma bicarbonate and pH are lowered. On the other hand, plasma bicarbonate content can be made greater than normal by loss of acid or by increased ingestion of alkalis. Disturbances of acid–base control can also occur by a primary decrease or increase in the pulmonary excretion of CO_2, that is, by changes in the concentration of free CO_2 in the plasma. The plasma pH will remain within normal limits only if compensatory adjustments can be made in the ratio of CO_2 to HCO_3^-. If, for example, the bicarbonate level falls to 18 mEq/liter, compensation by hyperventilation can bring pH to normal.

Since the bicarbonate of plasma is negatively charged, it is only fitting to consider the interaction of acid–base and anion–cation balance. Alterations in the ratio of sodium to chloride can have a marked effect on the availability of bicarbonate and can therefore influence the plasma pH. In clinically observed dehydration, a relative decrease of chloride (Cl^-) permits a large expansion of plasma bicarbonate, thereby inducing a critical state of alkalosis (Hoffman, 1970). Conversely, if a relative excess of chloride is present in plasma, the anion–cation balance is readily established by reducing the available bicarbonate concentration at the expense of producing an acid plasma. Therefore, the composition of fluids used in dehydration therapy must be designed to maintain the plasma in a proportional electrolyte balance.

II. The Effects of Dehydration on Muscular Performance

It is readily apparent that some athletic events grant a performance advantage to participants who reduce their body weight via voluntary dehydration. Athletes involved in 150-lb football, light-weight crew, wrestling, and boxing frequently "make weight" by acute body water losses. Sweat losses stimulated by exercise and environmental heat stress constitute the principal methods for depleting the body fluids, thereby lowering body weight.

This practice has received heavy criticism from medical and health authorities. Certainly coaches and athletes unite in their dislike of this process, but they are compelled to utilize it in order to insure equal advantage in height, weight, reach, strength, and leverage. Excessive weight reduction has been one of the chief targets of criticism toward amateur wrestling and has been cited frequently as an effective argument against the introduction of the sport into the scholastic athletic program.

Despite the extensive volume of research that has been amassed on this topic, the ergogenic value of voluntary dehydration is equivocal. The purpose of the following discussion is to review the effects of dehydration in terms of physiological responses and the performance of selected motor skills.

A. Physiological Responses

During muscular activities lasting more than a few minutes, the circulatory systems plays a crucial role in transporting nutrients to the active tissues, removing metabolic waste materials, and transporting heat from the active tissues to the body surface, where it can be dissipated. Any reduction in the extracellular fluids with dehydration might be expected, therefore, to impair the circulatory system's ability to perform these essential tasks.

Studies by Kozlowski and Saltin (1964) have demonstrated that the circulatory system's responses to dehydration are dependent on the methods utilized to promote heavy sweating. It was found that sweat loss during exposure to environmental heat stress (thermal dehydration) resulted in a decrease in plasma and interstitial fluid volumes. In contrast, Astrand and Saltin (1964) found no decrease in plasma volume after prolonged, severe exercise (metabolic dehydration) that caused a water deficit of about 4 liters. Thermal dehydration, therefore, produced a marked decrease in blood volume, while exercise dehydration significantly reduced the intracellular fluid volume without altering blood volume.

The duration of work at a maximal load was found to be reduced after thermal and metabolic dehydration (Saltin, 1964a). Comparisons between the two types of dehydration showed the largest reduction after metabolic dehydration. At present, the available data are insufficient to permit a complete explanation for this phenomenon.

With a reduction in body weight of 5.2% by thermal dehydration, Saltin (1964a) noted a reduction in plasma volume of up to 25%. After dehydration, the changes in the hemodynamic responses to submaximal work are characterized by a decrease in stroke volume (Saltin, 1964b) with a compensatory increase in heart rate (Palmer, 1969; Ribisl and Herbert, 1970) to maintain the cardiac output (Saltin, 1964b). When the severity of the exercise was increased the subject's maximal stroke volume, heart rate, and cardiac output were found to be similar to the maximal measurements made prior to dehydration. Despite the fact that there was no adverse effect on the observed circulatory functions during maximal exertion after dehydration, there was a marked decrease in maximal work time.

This inability to perform exhaustive exercise following dehydration does not appear to be related to a decrement in either circulatory function or oxygen transport. Buskirk *et al.* (1958), Elfenbaum (1966), Bock *et al.* (1967), and Saltin (1964a) observed no alteration in the maximal ability to consume oxygen following dehydration. However, in each investigation the subject's work time to exhaustion was significantly lower in the dehydrated state. Measurements of blood lactic acid following these maximal exercise bouts seem to suggest that dehydration may impair lactate production and the ability to perform anaerobic work (Saltin, 1964a).

Associated with the circulatory alterations during dehydration is an inability to dissipate body heat. Adolph's (1947) classic studies of men in the desert showed that during moderate exercise rectal temperatures were increased by 0.35°–0.55° for each percent body weight lost through sweating. Intuitively, one might expect dehydration to elicit a reduction in sweating, thereby impairing one's ability to dissipate body heat. However, several investigations have shown that dehydration affects neither sweating rates nor cutaneous blood flow (Adolph, 1947; Hertzman and Ferguson, 1960; Senay and Christensen, 1965). Adolph (1947) observed that sweat losses were approximately as fast at 9–11% deficits as at 3–5% dehydration. The explanation for the rise in body temperature during dehydration, therefore, appears to be complex and obscure at this time. Nevertheless, under conditions of heat stress and/or prolonged muscular activity, dehydration may impair performance by impairing one's capacity to dissipate body heat.

B. Muscular Strength, Speed, and Reaction

Over the past 30 years, numerous studies have examined the effects of rapid dehydration on muscular performance. Gillum, in 1940, observed that wrestlers who reduced their body weight by 2–4 lb tended to increase their strength and speed. While the method of weight reduction was not controlled in these experiments, the wrestlers showed a 5-point gain in the Rogers Physical Fitness Index after weight losses ranging from 2 to 13.5 lb over a 5-day period.

More recent research has failed to support these gains in strength and speed with dehydrative weight losses. To the contrary, Bosco *et al.* (1968) noted that isometric strength of elbow flexion was significantly reduced following a 3.1% hypohydration. In 1943, Tuttle studied five wrestlers who were dehydrated 3.6–4.9%. Eighteen measurements were made to assess the neuromuscular, cardiovascular, and respiratory responses before and after weight loss. It was concluded that up to 5% of body weight could be lost without significantly affecting any of the variables measured.

Edwards (1951) and Doscher (1944) have both found muscular strength, as measured by push-ups, pull-ups, and a hand dynamometer, to be unaffected by dehydration weight losses of up to 7%. These findings were supported by Byram (1953), who observed that weight reductions of 5% had no detrimental effects on muscular strength and endurance.

Nichols (1957) administered a battery of motor performance tests (Bass Stepping Stone Test, hand grip, vertical jump, and meter-stick chronoscope) to evaluate the effects of rapid weight reduction on balance, reaction time, strength, and power. The amount of weight lost by the 42 subjects varied from 3 to 18 lb, or from 1.67 to 11.11% (average, 6.8%) of body weight. It was concluded that performance of the tests measured was not significantly affected by a rapid weight loss up to 10% of body weight.

Williams *et al.* (1965) studied the effects of dehydration–starvation on

21 male subjects, who lost 3–5% of their body weight within a 24-hour period. While strength was found to be impaired by dehydration, reaction time, steadiness, and coordination were unaltered.

Singer and Weiss (1968) and Elfenbaum (1966), on the other hand, reported that strength was unaffected by dehydration of up to 9.3% of body weight. In addition, a significant improvement in reaction time was noted following dehydration (Singer and Weiss, 1968). With few exceptions, therefore, most investigators concur that dehydration has little or no effect on strength, muscular endurance, speed, and reaction time. It should be noted, however, that these results may be specific to the skills measured. The application of these findings to sporting and occupational situations seems difficult.

C. Summary

It appears that dehydration has varied effects on man's capacity to work. Under conditions of heat stress and prolonged exertion, body water losses of as little as 2% can impair circulatory and thermoregulatory functions. Such problems are typified by the frequency of industrial absenteeism that is common among foundry workers. Large daily sweat losses make repeated exposure to the heat of the foundry unbearable and circulatory embarrassment habitual.

Since some athletic events necessitate a high rate of energy expenditure under heat stress conditions, the risk of heatstroke and circulatory collapse are compounded by dehydration. Events such as football and distance running seem to be most strongly affected. Under these conditions adequate fluids should be ingested to minimize the debilitating consequence of dehydration.

Activities that are limited to brief bouts of maximal muscular exertion, e.g., weight lifting, seem to be little affected by dehydration. It is difficult to apply these research findings to the sport of wrestling, since the duration of this activity is such that muscular and circulatory endurance contribute to the athlete's working capacity. However, if by dehydrating the wrestler is permitted to compete against a smaller opponent, his diminished working capacity might be nullified by psychological, strength, and leverage gains. Morgan (1970), however, has shown that neither ergogenic nor harmful psychological effects result from a weight loss of 4% in college wrestlers. Additional research seems warranted to describe the effects of conditioning and repeated exposure to dehydration on the performance of men participating in selected physical activities.

III. Fluid Ingestion and Physical Activity

The function of thirst is to secure for the body sufficient water to balance all losses. Adolph (1947) noted that, for the most part, this sensation adequately fulfilled its function to the extent that while in the desert men generally recovered their water balance every night. In differing circumstances thirst has been found wholly inadequate. Despite large sweat losses men may feel little or no desire for fluids immediately following heat exposure or physical activity and may thereby remain in a dehydrated state for several hours. As previously mentioned, body water losses exceeding 2% of body weight can impair performance and endanger one's health. For this reason, numerous investigations have assessed the ergogenic effects of fluid ingestion before, during, and following physical activity or performance. The following discussion will attempt to assess the efficacy of various schedules for water ingestion in preventing dehydration and improving performance.

A. Hyperhydration and Performance

Fluid ingestion prior to and during physical activity is frequently criticized on the grounds that it distends the stomach, thereby impairing respiratory mechanics and muscular effort. Little *et al.* (1949) studied the effects of ingesting 1.0–1.5 liters of water 5 minutes before exercise. No adverse effects were found on heart rate or minute volume of ventilation during treadmill running. Similar findings were reported for performance times in 50- and 200-yd swims and a 220-yd run. These findings were supported by Coffin (1954), who studied the effects of ingesting 12 oz of water before performing a 200-yd dash. When compared to control tests, without water intake, no significant difference was found.

Like Coffin (1954), Blank (1959) studied the effect of water ingestion on performance in the 220-yd dash. Thirty-three collegiate track men ran 27 individual 220-yd time trials under three alternating conditions: (a) no liquid consumption within the hour preceding the trial, (b) consumption of 16 oz of water 5 minutes before the trial, and (c) free consumption of water 5 minutes prior to the run. Preexercise water ingestion was found to have no influence on performance in the 220-yd dash.

When performance was assessed in terms of the physiological effects of water balance on prolonged running, Blyth and Burt (1961) reported that running time to exhaustion was significantly increased by consuming 2 liters of fluid (1 liter of saline and 1 liter of water) in the 30-minute period preceding the run. Heart rates, rectal temperatures, and sweat losses did not differ within the experimental design of their study.

Moroff and Bass (1965) studied soldiers walking on a treadmill and observed that when 2 liters of water was consumed prior to the activity rectal temperatures and heart rates were significantly lower. In addition, sweating rates were significantly higher when the exercise was preceded by fluid ingestion. These findings are in agreement with the earlier data of Ladell (1955), who examined the effects of water, salt, and water and salt (saline) on exercise tolerance. Working tolerance was greatest following both water and saline ingestion. The rise in body temperature and heart rates was least for subjects who consumed water and salt. However, sweating rates were lowest for the saline condition.

Londeree *et al.* (1969) studied the application of fluid ingestion to the heat stress problems associated with football. Attired in football equipment, 10 well-conditioned men ran on a treadmill in an environment of 90°F with a relative humidity of 70%. Four 1-liter water ingestion schedules were assessed in terms of rectal temperature, heart rate, pulse pressure, sweat losses, and the specific gravity of whole blood and plasma. The results demonstrate that cold water consumed early in the exercise session combated the effects of heat stress better than late administration. However, this advantage dissipated toward the end of the exercise.

Based on the preceding review, it is quite apparent that, while the intake of fluids prior to exercise is effective in reducing the hyperthermic and cardiac stress associated with prolonged exertion in the heat, it probably offers little if any advantage to men during short-term effort. On the other hand, there is no physiological or performance data that would justify the restriction of fluids prior to muscular effort. To the contrary, under environmental heat stress participants should be encouraged to consume cold fluids in excess of thirst demands.

B. Fluid Intake during Exercise

Extensive research by Saltin (1964a) and others (Fordtran and Saltin, 1967; Saltin and Hermansen, 1967) has demonstrated that water and salt loss in sweat is a major cause of fatigue and impaired performance during severe exercise of long duration. Extensive research has been conducted to determine the contributions of water and electrolyte replacement during activity to performance. Efforts to match the large sweat losses associated with prolonged activity in the heat are complicated by the limited rate of gastric emptying.

Early research showed that moderate to heavy exercise inhibits the ability of the stomach and small intestine to empty (Campbell *et al.*, 1928; Hellebrandt and Tepper, 1934). Costill *et al.* (1970a) observed that during a 2-hour treadmill run men lost body fluids at a rate of 1.67 liters/hour but could replace only 0.82 liter/hour via oral ingestion. It is known that gastric emptying is dependent in a major way on the composition and volume of the solution ingested. While water is easily absorbed from the stomach, an isotonic saline solution (water plus 0.85% sodium chloride) empties even more rapidly (Fordtran and Saltin, 1967). Recent studies, however, showed that nearly identical volumes of water and an isotonic solution were emptied from the stomach when 100-ml feedings were made every 5 minutes during 2 hours of running (Costill *et al.*, 1970a). It is apparent, therefore, that despite one's efforts to achieve a balance between fluid loss and fluid replacement a significant water deficits is likely to occur during prolonged, exhaustive exercise in a hot environment. This fact was well illustrated by Greenleaf and Sargent (1965), who studied sweat loss and unrestricted water intake during exercise and heat exposure.

When forced to replace hour by hour the water lost in sweat, men work more efficiently and are less likely to become exhausted (Pitts *et al.*, 1944). Johnson *et al.* (1942) reported that water intake aided in maintaining homeostasis, but water taken in excess of thirst demands was even more effective. More recently, Gillis (1965) studied the administration of various volumes of water (1, 2, and 3 pints) to subjects exercising on a bicycle ergometer. He found that 3 pints of water resulted in significantly lower heart rates and rectal temperatures than did either 1 or 2 pints.

Costill *et al.* (1970a) studied cold fluid ingestion (water and a glucose–electrolyte solution) during distance running. As illustrated by Fig. 3, cold fluids produced a leveling of rectal temperature after 45 minutes. On the other hand, no thermal equilibrium was observed at the end of 120 minutes, when the subjects abstained from replacing fluids. This increased ability to achieve a thermal balance was unrelated to sweating rates and was attributed to the cold nature of the fluids (7°–9°C). Unlike Gillis' (1965) findings, heart rates were unaffected by the ingestion of fluids during exercise. Under competitive conditions, marathon runners have been shown to be incapable of replacing sweat losses during the race (Costill *et al.*, 1970a; Wyndham and Strydom, 1969). Despite fluid losses in excess of 6.1 kg (13.4 lbs), the average total fluid ingestion during the race was only 0.14 kg. It is obvious, there-

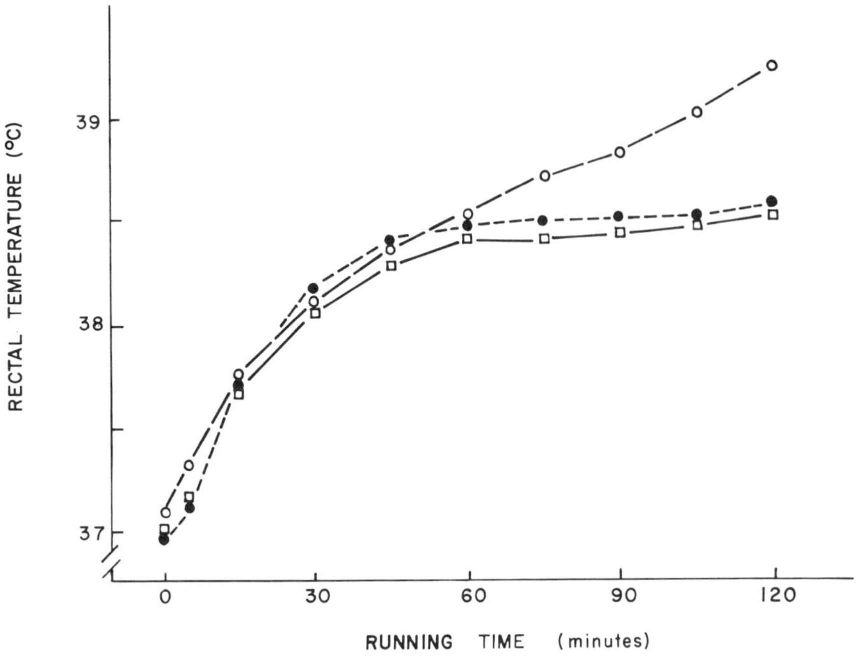

Fig. 3. Rectal temperature responses during 120 minutes of running with and without fluid ingestion. Legend: ●, electrolyte solution; ○, no fluids; □, water. (From Costill *et al.*, 1970a.)

fore, that during the strenuous effort of distance running severe dehydration is inevitable and often dangerous (Wyndham and Strydom, 1969).

Pitts *et al.* (1944) compared three water replacement conditions during intermittent marching and resting in a 100°F environment (relative humidity 35–45%). Without water the rectal temperature rose steadily to high levels and showed no signs of reaching a steady state. When enough water was consumed to keep thirst quenched, the rectal temperature was steady at about 101°F until about 4.5 hours. Finally, when water was consumed at a rate that matched the sweat losses, the body temperature remained very low. These findings are illustrated in Fig. 4. It is also interesting to note that subjectively the men experienced physical distress in proportion to their rectal temperatures. That is to say, the marching was easiest during the complete water replacement condition and most difficult when no water was consumed.

Even during prolonged sporting and industrial activities that are more intermittent in nature, the ability to keep pace with sweat loss is far from effortless. Few occupations place greater demand on the temperature-regulating responsibilities of sweating than does foundry work. In

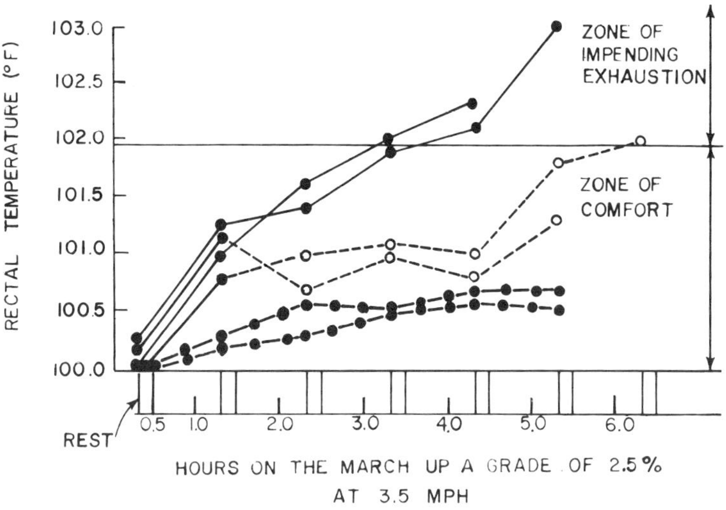

Fig. 4. Effects of water consumption on rectal temperature during marching in the heat. Legend: —, no water; - - - -, water *ad lib.;* ●—●, water equals sweat. (From Pitts *et al.,* 1944.)

1969 Passmore and Costill studied the influence of electrolyte and fluid replacement on dehydration of men at work in the 118°–126°F environment of a steel mill. In spite of the opportunity to drink fluids, the workers were 2.8–6.8 lb lighter after 8 hours of the work–heat exposure. Sweating rates appeared to be unrelated to either the composition or volume of fluids consumed.

While there seems to be significant value in the replacement of body fluids during prolonged severe effort, the rapid fluid losses, rate of gastric emptying, feeding habits, and inadequate thirst sensation make this practice largely ineffective. In addition, the rules of some athletic events prohibit free access to fluids. International marathon running competition, for example, forbids the drinking of water for the first 10 miles of the race. In view of the high rate of metabolic heat production and sweating, this ruling seems criminal and should be adjusted to reduce the risk of extreme dehydration and possible heatstroke. Hyperhydration prior to the race, however, might minimize the body water deficit incurred during the first 10 miles.

C. Fluid Administration following Dehydration

As previously mentioned, thirst serves to demand replacement for body fluid losses. In man, thirst sensations exhibit a characteristic time lag, which results in intermittent and inadequate drinking patterns (Adolph, 1947). If the ill effects of dehydration are to be eliminated, one must take fluids in excess of thirst demands. Despite the practical implications of rapid and complete rehydration, few researchers have examined this problem.

Eaves (1968) assessed the effects of ingesting three different commercially available fluids and water following 6% body weight losses. The subjects rehydrated 2% of their body weight within a 1-hour period. It was concluded that all of the liquids had equal effect on the endurance, as measured by the Balke Treadmill Test, of college wrestlers following dehydration. Since only partial fluid replacement was achieved, the full benefits of rehydration were not fully described by this study.

Palmer (1967) and Ribisl and Herbert (1970) have examined exercise heart rate responses before and after a 5% dehydration and again after rehydration. Figure 5 demonstrates that heart rate responses during and following a standard treadmill run were elevated by 12–15 beats/minute during dehydration (5%) but returned to the predehydration level when the men consumed enough fluids to equal their sweat losses. Measurements of physical working capacity (PWC—170) before and after the 5% dehydration and after a 5-hour period of rehydration indicates complete circulatory recovery with rehydration. However, heart rate alone seems to provide a limited view of the circulatory responses during rehydration.

During an investigation of rehydration following a 4% body weight loss, Costill and associates (1969, 1970b) assessed the value of ingesting solutions with varied osmolalities. The three experimental solutions contained sodium (22 mEq/liter), chloride (11.5–17.2 mEq/liter), potassium (2.6 mEq/liter), phosphate (3.9–22.9 mEq/liter), and glucose (3.88–7.67 gm/liter) with osmolalities of 289, 315, and 444 mOsm/liter. The periods of rehydration were compared to a water rehydration and a fifth condition during which the subjects did not rehydrate. Fluids equal to the weight loss during dehydration were consumed in 13 equal volumes during the first 3 hours of rehydration.

Plasma volume was found to return to normal more rapidly with the hypertonic solutions (315 and 444 mOsm/liter) than with either the isotonic solution (289 mOsm/liter) or water. These responses are illustrated in Fig. 6. Heart rate responses during a standard treadmill run were markedly lower during all rehydration conditions, but no significant advantage could be awarded to any of the test solutions.

The osmotic concentration of the extracellular fluid is normally maintained within limits of 283 ± 11 mOsm/liter, primarily by the regulation of water intake and excretion. Pitts *et al.* (1944) found no change

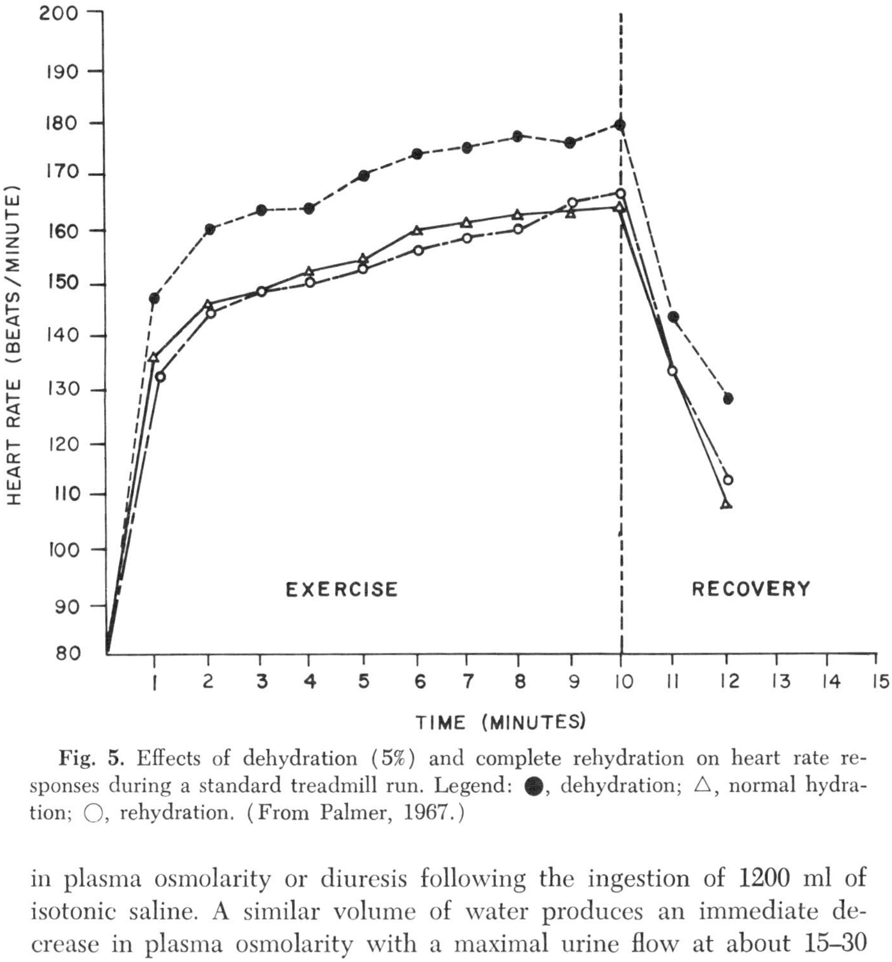

Fig. 5. Effects of dehydration (5%) and complete rehydration on heart rate responses during a standard treadmill run. Legend: ●, dehydration; △, normal hydration; ○, rehydration. (From Palmer, 1967.)

in plasma osmolarity or diuresis following the ingestion of 1200 ml of isotonic saline. A similar volume of water produces an immediate decrease in plasma osmolarity with a maximal urine flow at about 15–30 minutes after the peak-low plasma osmolarity has been attained. Despite the body water deficits of dehydration and the isotonicity of one experimental solution (289 mOsm/liter), Costill *et al.* (1970b) noted that rapid rehydration produced a mild decrease in serum osmolality and a large diuresis (Fig. 7). Efforts to completely rehydrate men within a short 3- to 4-hour period seemed to be only partially successful. Although still dehydrated by 1.5–2% of body weight, the ingested fluids failed to be distributed adequately and the extracellular excess was lost as urine.

Current collegiate wrestling rules require that competitors "weigh in" 5 hours before competition. This interval allows the dehydrated athlete an opportunity to replenish his body water losses. This situation has been examined by Herbert and Ribisl (1971). They found that wrestlers

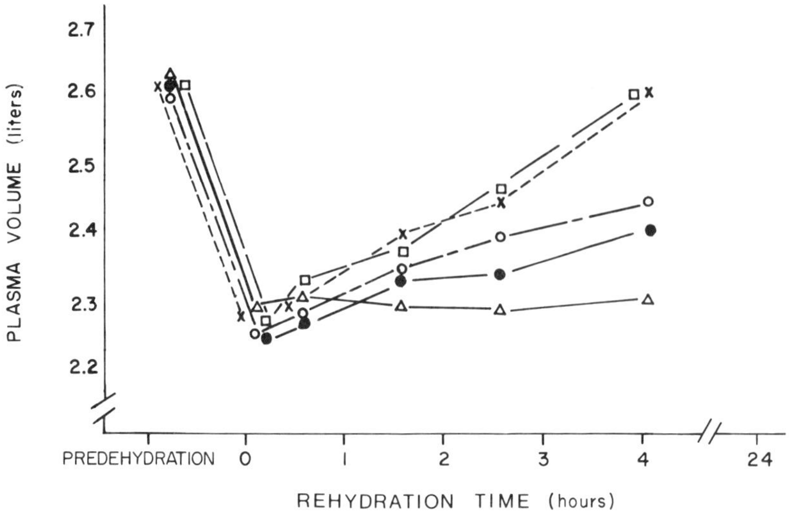

Fig. 6. Plasma volumes during rehydration with selected fluids. Subjects experienced a 4% dehydration, and fluids were replaced at 15-minute intervals during the first 3 hours of rehydration. Legend: △, no fluids; ○, solution A (289 mOsm/liter); ×, solution B (315 mOsm/liter); □, solution C (444 mOsm/liter); ●, water. (From Costill *et al.,* 1970b.)

were still 2.2% below their normal body weight following rehydration, suggesting that fluid replacement was not complete. As a result, the wrestler's physical working capacity was still significantly impaired at the time of competition. It was concluded that only with more complete rehydration can wrestlers hope to recover fully their normal physical working capacity.

Absenteeism among men who must work under extreme thermal stress has long been recognized as a major problem for industrial productivity (Dill *et al.* 1936). Daily exposure to high environmental temperatures, large sweat losses, and inadequate fluid replacement can result in a daily accumulating water deficit. Some workers, however, seem to compensate for their occupational water losses by consuming large fluid volumes each evening. A survey of their evening rehydration habits has shown that many of these workers consume copious volumes of beer with very little diuretic effect (Costill, 1970, unpublished data). Similar observations have been made among marathon runners, who run 15–30 miles each day and incur a 6–11% body weight loss (Costill, 1969). Prior to each training bout, the runners seemed to make a conscious effort to regain any fluid lost during a preceding exercise session.

The rapid administration of fluids following dehydration appears to

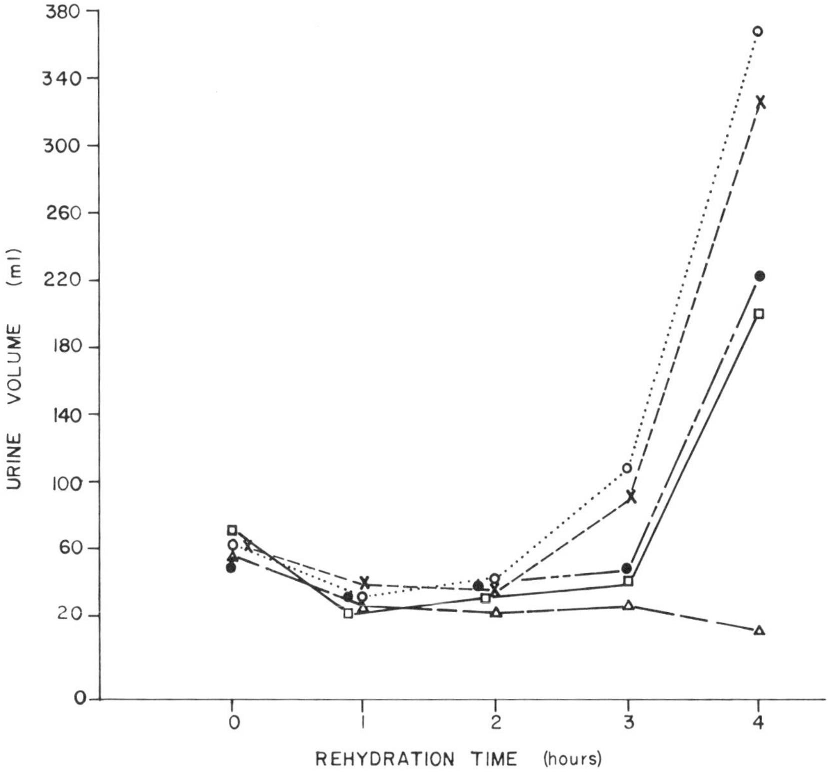

Fig. 7. Urine volumes during rehydration with selected fluids. For legend, see caption to Fig. 6. (From Costill *et al.*, 1970b.)

be regulated ineffectively by thirst. Voluntary rehydration during a 3- to 5-hour period has been found to be incomplete and physical working capacity impaired. When men replace all of their dehydration weight losses within 3–5 hours, working capacity and exercising heart rates are returned to normal. However, such rapid fluid replacement is seldom distributed in proportion to the needs of the body fluid compartments, which results in a sizable loss via the kidney. On the other hand, men who are dehydrated every day seem to adapt their rehydrative techniques to insure nearly normal hydration before each subsequent weight loss.

D. Summary

On the basis of the preceding review of research concerned with fluid ingestion and physical activity we can conclude that muscular performance, while impaired by dehydration, can be maintained near normal so long as body fluids are equal to or greater than normal. Hyperhydrating prior to physical activity seems to have little if any ergogenic effect during short-term work, but it does provide a reserve to combat dehydration and decrements in exercise tolerance during work in the heat. Efforts to replace fluids during physical activity have been found useful in preventing hyperthermia and dehydration but seem to be ineffective and often impractical during endurance athletics. Rapid fluid replacement following dehydration is most effective when men are required to ingest a fluid volume equal to the body water lost. Voluntary rehydration from a 4–7.5% dehydration is nearly complete within 24–36 hours and is easily monitored by recording body weight.

IV. Insufficient and Excess Electrolytes

Unfortunately little empirical evidence has been amassed to explain the effects of insufficient and excess electrolytes on muscular performance. Much of the information dealing with this problem has been based on skeletal muscle responses among individuals with clinically abnormal electrolyte balance. These findings are seldom applicable to normally active men. The following discussion, therefore, will review the research that has practical implications for men who develop an electrolyte deficit via profuse sweating and who accumulate an excess of electrolytes by oral ingestion.

A. Review of Literature

As previously mentioned, the electrolyte concentration of sweat is lower than that of the extracellular fluids. During heavy sweating, therefore, the total body electrolyte content is decreased but the concentration of extracellular sodium and chloride tends to increase. This sudden water–electrolyte imbalance is quickly reversed by the ingestion of water. Under these conditions a balance can be achieved only by ingesting a solution containing small quantities of electrolytes (Costill *et al.*, 1969). Figure 8 demonstrates the effects of fluid replacement on the serum electrolytes following a 4% dehydration. However, it is questionable whether the small electrolyte deficits or excesses seen in Fig. 8 are large enough to affect muscular performance.

When subjected to repeated sessions of heat and/or prolonged exercise stress, men frequently develop a salt deficit (Adolph, 1947). Johnson

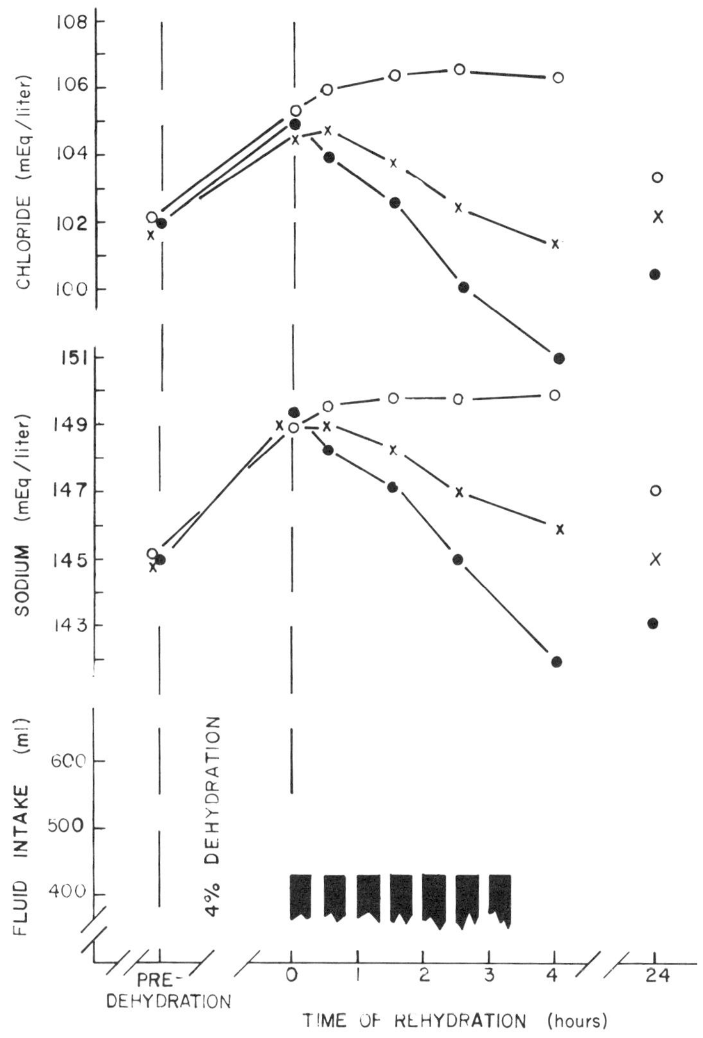

Fig. 8. Sodium and chloride changes during dehydration and rehydration. Legend: ○, no fluids; ●, water; ×, electrolyte solution.

et al. (1942) found that with a sweat rate of 1 liter/hour, the salt loss was about 2 gm/hour. Still, it should be noted that, although normal sweat contains 3 gm of salt per liter, the sweat of a heat-acclimatized man may contain as little as 1 gm/liter of sweat (Nahum, 1963).

Rose *et al.* (1970) attributed an observed decrease in serum magnesium following marathon competition to losses in sweat. In view of magnesium's involvement in muscular contractility, it was recommended that the fluids employed for rehydration purposes should contain magnesium as well as other electrolytes.

When the salt intake of healthy men is reduced by fasting, excessive sweating, or consuming salt-poor food, it is generally conceded (Marriott, 1950) that the kidneys nearly stop excreting sodium and chloride although the level of these electrolytes may remain unaffected during several weeks of such experiments. Thus, it is difficult to deplete the body of its sodium and chloride content unless the deprivation is severe and prolonged. Likewise, it is difficult to overload the body with sodium chloride provided the amount of water ingested is adequate.

Knochel and Vertel (1967) have pointed out that military recruits and football players undergoing training in hot environments constitute high-risk groups for potassium depletion. Traditional methods of preventing heat stress call for the use of salt tablets. Knochel and Vertel (1967) pointed out that salt loading through indiscriminate administration of salt tablets to heat-acclimatizing persons probably leads to serious potassium depletion. Schamadan and Snively (1967) noted a significant relationship between potassium depletion and heat distress among otherwise healthy football players in preseason training.

It seems generally agreed that either excesses or deficits in electrolytes can prove detrimental to muscular performance. For example, Ladell (1955) has shown that sweat rate and salt concentration of sweat are inversely related to the serum sodium and chloride levels. Men exercising in the heat showed less rapid increases in rectal temperature and heart rate when they consumed a saline solution. Similar findings were reported by Lee *et al.* (1941), who found that saline produced a more complete hydration than did water.

Taylor *et al.* (1944) studied the effects of three salt intake levels (6, 15, and 30 gm/day) on selected physiological variables during 3 days of exposure to a hot, dry environment. While sweat rates varied from 5 to 8 liters/day, the intake of 6 gm of salt per day caused heat exhaustion along with nausea, vomiting, tachycardia, hypotension, vertigo, dehydration, and collapse. There was no difference between the 15- and 30-gm/day groups, but both experienced fewer symptoms of heat exhaustion than the 6-gm/day subjects. It was concluded that a sweat rate of 5–8 liters/day produced a need for 13–15 gm of salt.

Laborit and associates (1957, 1958) have reported beneficial effects of aspartate (potassium and magnesium salts of aspartic acid) as a means of reducing fatigue at the neuromuscular level. It was postulated that aspartic acid, which functions in an intermediate position of the Krebs cycle, should provide a suitable substrate for the increase of metabolic efficiency and delay exhaustion. The value of aspartic acid salts was tested using swimming rats (Rosen *et al.*, 1962). The onset of exhaustion was significantly and consistently delayed by the administration of the aspartic acid salts.

Agersborg and Shaw (1961) have studied the effects of aspartate in more than 2000 patients and have reported that 80% felt that they had experienced subjective signs of relief from fatigue. Similar findings have been reported by Kruse (1961) and Taylor (1961). However, these studies were of a subjective nature, on patients who complained of chronic fatigue.

Consolazio *et al.* (1964) administered 2 gm of magnesium and potassium salts of aspartic acid daily for 5 weeks. No significant advantage was seen that would encourage the use of aspartate to obtain relief from fatigue. Additional research seems warranted to explain conclusively the influence of aspartic acid salts on exhaustive muscular effort.

At this point, some consideration should be given to the frequency of salt administration. Johnson *et al.* (1942) found no advantage in giving excess salt during work. They suggested that salt was best taken with food and drink during prolonged rest intervals. Considering the electrolyte content of the normal daily diet and kidney function, the problems attributed to electrolyte excess and lack are probably over emphasized. Nevertheless, men who incur large sweat losses each day are wise to rehydrate with fluids containing electrolytes in proportion to those normally lost in sweat.

B. Summary

Unfortunately very little information is available to describe fully the importance of electrolytes on muscular performance. Based on clinical observations, it is apparent that extreme distortions of the serum electrolytes can lead to abnormal neuromuscular responses. These conditions are seldom seen in healthy individuals. The indiscriminate administration of salts should be prohibited to prevent excess potassium losses and possible heat injuries. In the process of rehydration from a large body fluid loss, it seems prudent to consume a salinelike solution to insure sufficient replacement of electrolytes.

V. Conclusion

It is obvious from the preceding review of the research literature that water and electrolytes can serve as ergogenic aids to muscular performance under selected conditions. While both circulation and temperature regulation are impaired by 1–2% dehydration, optimal endurance performance can be maintained so long as body fluids are kept near normal levels. Ingesting fluids prior to short-term effort seems to have little ergogenic benefit, but it does provide a reserve to limit dehydration during prolonged exertion in the heat. Following large sweat losses, water and electrolyte administration can rapidly rectify the circulatory impairment achieved in the course of dehydration. However, rehydration within a 3- to 5-hour period is usually only 60% complete when fluids are administered *ad libitum*. The intake of electrolytes in excess of bodily needs seems to be of little ergogenic advantage. To the contrary, ingesting salt prior to physical activity can reduce sweating and induce excess potassium losses.

In spite of numerous research efforts, many questions relative to the role of water and electrolytes in muscular activity remain unanswered. Additional information is needed to explain the long-term effects of repeated bouts of dehydration on physical growth. Also, it would seem valuable to compare the effects of dehydration on trained and untrained individuals and to determine if an adaptative process is associated with repeated bouts of dehydration and rehydration. In view of the intellectual and physical stress placed on high school and college athletes, an examination of the psychological impact of dehydration on wrestlers seems warranted. Finally, more studies are needed to explain the role of selected electrolytes in the performance of muscular work. Only after these and other problems have been solved can we fully understand the ergogenic contributions of water and electrolytes.

References

Adolph, E. F. (1947). "Physiology of Man in the Desert." Wiley (Interscience), New York.

Agersborg, H. P. K., and Shaw, D. L., Jr. (1961). Presented at the Amer. College of Sports Medicine Meeting, Norristown, Pennsylvania.

Andersson, B. (1962). *Proc. Int. Congr. Physiol. Sci. 22nd* **1**, 661.

Astrand, P. O., and Saltin, B. (1964). *J. Appl. Physiol.* **19**, 829–832.

Blank, L. B. (1959). *Res. Quart.* **30**, 131–135.

Blyth, C. S., and Burt, J. J. (1961). *Res. Quart.* **32**, 301–307.

Bock, W., Fox, E. L., and Bowers, R. (1967). *J. Sports Med. Phys. Fitness* **7**, 67–72.

Bosco, J. S., Terjung, R. L., and Greenleaf, J. E. (1968). *J. Sports Med. Phys. Fitness* **8**, 81–86.

Brønsted, J. N. (1923). *Rec. Trav. Chim.* **42**, 718.

Bullard, R. W., Dill, D. B., and Yousef, M. K. (1970). *J. Appl. Physiol.* **29**, 159–167.

Buskirk, E., Iampietro, P., and Bass, D. (1958). *J. Appl. Physiol.* **12**, 189–194.

Byram, H. M. (1953). Master's thesis, State Univ. of Iowa, Iowa City.
Campbell, J. M., Mitchell, G. O., and Powell, A. T. W. (1928). *Guy's Hosp. Rep.* **78**, 279–93.
Coffin, W. A., Jr. (1954). Master's thesis, Univ. of Kansas, Lawrence.
Consolazio, C. F., Nelson, R. A., Matoush, L. O., and Isaac, G. J. (1964). *J. Appl. Physiol.* **19**, 257–261.
Costill, D. L. (1969). "Limitations of Human Endurance with Special Reference to Age." Ball State Univ. Press, Muncie, Indiana.
Costill, D. L., McClements, L., and Fisher, A. (1969). Royal Crown Cola Co. Report 1.
Costill, D. L., Kammer, W. F., and Fisher, A. (1970a). *Arch. Environ. Health* **21**, 520–525.
Costill, D. L., Sparks, K. E., Fisher, A., Gregor, R., and Warner, P. (1970b). Royal Crown Cola Co. Report 3.
Dill, D. B. (1938). "Life, Heat and Altitude." Harvard Univ. Press, Cambridge, Massachusetts.
Dill, D. B., Bock, A. V., and Edwards, H. T. (1936). *J. Ind. Hyg. Toxicol.* **18**, 417–431.
Doscher, N. (1944). *Res. Quart.* **15**, 317–324.
Eaves, C. G. W. (1968). Doctoral dissertation, Ohio State Univ., Columbus.
Edwards, J. B. (1951). Master's thesis, Univ. of North Carolina, Charlotte, North Carolina.
Elfenbaum, L. (1966). Doctoral dissertation. Ohio State Univ., Columbus.
Elkinton, J. R., and Danowsky, T. S. (1955). "The Body Fluids: Basic Physiology and Practical Therapeutics." Williams & Wilkins, Baltimore, Maryland.
Fordtran, J. S., and Saltin, B. (1967). *J. Appl. Physiol.* **23**, 331–335.
Gillis, R. J. (1965). Doctoral dissertation, Springfield College, Springfield, Massachusetts.
Gillum, O. C. (1940). Master's thesis, Ohio State Univ., Columbus.
Greenleaf, J. E., and Sargent, F. (1965). *J. Appl. Physiol.* **20**, 719–724.
Guyton, A. C. (1961). "Textbook of Medical Physiology," pp. 37–40. Saunders, Philadelphia, Pennsylvania.
Hellebrandt, F. A., and Tepper, R. H. (1934). *Amer. J. Physiol.* **107**, 355–363.
Herbert, W. G., and Ribisl, P. M. (1971). *Res. Quart.* In press.
Hertzman, A. B., and Ferguson, I. D. (1960). *U. S. Armed Forces Med. J.* **11**, 542–560.
Hoffman, W. S. (1970). "The Biochemistry of Clinical Medicine." Yearbook Publ., Chicago, Illinois.
Johnson, R. E., Belding, H. S., Consolazio, F. C., and Pitts, G. C. (1942). Harvard Fatigue Laboratory Report 13, Cambridge, Massachusetts.
Kaufman, H. E., and Rosen, S. W. (1956). *Surg. Gynecol. Obstet.* **103**, 101.
Knochel, J. P., and Vertel, R. M. (1967). *Lancet* **1**, 659–661.
Kozlowski, S., and Saltin, B. (1964). *J. Appl. Physiol.* **19**, 1119–1124.
Kruse, C. A. (1961). *Northwest Med.* **60**, 597–603.
Laborit, H., Moynier, R., Trzebski, A., Guiot, G., and Baron, C. (1957). *C. R. Soc. Biol.* **151**, 1383–1386.
Laborit, H., Weber, B., Niaussat, P., Jouany, J. M., Guiot, G., Zawadowski, J., and Baron, C. (1958). *Anesth. Analg. Reanim.* **15**, 480–494.
Ladell, W. S. S. (1955). *J. Physiol.* **127**, 11–46.

Ladell, W. S. S. (1965). "The Physiology of Human Survival." Academic Press, New York.
Lee, D. H. K., Murray, R. E., Simmonds, W. J., and Atherton, R. G. (1941). *Med. J. Aust.* **2**, 249–258.
Little, C. C., Strayhorn, H., and Miller, A. T. (1949). *Res. Quart.* **20**, 298–401.
Londeree, B. R., Updyke, W. F., and Burt, J. J. (1969). *Res. Quart.* **40**, 725–732.
McGee, W. J. (1906). *Interest. Med. J.* **13**, 279.
Marriott, H. L. (1950). "Water and Salt Depletion." Blackwell, Oxford.
Morgan, W. P. (1970). *Med. Sci. Sports* **2**, 24–27.
Moroff, S. V., and Bass, D. E. (1965). *J. Appl. Physiol.* **20**, 267–270.
Nahum, L. H. (1963). *Conn. Med.* **27**, 495–497.
Nichols, H. (1957). Doctoral dissertation, Univ. of Michigan, Ann Arbor.
Palmer, W. K. (1967). Master's thesis, Ball State Univ., Muncie, Indiana.
Palmer, W. K. (1969). *Res. Quart.* **39**, 1054–1059.
Passmore, J., Jr., and Costill, D. L. (1969). Royal Crown Cola Co. Report 4.
Pitts, G. C., Johnson, R. E., and Consolazio, F. C. (1944). *Amer. J. Physiol.* **142**, 253–259.
Pitts, R. F. (1963). "Physiology of the Kidney and Body Fluids." Yearbook Publ., Chicago, Illinois.
Pugh, L. G. C. E., Corbett, J. L., and Johnson, R. H. (1967). *J. Appl. Physiol.* **23**, 347–352.
Ribisl, P. M., and Herbert, W. G. (1970). *Res. Quart.* **41**, 536–541.
Robinson, J. R. (1954). "Reflections on Renal Function," p. 55. Blackwell, Oxford.
Robinson, S. (1949). *In* "Physiology of Heat Regulation and the Science of Clothing" (L. H. Newburg, ed.), pp. 212–231. Saunders, Philadelphia, Pennsylvania.
Rose, L. I., Carroll, D. R., Lowe, S. L., Peterson, E. W., and Cooper, K. H. (1970). *J. Appl. Physiol.* **29**, 449–451.
Rosen, H., Blumenthal, A., and Agersborg, H. P. K. (1962). *J. Pharm. Sci.* **51**, 592–593.
Saltin, B. (1964a). *J. Appl. Physiol.* **19**, 1125–1132.
Saltin, B. (1964b). *Acta Physiol. Scand. Suppl.* **62**, No. 230, 52.
Saltin, B., and Hermansen, L. (1967). *In* "Nutrition and Physical Activity" (G. Blixt, ed.), Vol. 4. Almqvist & Wiksell, Stockholm.
Schamadan, J. L., and Snively, W. D., Jr. (1967). *Ind. Med. Surg.* **36**, 785–788.
Schmidt-Nielsen, K. (1964). "Desert Animals: Physiological Problems of Heat and Water," Chap. 5. Oxford Univ. Press, Oxford.
Senay, L. C., and Christensen, H. L. (1965). *J. Appl. Physiol.* **20**, 278–282.
Singer, R. N., and Weiss, S. A. (1968). *Res. Quart.* **39**(2), 361–369.
Stein, L. (1963). *Science* **139**, 46.
Stein, L., and Seifter, J. (1962). *Amer. J. Physiol.* **202**, 751.
Taylor, B. B. (1961). *West. Med.* **2**, 535.
Taylor, H. L., Henschel, A. F., Mickelson, O., and Keys, A. (1944). *Amer. J. Physiol.* **140**, 439–451.
Tuttle, W. W. (1943). *Res. Quart.* **14**, 158–166.
Williams, W. R., Blyth, C. S., and Jamerson, R. E. (1965). *In* "Proceedings of the AAHPER Convention, Dallas, Texas."
Wyndham, C. H., and Strydom, N. B. (1969). *S.A. Med. J.* **42**, 893–896.

Chapter 11

Oxygen

Jack H. Wilmore

I. Introduction

A. Historical Overview

The specific use of oxygen as a potential ergogenic aid probably dates back several centuries, although this is not documented in the literature. After having isolated "pure air," or oxygen as we know it now, Priestley wrote in 1775: "The feeling of it in my lungs was not sensibly different from that of common air; but I fancied that my breast felt peculiarly light and easy for some time afterwards. Who can tell but that, in time, this pure air, may become a fashionable article in luxury. Hitherto only two mice and myself have had the privilege of breathing it" (Bean, 1945).

The initial attempts to scientifically investigate oxygen as a potential ergogenic aid began in the first decade of this century (Douglas and Haldane, 1909; Hill and Flack, 1909, 1910; Hill and MacKenzie, 1909). However, the use of oxygen as an ergogenic aid in athletics was not established until the 1932 Olympic Games, when Japan won great victories in swimming. Many interpreted their success to the fact that the Japanese swimmers breathed pure oxygen prior to competition (Karpovich, 1960). Considerable research has been reported since that time and has clarified considerably the basic question as to whether oxygen can be justifiably classified as a true ergogenic aid. Unfortunately, additional research is necessary to provide sound physiological explanations for the phenomena that have been observed in these various studies.

B. Theoretical Considerations

Before reviewing in detail the literature on oxygen as an ergogenic aid, it is first necessary to consider the appropriate physiological mechanisms through which oxygen could have an influence as a work-producing or performance-enhancing agent. One of the major limitations to the individual's maximal tolerance for work, i.e., physical working capacity, is the oxygen transport system. Oxygen supply to the exercising muscles is controlled largely by the following factors (Christensen *et al.*, 1934): (a) pulmonary ventilation or the transportation of oxygen from the atmosphere to the alveoli, (b) pulmonary diffusion of oxygen from the alveoli to the pulmonary capillary blood, (c) cardiac output or minute volume of the heart, (d) peripheral blood flow to and through the muscles, and (e) oxygen diffusion from the muscle capillaries to the active tissue. While each of these five factors can be responsible for limiting one's performance in specific circumstances, only a, b, and e appear to be influenced by supplementing the oxygen supply during exercise.

Because of the combination of the above factors, each individual is limited as to the greatest quantity of oxygen he can deliver to the tissues during maximal exercise. This limit is referred to as the maximal oxygen uptake, a well-defined and reproducible end point that represents the individual's aerobic capacity for endurance work. Increasing this maximal oxygen consumption through supplemental oxygen breathing would certainly result in increased physical capacity and performance.

It is possible that oxygen supplementation could also enhance the so-called anaerobic aspect of the individual's work performance. The area of anaerobic metabolism is much more difficult to evaluate, unfortunately, as there is presently a great deal of conflict and confusion concerning the various biochemical processes at the cellular level and their relative importance to the work capacity of the total organism. However, it is possible to speculate that the administration of oxygen could increase the tissue oxygen storage capacity and could influence both the production and removal of lactic acid. In both circumstances, what is measured as the anaerobic capacity would certainly be enhanced.

C. Definition of the Problem

Again, before reviewing the literature, it is important to have in mind the objectives of this review. First, it is necessary to establish whether oxygen is an ergogenic aid, i.e., whether it clearly enhances one's physical performance. Second, providing that oxygen is demonstrated to be an ergogenic aid, it then becomes necessary to determine the basic physiological mechanism(s) through which it exerts its effect.

Several factors have an important bearing on the interpretation of the literature. First, the method of supplementing oxygen to the individual is important. Increasing the oxygen tension (pO_2) in the inspired gas can be accomplished in three ways (Bean, 1945): (a) using hyperoxygenated air or pure oxygen at normal atmospheric pressure, (b) using normal air under compression, and (c) using hyperoxygenated air or pure oxygen under compression. Under the first condition, it is possible to increase the oxygen tension up to 1 atm or 760 mm Hg, while oxygen tensions in excess of 1 atm may be obtained under the second and third conditions.

Last, the sequence of oxygen supplementation greatly influences the results and subsequent interpretations of the various research studies. It makes a great difference when interpreting the results of these studies to ascertain when the oxygen was administered: before, during, or following the exercise period. Because of this, the following review has been separated into three phases: oxygen administration prior to, during, and following exercise.

II. The Administration of Oxygen Prior to Exercise

A. Literature Review

Much of the early research was confined to observing the influence of oxygen administered prior to the performance of exercise. Douglas and Haldane (1909) investigated the effects of (a) forced breathing for 3 minutes and (b) quiet oxygen inhalation for 3 minutes on the subsequent performance of running up and down a 40-ft stairway twice. They found that oxygen breathing had only a slight effect on the postexercise pulse rate or ventilation volume values when compared to the control conditions of forced breathing. Hill and MacKenzie (1909) took opposition to the results of Douglas and Haldane (1909). They demonstrated nearly a fivefold increase in the number of times their subjects could pull a 60-lb weight 19 in. high while breath holding immediately following forced oxygen breathing as opposed to quiet air breathing for 3 minutes. When quiet air breathing and forced oxygen breathing were compared, forced oxygen breathing resulted both in substantially more work being performed and in almost a twofold increase in breath-holding time. They also noted improvement in running performance (250 and 880 yd) following oxygen breathing.

Hill and Flack (1909) observed pulse rate, blood pressure, and respiration responses following running up and down a flight of 26 stairs, 8–9 times, as fast as possible. The run was preceded by either air or oxygen breathing for a period of 5 minutes. They found that, after oxygen breathing, the individual's running time was improved, the recovery pulse rate lowered, and there was a relief from the feeling of dyspnea, while respiration rate and ventilation volume were essentially unchanged. In another series of tests on boxers, they found that oxygen breathing greatly restored the "vigour" of the individual. They concluded by stating, "Oxygen given at the end of the third round to a 'done' man sends him back to the ring full of fire and energy."

In a later study, Hill and Flack (1910) investigated the effects of oxygen breathing prior to (a) working against a 60-lb weight with both arms and one foot, (b) running back and forth along a 30-yd runway, and (c) putting one foot on a chair and lifting the body weight up to seat height a number of times in succession. In all cases, the work was performed during breath holding up to the breaking point, after the deep breathing of either air or oxygen. They found that the amount of work performed was substantially greater following oxygen breathing. They concluded that preliminary breathing of oxygen is beneficial in the first part of a race and is more effective in races of 880 yd or less than in races of longer distance. The beneficial effect was attributed to both an increased tolerance to CO_2 accumulation and an increased storage of oxygen within the body.

Karpovich (1934), stimulated by these earlier studies and by the success of the 1932 Japanese Olympic swimming team, who breathed oxygen prior to competing, studied the effects of oxygen inhalation on swimming performance. He first had his subjects take two deep inspirations of oxygen prior to holding their breath and diving into the water. In 11 out of 17 cases, the individuals broke their own unofficial records after oxygen breathing. In two cases, they bettered their usual time, and the remaining four made their usual time. In a second series of tests, he found that 3–5 minutes of oxygen breathing 4–5 minutes before a 100-yd swim had no noticeable effect on the speed of swimming.

In a third series of tests, the subjects inhaled oxygen immediately before, and up to 1, 2, and 3 minutes before, running in place while breath holding. When compared with breathing air for the total period prior to the running in place, the oxygen breathing immediately before and up to 1 minute before resulted in marked increases in running time to the breaking point. The data for the 1-minute interval are presented in Table I. The 2-minute time interval showed only a slight effect, and no differences were noted in time intervals of 3 minutes or greater. Thus, the oxygen must be administered within 1 minute of the performance to have a substantial effect. In his conclusions, Karpovich remarks that the effect of preliminary oxygen breathing is more noticeable in 100- and 200-yd swims. The 50-yd swim is adequately handled by anaerobic mechanisms, and distances of 440 yd or greater would not be sufficiently influenced. Unfortunately, the subjects in this study knew they were breathing oxygen and therefore the results could have been influenced by psychological as well as physiological factors.

TABLE I

THE PERFORMANCE IN RUNNING 1 MINUTE AFTER TAKING OXYGEN[a,b]

	Times of the subjects (seconds)[c]								
Condition	A	B	C	D	E	F	G	H	Mean
Without O_2	29	33	38	38	49	38	41	40	38.5
With O_2	52	36	48	49	62	68	80	51	55.8

[a] The exercise used was a running in place holding the breath.
[b] Adapted from Karpovich, 1934.
[c] The figures represent the average time of several trials.

Elbel *et al.* (1961) used athletes in good physical condition, having them breathe oxygen during 6 minutes of rest, air during 5 minutes of level treadmill running at 8 mph and then oxygen during 19 minutes of recovery. In the control test, the subjects breathed air throughout. The oxygen breathing prior to the run resulted in a lower pulse rate at rest and during the first 2 minutes of exercise. The respiratory rate was greater during the preexercise rest period and the oxygen saturation was increased during the resting period.

B. Summary

It appears that the preliminary inhalation of oxygen prior to exercise has a limited effect on the performance of that exercise. The amount of work performed or rate of work in a maximal exercise of short duration is substantially increased as a result of oxygen breathing immediately before exercising. The performance of a submaximal exercise is also facilitated by oxygen breathing, in the sense that the exercise is performed more economically, e.g., lower pulse rate. However, the benefits obtained from preliminary oxygen breathing do appear to be limited in two respects. First, the interval between the cessation of oxygen breathing and the beginning of exercise should probably be no greater than 2 minutes. Second, the effect of oxygen breathing appears to diminish for exercises in excess of 2 minutes. The reasons for this will be discussed later in this chapter.

III. The Administration of Oxygen during Exercise

A. Literature Review

In 1911, Feldman and Hill reported the results of their investigation on the effects of oxygen inhalation before and during various exercises on the subsequent lactic acid production as measured in the urine. Oxygen breathing, as compared to air breathing, was shown to reduce lactic acid production resulting from exercise. It was concluded that increased production of lactic acid is due to oxygen want.

Briggs (1920) studied both fit and unfit men while performing on a bicycle ergometer, walking and running on a flat surface, and climbing an incline of 21° slope. He found that oxygenated air made work easier for unfit men but not for fit men. Enrichment above 60% oxygen had no additional effect over what was observed for mixtures below 60%. On the bicycle ergometer, the subjects were able to perform low levels of work at lower oxygen uptakes when breathing oxygen-enriched mixtures. However, very little difference resulted from oxygen breathing when the subjects were walking, running, or climbing the 21° slope. In heavy exertion with oxygen breathing, Briggs concluded, "even the fittest man derives benefit."

Hill *et al.* (1924b) undertook an investigation of factors that limit oxygen uptake. They compared air breathing with the breathing of mixtures of both higher and lower oxygen percentages. Their subjects ran in place to maximal or near maximal levels. They found that breathing mixtures of high oxygen content enabled their subjects to attain considerably higher oxygen uptakes. When 50% oxygen, rather than air, was breathed the oxygen uptakes increased from 9 to 35%.

Benedict *et al.* (1935) observed respiratory exchange, respiratory rate, and heart rate responses before, during, and after a bicycle ergometer ride in which subjects breathed air, 40, 60, and 90% oxygen. Oxygen breathing had no effect on respiration rate during rest or work. The heart rate was lower during both rest and work when the oxygen-enriched mixtures were breathed. Oxygen consumption was not influenced during rest, work, or recovery by the breathing of any of the increased oxygen mixtures. It is important to note, however, that the level of work used in this study required an oxygen consumption of only 1400 ml/minute.

Christensen *et al.* (1934), in a series of preliminary experiments, found that oxygen absorption and the rate of maximal work can be increased by the breathing of a 45% oxygen mixture. The effect of oxygen was not apparent in brief periods of work of 1 minute or less, but oxygen facilitated work of 2 minutes or more. They attributed this fact to a lag in the time it takes the circulation to reach its maximal rate. This lag time thus becomes the limiting factor for oxygen supply to the tissues during the initial stages of maximal work.

Nielsen and Hansen (1937) demonstrated that in heavy work ventilation can be substantially lowered when subjects breathe oxygen-enriched air. A similar effect was not found at lower work intensities. In 1946, Asmussen and Nielsen investigated this problem in greater depth. They found that at oxygen uptakes greater than 1.1 liters/minute the ventilation volumes during oxygen breathing were lower than during air breathing. This difference increased up to the maximal oxygen uptake, where oxygen breathing was 30 liters/minute or 31% lower than air breathing. In the same series of experiments, they also observed the alveolar CO_2 tensions and blood lactate responses to the oxygen- and air-breathing exercises. Beyond an oxygen uptake of 1 liter/minute the alveolar CO_2 tension with oxygen breathing began to rise substantially above the values obtained for air breathing, up to a peak value of approximately 47 mm Hg. Blood lactate values were lower in the oxygen-breathing experiments starting at about 1.2 liters/minute oxygen uptake, with the differences becoming progressively larger with increasing oxygen uptakes, e.g., 40% lower at 3.6 liters/minute.

Asmussen and Nielsen (1946) had their subjects breathe oxygen mixtures of 21, 30, 60, and 100% while bicycling at a constant load of 1440 kg/minute. Their ventilation and blood lactate responses are shown in Figs. 1 and 2. Without exception, with increasing oxygen content of the inspired air, there is a stepwise lowering of the blood lactate curves and a corresponding decrease in ventilation for the same amount of work. They concluded that oxygen breathing acts both on the respiratory center and on the chemoreceptors. These conclusions were substantiated in later experiments (Asmussen and Nielsen, 1950; Asmussen, 1950).

Lundin and Strom (1947) studied blood lactic acid levels in subjects working on a bicycle ergometer while breathing nitrogen–oxygen mixtures with varying percentages of oxygen. They found the blood lactate values to have an inverse proportional relationship to the partial pressure of oxygen in the inspired gas mixture.

Hickam *et al.* (1951) studied the effects of high and low oxygen concentrations on various physiological parameters during treadmill exercise

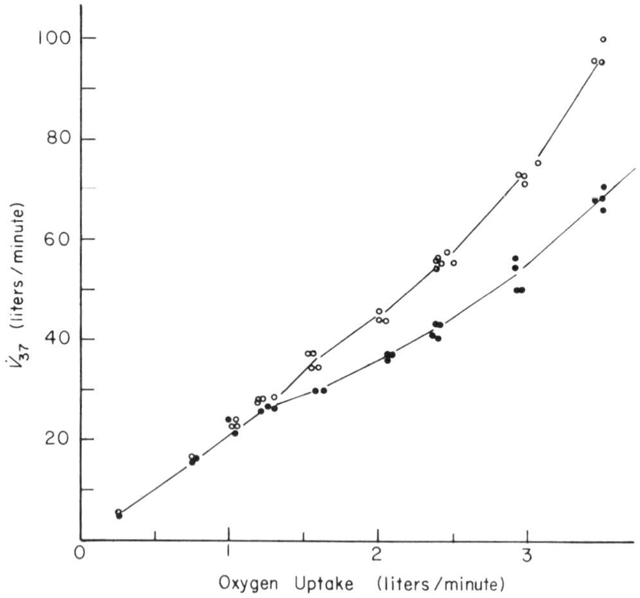

Fig. 1. Ventilation (37°C, prevailing barometric pressure, saturated) in relation to oxygen uptake: ○, in air; ●, in 100% oxygen. (From Asmussen and Nielsen, 1946.)

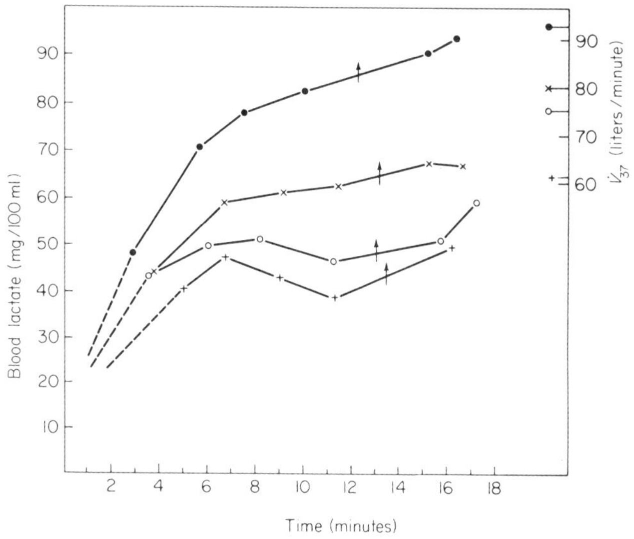

Fig. 2. Blood lactate concentration during work with the legs (1440 mkg/minute) while breathing air, ●; 30% oxygen, ×; 60% oxygen, ○; and 100% oxygen, +. At the right ordinate are shown the corresponding ventilations ($\dot{V}_{37}$) determined at the points of time indicated by the arrows. (From Asmussen and Nielsen, 1946.)

at 5.1 mph on a 3.5% grade. The subjects breathed either air, 15% oxygen in nitrogen, or 99.5% oxygen. When breathing 99.5% oxygen as compared to room air, there was a significant decrease in ventilation from 55.8 to 47.4 liters/minute, an increase in arterial saturation, an increase in arterial pCO_2, and a decrease in arterial pH. Each of these changes could be considered facilitative with regard to physiological economy in performing the exercise.

Asmussen *et al.* (1948) reported a progressively greater endurance capacity in their subjects when breathing 12, 21, and 100% oxygen, respectively. The maximal oxygen uptake was much greater at 21 compared with 12% oxygen. Unfortunately, maximal oxygen uptake was not measured in subjects breathing 100% oxygen for reasons that will be discussed later.

Miller (1952) examined the effects of oxygen breathing before, during, and after exercise on the treadmill at both heavy and exhaustive levels of work. He found that the heart rate and blood pressure response to exercise were not altered by the administration of oxygen before, during, or after the exercise. There were, however, significantly lower blood lactate levels when oxygen was breathed during exercise. This lactate response was not demonstrated in a group of sedentary subjects performing work of a moderate intensity. In the exhaustive runs, the time to exhaustion increased from a mean of 7.3 to 8.8 minutes as a result of oxygen breathing, an increase in performance in excess of 20%.

Bannister and Cunningham (1954) investigated the influence of various oxygen mixtures on treadmill runs to exhaustion. They selected an intensity of exercise that would bring on exhaustion within 6–9 minutes when air was breathed. The subjects then ran to exhaustion while breathing 33, 66, and 100% oxygen. Unfortunately, no attempt was made to control the psychological effect; i.e., the subjects knew which mixtures they were breathing. As can be seen from Table II, in all cases the addition of oxygen to the inspired air increased the time required to reach the breaking point (exhaustion). The improvement was greater at 66 and 100% oxygen than at 33% oxygen. At 66% oxygen, the time to exhaustion was at least doubled, and in two cases tripled. Performance was generally better at 66 compared to 100% oxygen. The pulmonary ventilation was decreased as was the blood lactate response when the oxygen-enriched mixtures were breathed, while the alveolar pCO_2 increased to higher levels. Almost as dramatic as these physiological alterations were the responses of the subjects who generally felt the run to be much easier when breathing the 66% oxygen mixture.

Asmussen and Nielsen (1955) studied subjects' cardiac output during submaximal work while they breathed low (approximately 12%) and high (approximately 99%) oxygen mixtures compared with air. When low oxygen mixtures were breathed, the cardiac output was from 10% to 20% higher and the arteriovenous difference from 10 to 20% lower than when air was breathed. The cardiac output increase was the result of an increased pulse rate, as the stroke volume actually decreased as much as

TABLE II

DURATION OF EXERCISE DURING THE INHALATION OF DIFFERENT AIR–OXYGEN MIXTURES[a,b]

	21% O_2		33% O_2		66% O_2		100% O_2	
Subject	minutes	seconds	minutes	seconds	minutes	seconds	minutes	seconds
A (1)	8	45	8	45	17	15[c]	16	32[c]
A (2)	8	26	15	17	23	40	20	40
B	8	58	11	20	24	48[c]	20	45
C	6	35	13	25	23	0[c]	17	18
D	6	25	10	15	13	50	11	55

[a] Adapted from Bannister and Cunningham (1954).
[b] Speed in all experiments was 6¼ mph.
[c] Denotes breaking point not reached.

11%. When pure oxygen was breathed, the cardiac outputs and arteriovenous oxygen differences were nearly the same as they were when air was breathed, although the pulse rate showed a slight decrease, averaging about 6%.

Velasquez and Reynafarje (1966) used oxygen–nitrogen mixtures of 16.2, 20.9, 35.8, and 100% during submaximal treadmill exercise at 12 km/hr and 5.8% grade. This part of the study was conducted at 14,900 ft (PB = 446 mm Hg); thus, the 35.8% mixture was comparable to breathing air at sea level (pO_2 would be 143.6 and 146 mm Hg, respectively). When comparing the 35.8% oxygen breathing with breathing room air, there was no difference in ventilation volume or oxygen debt. However, the higher oxygen concentration resulted in a 12% greater $\dot{V}O_2$ and a reduction in the accumulation of blood lactate. These results are illustrated in Fig. 3.

Cunningham (1966) studied the effects of breathing high concentrations of oxygen on treadmill runs to exhaustion. The mean performance time was increased from 243 seconds with air breathing to 384 seconds as a result of oxygen breathing (70–73% oxygen in nitrogen). Maximal heart rate was not changed, but oxygen debt was significantly reduced during the first minute of recovery and the peak excess blood lactate value was lower after the breathing of oxygen during the exercise. Even

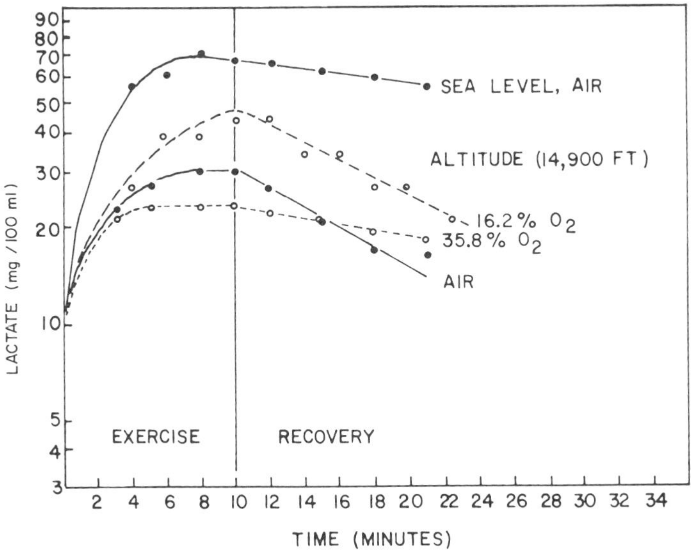

Fig. 3. Lactate accumulation and disappearance from peripheral blood during exercise and recovery, breathing of high and low oxygen mixtures, at 14,900 ft, 12 km/hr, and 5.8% grade. (From Velasquez and Reynafarje, 1966.)

though the subjects performed more work during oxygen breathing, it appeared as though they did not attain the same degree of anaerobic work as they did when breathing air. Therefore, Cunningham suggested that lactic acid accumulation may not be a limiting factor in work.

Hagerman *et al.* (1968) reported on the effects of breathing 100% oxygen on resting, exercise, and recovery oxygen consumptions, pulmonary ventilation volumes, and heart rates. The subjects rode a bicycle ergometer for 5 minutes at a load that elevated the mean heart rate above 170 beats/minute. Their results indicated a marked increase in resting oxygen consumption, a decrease in resting ventilation volume, a marked decrease in exercise and recovery ventilation volumes, and an insignificant reduction in the energy cost of the exercise with oxygen breathing. Unfortunately, the experiment was carried out on only six subjects, and in some cases where substantial mean differences did occur, e.g., increases less than 25%, the t value was not high enough to attain statistical significance. In addition, it is exceptionally difficult to accurately assess oxygen uptake and energy cost during the breathing of mixtures of oxygen in excess of 21%. The reason for this will be discussed later.

Hughes *et al* (1968) studied the influence of breathing varying oxygen concentrations on the cardiopulmonary and metabolic responses to submaximal and maximal exercise on a bicycle ergometer. The subjects breathed concentrations of 11, 16, 21, and 33% oxygen. At the submaximal work loads, the ventilation volumes, heart rates, and cardiac outputs were lower at the higher oxygen concentrations, although the maximal values were similar. The peak lactate values attained were lower when 33% oxygen was breathed compared to 21% oxygen. The blood pH was substantially lower when 33% oxygen was breathed, and three of the four subjects attained their greatest work capacity at this concentration.

Taunton *et al.* (1970) investigated physical working capacity in hyperbaric environments and under conditions of hyperoxia. Two subjects performed on a bicycle ergometer at work rates of 1000, 1300, 1500, and 1800 kpm/minute for 5 minutes while breathing air at 1 and 2 atm and while breathing oxygen at 2 atm. The results of this study are illustrated in Fig. 4. It was demonstrated that the greater the pO_2 of the inspired air, the lower the heart rate, ventilation volume, and ventilatory equivalent for each work load. The oxygen consumption and carbon dioxide production exhibited the opposite response. There was a general absence of undesirable effects from severe exercise at 2 atm oxygen, which is of practical significance in work under hyperbaric conditions.

Banister *et al.* (1970) also studied the effects of breathing oxygen at 2 atm, compared to normal air, on the performance of a heavy bicycle

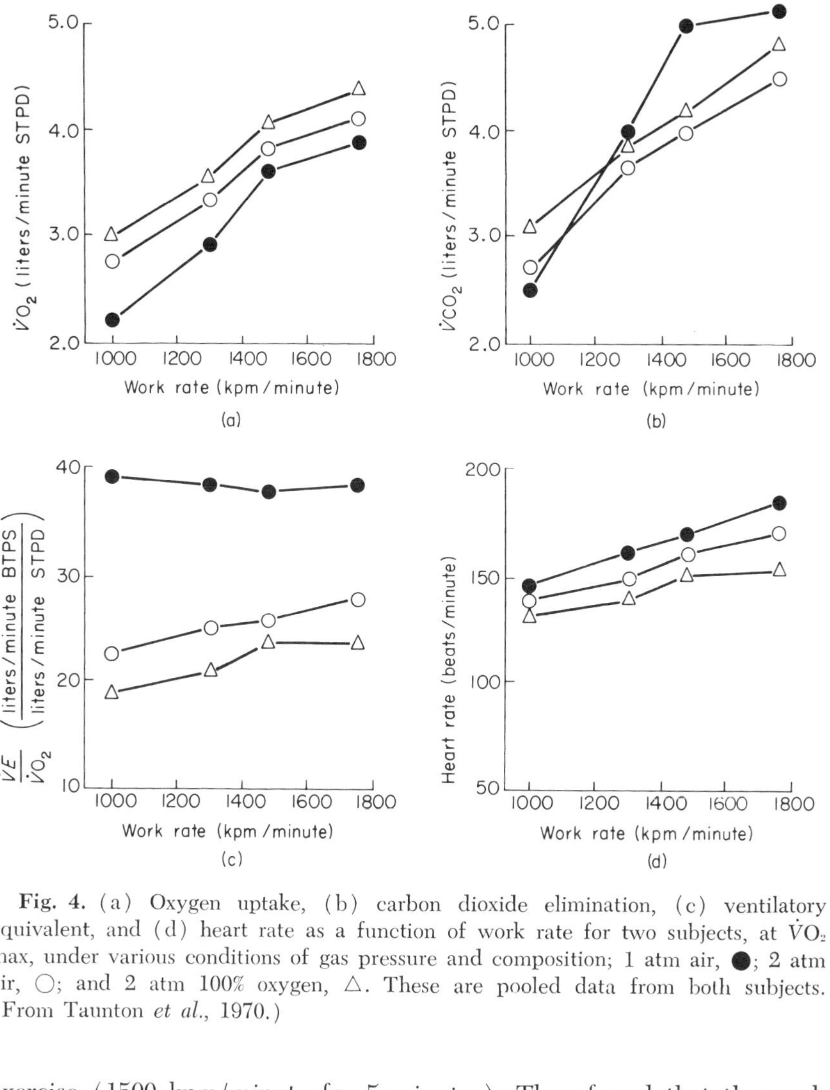

Fig. 4. (a) Oxygen uptake, (b) carbon dioxide elimination, (c) ventilatory equivalent, and (d) heart rate as a function of work rate for two subjects, at $\dot{V}O_2$ max, under various conditions of gas pressure and composition; 1 atm air, ●; 2 atm air, ○; and 2 atm 100% oxygen, △. These are pooled data from both subjects. (From Taunton *et al.*, 1970.)

exercise (1500 kpm/minute for 5 minutes). They found that the peak heart rate decreased from 173 to 159 beats/minute as a result of oxygen breathing at 2 atm for 2 hours before and during the exercise. A reduction was also noted in the pulmonary ventilation, which dropped from a value of 138 liters/minute during air breathing to 95 liters/minute as a result of oxygen breathing at 2 atm. Carbon dioxide production was decreased and oxygen uptake increased when oxygen was breathed. Exercise with oxygen breathing also resulted in substantially lower lactic acid levels and a higher blood pH. The authors concluded that the changes found with oxygen breathing at 2 atm are attributable to the variation in importance of high arterial and tissue oxygen tension during oxygenation and to the possible toxic effects of oxygen on enzyme systems in glycolysis.

Wyndham *et al.* (1970) observed the effects of acute changes in altitude in a deep mine on maximal oxygen uptake. Maximal oxygen uptake was determined at ground level (1763 m above sea level) and immediately after descent in a deep mine to 1828 m, which approximated sea level. A second group of subjects went through the same base-line testing at ground level and were then tested immediately after descending to a depth of 3033 m, or 1270 m below sea level. The barometric pressures at these sites were 630 mm Hg at ground level, 765 mm Hg at 1828 m depth, and 865 mm Hg at 3033 m depth. Exercising at the greatest depth would be approximately the equivalent of exercising while breathing a 24% oxygen mixture.

The results showed that the men were able to run 0.8 km faster at 1828 m below surface than on the surface and 1.6 km faster at 3033 m below the surface than on the surface. The mean maximal oxygen uptake at 1828 m depth was 49.7 ml/kg × minute compared to 44.7 ml/kg × minute on the surface for the first group, while the mean was 52.5 ml/kg × minute at a depth of 3033 m and 44.7 ml/kg × minute on the surface for the second group. The mean heart rates at the point of maximal oxygen uptake were significantly higher at both 1828 and 3033 m compared to the surface values. Likewise, the pulmonary ventilation volumes (STPD) were substantially greater at the lower depths. There were, however, no differences in the BTPS ventilation volumes.

B. Summary

Evidence supports the contention that oxygen is an ergogenic aid when administered during exercise. The amount of work performed in exhaustive tests and the rate of work are substantially increased by oxygen breathing during the exercise period. In submaximal exercise, the work is performed more economically or efficiently, i.e., at a lower physiological cost to the individual. This is evidenced by the fact that the work can be performed at lower heart rates, lower ventilation volumes, and with lower lactate production. There is also the possibility that the aerobic capacity (maximal oxygen uptake) is increased by oxygen breathing, but this is open to some question for reasons to be discussed later.

IV. The Administration of Oxygen during Recovery

A. Literature Review

For many years it has been common to observe the athletic trainer run to fetch the oxygen mask when the star performer comes off the field in an exhaustive daze. More often than not, the individual is back in the game within a few minutes, fully recovered. Is this a direct result of the administration of oxygen, or are there other explanations?

Miller (1952) studied the influence of oxygen administration on specific cardiovascular variables before, during, and following treadmill exercise of submaximal and maximal intensity. When the oxygen was administered during the recovery period, no alterations were found in the speed of recovery of the heart rate or blood pressure or in the postexercise blood lactate levels. Elbel *et al.* (1961) found somewhat conflicting results when their subjects breathed oxygen during the recovery period following a moderately heavy treadmill exercise. Their postexercise recovery pulse rates were consistently lower and respiratory rates consistently higher with oxygen breathing. There was, however, no difference in the payment of the oxygen debt.

Bjorgum and Sharkey (1966) analyzed the effects of oxygen inhalation following treadmill running on recovery from the exercise. This study used compressed air and normal air as the control conditions. Their findings indicated that postexercise oxygen inhalation was of no physiological aid to recovery. This was reflected in a lack of differences in pulse rate decrease, postexercise oxygen uptake, and pulmonary ventilation rate.

Hagerman *et al.* (1968) observed the effects of breathing oxygen during rest, exercise, and recovery on the performance of and recovery from 5 minutes of heavy work on a bicycle ergometer. They found no significant difference between oxygen and air breathing during recovery with regard to recovery pulse rate, although a definite trend favored oxygen breathing. Similar findings were reported for ventilation volumes. Again, the exceedingly small number of subjects in this study makes a statistical interpretation extremely difficult.

B. Summary

Unfortunately, too few studies have been conducted in this area to allow an unequivocal statement to be made relative to the merits of oxygen administration in facilitating recovery from exercise. It appears, however, that if there is an effect from postexercise oxygen breathing, its magnitude is small and probably inconsequential in regard to subsequent performance. Since none of these studies observed maximal, exhaustive exercise, it is possible that a real effect may have been masked by the lack of a sufficient exercise stress.

V. General Physiological Interpretations and Implications

A. Interpretations

Most of the data reviewed in the preceding sections appear to be accurate and the interpretations sound. However, it is obvious that many of the studies failed to control for the "psychological effect." Miller (1952) touched on this briefly. He gave a different set of subjects air in both of two different exercise periods; however, the subjects were told that one of the administrations was oxygen, and they were told in which test the "oxygen" was given. He found an almost invariable improvement with "oxygen" and concluded that "we are inclined to explain most of the reported benefits of oxygen administration to athletes on this basis" (Miller, 1952, p. 168). He certainly raised a most valid point, but the degree to which this factor has influenced these previous studies will never be known. This certainly dictates the inclusion of psychological controls in future studies.

Another type of error may have influenced the accuracy of several of the previous studies. Unfortunately, when gas mixtures in excess of 20.9% oxygen are breathed, potential errors of serious magnitude influence the calculation of oxygen uptake. Hill *et al.* (1924a) have presented a very thorough and concise review of this problem. First, when measuring oxygen uptake, it is necessary to know both the inspired and expired volumes of oxygen. Since the former is cumbersome, most investigators measure either the expired or inspired volume and estimate the other volume. This estimation is made on the basis that the volume of nitrogen inspired equals the volume of nitrogen expired. The expired air volume is known, the percentage of nitrogen in the inspired air is known since it is relatively constant, and the expired nitrogen concentration can be obtained by subtracting the sum of the oxygen and carbon dioxide fractions from unity. Unfortunately, as the nitrogen concentration is reduced in the inspired air, i.e., through increased percentages of oxygen, the error of estimation increases greatly. Hill *et al.* (1924a) calculated that an error of 20 ml in oxygen uptake at 20% oxygen in the inspired air is equivalent to an error of 860 ml at 90% oxygen. The latter represents greater than a 20% error at a gross oxygen uptake of 4 liters/minute. Unfortunately, the direct measurement of both these volumes would not solve this problem. In fact, it has been shown that measuring both volumes at high oxygen pressures produces an even greater error, approaching 30% of the actual value (Hill *et al.*, 1924a).

A second potential problem associated with calculating oxygen uptake values at high oxygen pressure involves the loss of nitrogen from the body water. This occurs as a result of the lowered pressure of nitrogen in the inspired air and can amount to a substantial loss of accuracy in the calculation of oxygen uptake. In addition, the body takes up a substantial amount of oxygen in the tissues, which is not a true reflection of the actual oxygen used for metabolism over the same time interval. Both of these problems can be at least partially resolved by measuring the carbon dioxide production and by using an approximation of the respiratory exchange ratio, calculating the oxygen uptake from this value. Carbon dioxide production is far less affected by either of the above-mentioned problems. As an example

$$CO_2 \text{ production} = \dot{V}E \text{ expired} \times F_ECO_2 - \dot{V}E \text{ inspired} \times F_ICO_2$$

where $\dot{V}E$ represents the ventilation volume and F_ECO_2 and F_ICO_2 represent the fraction of carbon dioxide in the expired and inspired air. Since F_ICO_2 is relatively constant and approximately zero, and $\dot{V}E$ expired and F_ECO_2 are measured directly, the subsequent calculation of CO_2 production is relatively accurate. Several investigators have taken advantage of this technique (Taunton *et al.*, 1970; Banister *et al.*, 1970).

Even though the possibility of the errors mentioned above exists in the studies reviewed in this chapter, the overall magnitude of such error is probably small. Thus, it is necessary to explain why oxygen should have a facilitative or ergogenic effect on the performance of various tasks. Unfortunately, the physiological mechanisms involved are complex and are not easily interpretable.

The most obvious explanation would be in relating the increased performance or capacity associated with oxygen breathing to a lessening of arterial hypoxemia. Unfortunately, the literature is conflicting on this point. Mitchell *et al.* (1958) found the oxygen saturation of arterial blood during the last stage of exhaustive exercise to be only slightly lower than the resting values, i.e., 97.1% at rest compared to 94.7% at the end of exercise. Rowell *et al.* (1964) noted a substantially greater decrease in their subjects' arterial oxygen content and saturation during the final 15 seconds of a maximal run on the treadmill. They observed a group of athletes and a group of sedentary subjects both before and after an intensive conditioning program. The sedentary subjects, before training, responded in much the same manner as the subjects in the Mitchell *et al.* (1958) study. After training, however, the sedentary men showed a substantial reduction between resting and peak exercise values, going from a mean of 95.4 to 91.4%. The athletes exhibited even lower peak exercise values, reaching 85.2% saturation.

Even if the arterial saturation did drop to the lowest values reported by Rowell *et al.* (1964) for their athletic group, oxygen breathing would not appear to have too great an effect on increasing one's capacity for work, i.e., raising the saturation from 85% to 100%. It is important to remember, however, that it is not the degree of saturation as much as it is the partial pressure of oxygen that has the greatest significance relative to oxygen-delivering capacity.

When the blood is 97–98% saturated, the pO_2 of the arterial blood is approximately 100 mm Hg (Comroe *et al.*, 1962). At a saturation of 85%, the pO_2 of the arterial blood drops dramatically to about 56 mm Hg (Ganong, 1963). In other words, a reduction in the arterial saturation of only 12–13 percentage points results in a partial pressure drop to nearly half of the initial value. This is due to the rather flat aspect of the oxygen–hemoglobin disassociation curve at its upper end. When 100% oxygen is breathed, the pO_2 of the arterial blood is 640 mm Hg, over six times greater than when atmospheric air is breathed (Comroe *et al.*, 1962). The significance of this may not be readily apparent.

The ability to transport oxygen from the alveoli to the blood in the lung and from the capillary blood to the active tissues is directly a function of the differential in pressure between any two points. If the pO_2 of the active tissue fell to 20 mm Hg and the pO_2 of the arterial blood fell to 60 mm Hg during the latter stages of an exhaustive exercise, the pressure differential (ΔP) would be 40 mm Hg. However, if 100% oxygen were being breathed, the pO_2 of the arterial blood would be approximately 600 mm Hg and the resulting ΔP would be 580 mm Hg. Since the ΔP is the driving force behind oxygen transport or diffusion, the breathing of oxygen could greatly enhance the performance, as the ΔP would be increased nearly 15-fold above normal. The possibility of this being a primary factor in explaining the ergogenic effect of oxygen is not too remote. Buskirk *et al.* (1967) demonstrated that the decrease in maximal oxygen uptake associated with increasing altitudes is a linear function of the decrease in partial pressure of oxygen; the lower the pO_2 of the ambient air, the greater the decrease in maximal oxygen uptake from sea-level values (see Fig. 5). The phenomenon discussed

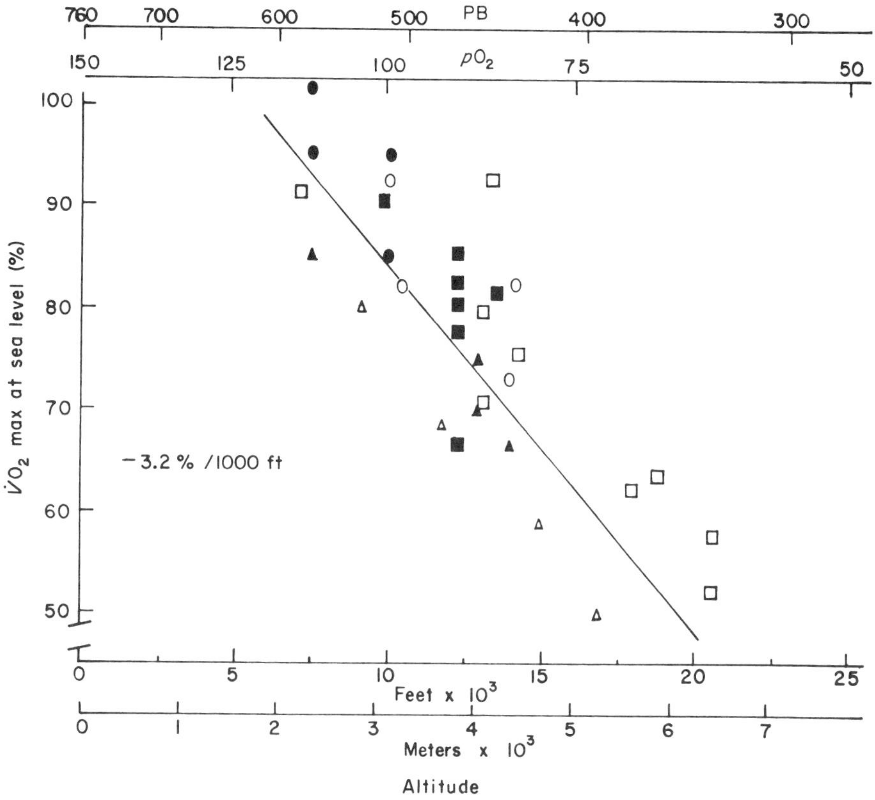

Fig. 5. Reduction in maximal oxygen intake ($\dot{V}O_2$ max) in relation to altitude, barometric pressure (PB), and the partial pressure of oxygen in the ambient air. Symbols represent data of various authors. (From Buskirk *et al.*, 1967.)

here relative to oxygen breathing would be on the opposite end of this continuum.

The above discussion certainly does not account for all of the improvement in performance found with oxygen breathing. It is well documented that there is a sixfold increase in the amount of oxygen transported in the dissolved state in the blood, although the total oxygen content of the blood is increased from only 19.8 to 22.0 ml/100 ml of blood as a result of oxygen breathing (Comroe *et al.*, 1962). It is also obvious that the reduction in ventilation volume associated with oxygen breathing is much more economical for the individual in terms of a basic conservation of energy, which can be redirected to the task at hand. Unfortunately, the final answers as to the specific mechanism(s) through which oxygen has its ergogenic effect will have to await additional research of a highly specific and controlled nature.

B. Implications

Oxygen has been demonstrated to be an effective ergogenic aid. The question now becomes one of a practical nature: How should it be used relative to athletic performances? It appears that significant improvements in performance can be obtained by breathing oxygen immediately prior to a contest or event, providing the exertion is maximal and of short duration. However, there are not too many instances in which this could be done. In track and swimming, which immediately come to mind, the time interval between the preparation for starting the race and the actual start approaches the length of time beyond which oxygen has no effect. This is true in almost all activities except possibly for wrestling and boxing.

Likewise, the application of oxygen during exercise has been proven beneficial in the performance of that exercise, but the translation of this research finding into a competitive situation is not too practical. There are few competitive situations of an endurance nature that would lend themselves to the administration of oxygen during the competition. Rowing or bicycling could be exceptions.

The administration of oxygen during the recovery period is after the fact and would be an important ergogenic aid only if the individual were going to immediately continue competition. This is the area where oxygen administration would be of greatest practical value but, unfortunately, it is not clear as to whether oxygen has an ergogenic effect during the postexercise period, despite the practices of many athletic teams today.

With regard to industrial or military situations it is quite possible that oxygen could be effectively used as an ergogenic aid. Certainly this would be true if work were being performed under less than ideal conditions, e.g., in the depths of mines or at extreme altitudes. The articles of Taunton *et al.* (1970), Banister *et al.* (1970), and Wyndham *et al.* (1970) have substantiated this in part. Unlike the typical athletic situation, there are few practical constraints that would limit the use of oxygen in either the industrial or military setting.

In conclusion, the material presented in this chapter has answered many questions. It has also posed many new questions. One big question that must certainly be answered before the results of these studies have any practical value concerns the ethics of administering oxygen to athletes to enhance their performance. Does this practice fall into the same category as that of dietary supplementation, e.g., increased minerals, vitamins, or carbohydrates? Or does this practice more closely follow the practice of administering drugs of an acute or chronic nature, such as amphetamines or anabolic steroids? The answer to this question is well beyond the scope of this chapter.

References

Asmussen, E. (1950). *Acta Physiol. Scand.* **20,** 133.

Asmussen, E., and Nielsen, M. (1946). *Acta Physiol. Scand.* **12,** 171.

Asmussen, E., and Nielsen, M. (1950). *Acta Physiol. Scand.* **20,** 79.

Asmussen, E., and Nielsen, M. (1955). *Acta Physiol. Scand.* **35,** 73.

Asmussen, E., and Nielsen, M. (1960). *Acta Physiol. Scand.* **50,** 153.

Asmussen, E., von Döbeln, W., and Nielsen, M. (1948). *Acta Physiol. Scand.* **15,** 57.

Banister, E. W., Taunton, J. E., Patrick, T., Oforsagd, P., and Duncan, W. R. (1970). *Resp. Physiol.* **10,** 74.

Bannister, R. G., and Cunningham, D. J. C. (1954). *J. Physiol.* **125,** 118.

Bean, J. W. (1945). *Physiol. Rev.* **25,** 1.

Benedict, F. G., Lee, R. C., and Strieck, F. (1935). *Arbeitsphysiologie* **8,** 266.

Bjorgum, R. K., and Sharkey, B. J. (1966). *Res. Quart.* **37,** 462.

Briggs, H. (1920). *J. Physiol.* **54,** 292.

Buskirk, E. R., Kollias, J., Piconreatigue, E., Akers, R., Prokop, E., and Baker, P. (1967). *In* "The Effects of Altitude on Physical Performance" (Roy F. Goddard, ed.), pp. 65–71. Athletic Institute, Chicago, Illinois.

Christensen, E. H., Krogh, A., and Lindhard, J. (1934). *Quart. Bull. Health Organ. League Nat.* **3,** 388.

Comroe, J. H., Forster, R. E., DuBois, A. B., Briscoe, W. A., and Carlsen, E. (1962). "The Lung." Yearbook Publ., Chicago, Illinois.

Cunningham, D. A. (1966). *Res. Quart.* **37,** 491.

Dill, D. B., Edwards, H. T., Folling, A., Oberg, S. A., Pappenheimer, A. M., and Talbott, J. H. (1931). *J. Physiol.* **71,** 47.

Douglas, C. G., and Haldane, J. S. (1909). *J. Physiol.* **39,** 1.

Dripps, R. D., and Comroe, J. H. (1947). *Amer. J. Physiol.* **149,** 277.

Elbel, E. R., Ormond, D., and Close, D. (1961). *J. Appl. Physiol.* **16,** 48.

Feldman, I., and Hill, L. (1911). *J. Physiol.* **42,** 439.

Ganong, W. F. (1963). "Review of Medical Physiology." Lange Publ., Los Altos, California.

Hagerman, F. C., Bowers, R. W., Fox, E. L., and Ersing, W. W. (1968). *Res. Quart.* **39,** 965.

Hickam, J. B., Pryor, W. W., Page, E. B., and Atwell, R. J. (1951). *J. Clin. Invest.* **30,** 503.

Hill, A. V., Long, C. N. H., and Lupton, H. (1924a). *Proc. Roy. Soc. London* **B97,** 84.

Hill, A. V., Long, C. N. H., and Lupton, H. (1924b). *Proc. Roy. Soc. London* **B97,** 155.

Hill, L., and Flack, M. (1909). *J. Physiol.* **38**, 28.
Hill, L., and Flack, M. (1910). *J. Physiol.* **40**, 347.
Hill, L., and MacKenzie, J. (1909). *J. Physiol.* **39**, 33.
Himwich, H. E., and Barr, D. P. (1923). *J. Biol. Chem.* **57**, 363.
Hughes, R. L., Clode, M., Edwards, R. H. T., Goodwin, T. J., and Jones, N. L. (1968). *J. Appl. Physiol.* **24**, 336.
Karpovich, P. V. (1934). *Res. Quart.* **5**, 24.
Karpovich, P. V. (1960). *In* "Exercise and Fitness," pp. 82–90. Athletic Institute, Chicago, Illinois.
Lundin, G., and Strom, G. (1947). *Acta Physiol. Scand.* **13**, 253.
Miller, A. T. (1952). *J. Appl. Physiol.* **5**, 165.
Mitchell, J. H., Sproule, B. J., and Chapman, C. B. (1958). *J. Clin. Invest.* **37**, 538.
Nielsen, M., and Hansen, O. (1937). *Scand. Arch. Physiol.* **76**, 37.
Rowell, L. B., Taylor, H. L., Wang, Y., and Carlson, W. S. (1964). *J. Appl. Physiol.* **19**, 284.
Taunton, J. E., Banister, E. W., Patrick, T. R., Oforsagd, P., and Duncan, W. R. (1970). *J. Appl. Physiol.* **28**, 421.
Velasquez, T., and Reynafarje, B. (1966). *Fed. Proc. Fed. Amer. Soc. Exp. Biol.* **25**, 1400.
Wyndham, C. H., Strydom, N. B., van Rensburg, A. J., and Rogers, G. G. (1970). *J. Appl. Physiol.* **29**, 552.

Chapter 12

Nutrition

Donald H. Horstman

I. Introduction

Man's search for ways to improve physical performance has taken him down many paths. Because of obvious relationships, ease of administration, and to some extent profit motivation, much of the search has been concerned with finding nutritional factors that will enhance physical performance. With the large amount of previous work in this area one could assume that the value of various nutritional factors as an aid to performance would be clarified. However, due to many factors, including individual bias, traditional beliefs and practices, and superstition, there still remains no definitive statement as to the role that various foodstuffs play in aiding performance.

The most prevalent conclusion drawn by authors who have reviewed the relationship between nutritional status and physical performance is that a well-balanced diet is all that is necessary to insure optimal performance (Mayer and Bullen, 1960; Bourne, 1968). In the mind of this author there is sufficient evidence to warrant the conclusion that optimal nutritional status for physical performance may be dependent on more than a well-balanced diet.

The primary concern of this chapter is to review the studies that have strongly suggested the ergogenic value of various nutritional factors. In summarizing the review of each nutritional factor, the author will attempt to make as positive a statement as possible, based on the available literature, relative to its effect on physical performance and its potential as an ergogenic aid.

Before considering the ergogenic role of specific nutrients, a brief discussion of caloric balance and patterns of eating seems appropriate in that these factors provide a framework in which any performance-improving nutrient must operate. Studies show that, under normal conditions, caloric intake in other than sedentary individuals is proportional to daily physical activity (Mayer *et al.*, 1956; Åstrand and Rodahl, 1970). Studies have also shown that caloric undernutrition, including starvation, results in debilitation of large muscles and concomitant decreases in work capacity (Kraut and Müller, 1946; Keys *et al.*, 1950; Taylor *et al.*, 1957). Suffice it to say that caloric balance (i.e., caloric intake equals caloric output) is a prerequisite to optimal physical performance.

Assuming that proper caloric balance is maintained, the pattern in which these calories are obtained is also, to some extent, relevant to performance. Haggard and Greenberg (1939) indicated that increased efficiency resulted from more frequent, smaller meals. This effect has more recently been attributed to the psychological effects of a rest period, with or without food administration (Hutchinson, 1952). It is still recommended that daily caloric intake be divided into at least three evenly spaced meals. The many studies of inclusion and omission of breakfast indicate the necessity of proper spacing of food intake for optimal physical performance. Breakfast is normally consumed 12–16 hours following the evening meal. Food deprivation for this time period resulted in the occurrence of hypoglycemia and decrements in work performance during the mornings when breakfast was omitted (Tuttle *et al.*, 1949, 1950, 1951; Daum *et al.*, 1950; Coleman *et al.*, 1953). Studies of the effects of varying the time interval (30 minutes to 3 hours) between eating and performance have demonstrated no significant differences in the performance times of various running and swimming events (Asprey *et al.*, 1963, 1964, 1965a,b, 1968; Ball, 1962). The general conclusion has been that food intake close to the time of performance has no deleterious effects on the subsequent performance.

II. Psychological Effect

Although a discussion of the psychological effects of diet on physical performance is not really within the scope of this chapter, perhaps a few words concerning this topic are in order before dealing with the more substantial facets of nutritional status and its relationship to performance. Athletes, and people in general, are usually convinced that certain foods are necessary in order for them to perform their best. Billy Casper has a buffalo steak before each golf match, and many people must have morning coffee before attempting to face the world. Only in very rare instances are the foods taken deleterious to performance. In some cases the food taken may be of benefit in optimizing the nutritional status for performance. For example, in the mid-1960's track athletes often consumed honey or tea laced with honey throughout the course of a track meet. The honey may have served to maintain elevated blood glucose levels and the tea may have prevented dehydration and ionic imbalances associated with the sugar ingestion, both of which may have contributed toward obtaining optimal nutritional status for performance. Regardless, the essential point is that if an athlete, or any individual, is convinced that a certain nutrient is necessary for a successful performance or a good day's work, then in all likelihood that nutrient is a necessity for that particular individual. Investigators who have studied the effects of diet on athletic performance agree that if an athlete is deprived of a nutrient which he considers essential for successful performance the chances are very good that he will not perform successfully (Van Itallie, 1968). It is hoped that this chapter will assist persons concerned with nutrition and muscular performance to distinguish between myth and fact.

III. Fuels for Performance

A. Protein

The relationship between protein intake and physical performance is usually dismissed in a few sentences as being nonexistent. However, a more in-depth coverage of this topic will be presented in this chapter. The reason is that, historically, foods containing large amounts of protein have often been most preferred by athletes, and, presently, many individuals are also using protein supplements in addition to normal dietary protein in an attempt to enhance physical performance. There is a question as to the value of protein intake greater than that found in the normal diet. It has been fairly well established that if other substrate sources are available, very little protein is used as fuel for muscular work (von Pettenkofer and Voit, 1866; Krogh and Lindhard, 1920; Cathcart and Burnett, 1926). More specific examples of this have been reported by Atwater and Benedict (1903) who found that nitrogen excretion was not raised significantly when daily energy metabolism was doubled from 2310 kcal at rest to 4556 kcal by 8 hours of moderate work, and by Hedman (1957), who found no significant differences in nitrogen excretion during rest and following 2.5 hours of hard skiing (oxygen consumption of 3.8 liters/minute). The nitrogen excretion was not elevated when exercise was continued following depletion of muscle glycogen stores.

Studies relating the level of protein intake to work performance have, for the most part, shown no beneficial effects when protein intake was increased above, nor any adverse effects when decreased below, recommended allowances. Darling *et al.* (1944) maintained three groups of subjects for 2 months on three different dietary protein regimens (low, 50 gm/day; normal, 100 gm/day; high, 160 gm/day). The subjects engaged in hard work throughout the experiment. No significant difference in physical performance among the three groups was evident. Pitts *et al.* (1944) studied three subjects with different daily protein intakes (75–150 gm/day). Physical performance was evaluated under both hot and temperate environmental conditions. Although performance did improve relative to training and acclimatization, no differences due to the varied protein intakes were observable under either environmental condition.

Rodahl *et al.* (1962) studied the effects of varying protein and/or caloric intake on physical work performance in a normal environment and during severe cold stress. Four diets were evaluated at the following daily intakes: Diet I: 3000 kcal, 70 gm protein; Diet II: 3000 kcal, 4 gm protein; Diet III: 1500 kcal, 70 gm protein; Diet IV: 1500 kcal, 4 gm protein. Base-line data were collected over several days with all subjects maintained at 22°C and consuming Diet I. Ten experimental days at 22°C on any of the remaining three diets did not result in significant changes in maximal oxygen uptake or total running time at 7.5 mph, 8.6% grade. Again following base-line measurements while subjects were maintained at 22°C on Diet I, all four diets were evaluated while subjects were exposed for prolonged periods at 8°C. No significant deterioration in physical work capacity was observed in two subjects living on Diet I for 9 days. Three subjects maintained on Diet IV showed marked deterioration and were unable to tolerate 8°C for longer than 5 days. Two subjects maintained on Diet II and two maintained on Diet III at 8°C for 3 days showed declines in maximal oxygen uptake and total running time. It was concluded that dietary stress, as caloric and/or protein deficiency, in conjunction with severe, prolonged cold stress caused a marked deterioration in physical work capacity within a few days.

In situations characterized by positive nitrogen balance and/or performance that is dependent to a great extent on muscular strength, protein intake could possibly play a role in aiding performance. Periods of normal growth in young people, athletic training in which increases in muscle mass occur, and of course the combination of the two, fit these criteria. Results of studies of protein supplementation under these conditions have varied. Kraut *et al.* (1953) submitted two subjects to 3 months of heavy physical conditioning. During this period caloric balance was maintained and the protein intake was 2 gm protein/day × kg body weight. At the end of this training period muscular strength had increased twofold and 8.3 kg of additional protein tissue was added. Physical conditioning was continued for 80 more days with a daily protein intake of 1 gm/kg body weight, resulting in an increase of protein tissue content of 1.5 kg. When physical conditioning was continued for an additional 49 days with a daily protein intake of 0.8 gm/kg body weight, nitrogen balance was attained concomitant with constant body weight and muscular strength. The authors concluded that both heavy exercise and increased protein intake were necessary for increased strength and protein tissue.

Rasch and Pierson (1962) placed 30 male college students on a weight-training program for 6 weeks. Very small protein supplementation (2.5 gm/day) was provided half the group; the other half received a placebo. At the end of 6 weeks of training both groups showed significant increases in muscular strength, with no significant difference between the increases of the protein-supplemented and placebo groups. No significant changes in body weight, arm volume, or upper arm girth occurred in either group.

Yamaji (1951a) noted that subjects being conditioned by heavy muscular work were in positive nitrogen balance. He further noted that the nitrogen retention with a daily protein intake of 2 gm/kg body weight was greater than with a diet providing 1–1.5 gm/kg body weight. Yamaji (1951b) also noted decreased levels of blood hemoglobin and albumin during the initial days of heavy physical conditioning. The actual decrease of these constituents was less and their rate of return to normal faster in the subjects with high levels of daily protein intake. The author concluded that if adequate dietary protein is not available during physical conditioning, blood proteins are used as the amino acid source for increased muscular protein.

Yoshimura (1965) has studied this latter phenomenon, which he has termed "sports anemia," in great depth. He has demonstrated a factor in the plasma following strenuous exercise that leads to an increase in erythrocyte fragility, which he has hypothesized as the cause of the decrease in blood hemoglobin. A decline in blood hemoglobin could limit physical work performance due to the decreased oxygen-carrying capacity of the blood. Sports anemia was always associated with hypoproteinemia, indicating a relationship to protein deficiency. Sports anemia did not appear in well-trained subjects and was avoided when conditioning untrained subjects by increasing the intake of low-quality protein to above 2 gm/day × kg body weight or by increasing the intake of high-quality protein (primarily meat and meat products) to above 1.2 gm/day × kg body weight. It was suggested that protein intake should conform to these levels when individuals are performing heavy work schedules.

Rasch *et al.* (1969) did not find any evidence of sports anemia in two groups of subjects who underwent vigorous physical conditioning. One group of subjects received a daily protein supplementation of an additional 1 gm/kg body weight, while the other received a placebo. These authors suggested that sports anemia is no more than simple dilution resulting from the increased plasma volume of the blood that normally accompanies physical training. In addition, physical performance as estimated from performance of pull-ups, squat thrusts, standing broad jump, and sit-ups was significantly increased in both groups following physical conditioning, although no difference between the groups was evident.

The average Western diet provides adequately for the protein requirement of the average Western man. During periods of heavy physical work or athletic conditioning the daily caloric intake is normally increased, often to as much as 5000 kcal. If the normal proportion of protein is maintained in the diet any requirement for normal growth, increased muscle tissue, or sports anemia should also be more than adequately provided. Therefore, it is doubtful that excessive protein intake or supplementation is of additional benefit to attaining an optimal nutritional level for performance.

B. Fat and Carbohydrate

With the discounting of protein, a balance of fats and carbohydrates is utilized as fuel for muscular performance. The proportional utilization of each is dependent on several factors, including severity of exercise, duration of exercise, diet, and physical fitness. The regulatory role of the diet in balancing the proportional utilization of fats and carbohydrates offers the most distinct possibility of a nutritional factor with the properties of an ergogenic aid.

Improved potential for performance can be related to certain forms of efficiency. Therefore, the three most prevalent ways in which efficiency has been defined must be considered. Storage efficiency may be defined as

Energy content (kilocalories)/unit weight of substrate (grams)

In terms of this definition of efficiency, fats are more efficient fuels than carbohydrates in that they contain about 9 kcal/gm while the latter contain only about 4 kcal/gm. Efficient substrate storage does not contribute to improving performance potential under most conditions. Mechanical efficiency, in the classical sense, may be defined as

Work output (kilocalories/minute)/oxygen consumption (kilocalories/minute)

Increases in mechanical efficiency contribute to the potential for performance as more work is accomplished per unit of energy produced. However, although dietary effects on mechanical efficiency have been reported, the mechanism involved is not well understood. Utilization efficiency may be defined as

Energy production (kilocalories/minute)/oxygen consumption (liters/minute)

The contribution of utilization efficiency to potential for performance becomes important at high work loads at which oxygen consumption is limited. More work may be accomplished from a greater energy yield per unit of oxygen consumed. There is a firm basis for dietary influences on utilization efficiency and, from the standpoint of more efficient utilization of oxygen, carbohydrate is the fuel of choice.

This can be explained by the following theoretical consideration of respiratory quotient (RQ), which is the ratio of the volume of CO_2 produced to the volume of O_2 consumed. From the equation for the oxidation of 1 mole of glucose,

$$C_6H_{12}O_6 + 6\ O_2 \rightarrow 6\ CO_2 + 6\ H_2O + 673\ \text{kcal}$$

one can see that the RQ-6 CO_2/6 O_2 = 1.00. Converting the 6 moles of O_2 to volume by multiplying by Avogadro's conversion (22.4 liters/mole), the oxidation of 1 mole of glucose requires 134.4 liters of O_2. Since the energy yield of 1 mole of glucose is 673 kcal and the oxygen required is 134.4 liters, the utilization efficiency of combusting glucose exclusively is 673 kcal/134.4 liters O_2, which equals 5.01 kcal/liter of oxygen. A similar figure is obtainable for other forms of carbohydrate. If we repeat the same procedure for the combustion of 2 moles of fat, each containing one palmitate and two stearate molecules, we find the following.

$$2(C_{55}H_{106}O_6) + 157\ O_2 \rightarrow 110\ CO_2 + 106\ H_2O + 16{,}353\ \text{kcal}$$
$$RQ = 110\ CO_2/157\ O_2 = 0.701$$
$$22.4\ \text{liters/mole} \times 157\ O_2 = 3516.8\ \text{liters of}\ O_2$$
$$16{,}353\ \text{kcal}/3516.8\ \text{liters}\ O_2 = 4.65\ \text{kcal/liter}\ O_2$$

The utilization efficiency of combusting this fat exclusively is 4.65 kcal/liter of oxygen, and again a similar figure is obtainable for other fats. The theoretical advantage of oxidizing carbohydrate exclusively is a 7–8% increase in the efficient utilization of oxygen. From the preceding we can also conclude that the relative contribution of fats and carbohydrates to energy production can be calculated from the nonprotein RQ. The relative utilization of carbohydrate increases as the RQ increases toward unity (1.00), while the relative utilization of fat decreases at the same time.

A note of caution is necessary since, in order to relate RQ to substrate utilization, the CO_2 measured in expired air must be a true representation of that actually produced from the oxygen consumed at that particular time (Åstrand, 1967). The CO_2 in expired air can be influenced by factors such as lactate production, hyperventilation, or hypoventilation, and measures of true RQ during exercise are contingent on the exercise being brought to a true steady state without influence from these factors.

That the severity of exercise influences the proportions of fat and carbohydrate utilized during exercise was first suggested by Bock *et al.* (1928). They attributed high RQ found during heavy exercise, as opposed to low RQ found during light exercise, to the preferential utilization of carbohydrate during heavy exercise. Christensen and Hansen (1939) also observed increased utilization of carbohydrate, as indicated by increased RQ, as the intensity of work was increased in subjects maintained on normal diets. Hermansen *et al.* (1967) estimated carbohydrate combustion from oxygen consumption and RQ, and directly measured muscle glycogen utilization in subjects performing 1 hour of exercise at three different relative work levels (28, 54, and 78% of maximal oxygen consumption). Glycogen utilization was a linear function of relative work load, and calculated carbohydrate combustion was a linear function of glycogen utilization. A shift to carbohydrate utilization during heavy exercise is a distinct advantage to the individual, since at this work level efficient utilization of oxygen is important to performance. At low and medium work loads, oxygen-delivery capabilities are not greatly taxed and more than sufficient oxygen is available for work performance. As the severity of exercise increases, the capacity to deliver oxygen is near the upper limit and the oxidation of a greater percentage of carbohydrate results in a greater energy yield per unit of oxygen consumed.

Having established the theoretical advantage of utilizing carbohydrate, as opposed to fat, during exercise we can now address ourselves to the factors that influence the availability of carbohydrate as substrate for exercise. Havel *et al.* (1963) measured both RQ and the oxidation of free fatty acids (FFA) directly, with radioisotopes, in human subjects performing moderate exercise. The subjects either were fasting or had previously been fed and given continued carbohydrate supplementation. The resulting respiratory quotients indicated that carbohydrate accounted for about 10% of the energy metabolism in the fasting subjects and about 80% in the previously fed subjects. The more direct measures of oxidation of FFA indicated that during the exercise FFA accounted for about 50 and 10% of energy metabolism, respectively, in the fasting and fed subjects. The implication is that, if carbohydrate is made available by simple ingestion, greater amounts of it will be utilized as substrate for exercise metabolism.

This potential for more efficient utilization of oxygen was realized in experiments in which dogs performed identical 40-minute runs (at approximately 45% of maximal oxygen consumption) on a motor-driven treadmill 1.5 and 24 hours following a high-carbohydrate meal. The rate of caloric expenditure was nearly equal under both conditions; however, the exercise oxygen cost per unit body weight 24 hours following feeding was about 10% greater than that at 1.5 hours following feeding (Young *et al.*, 1959). Horstman (1970, unpublished data) also found about 10% greater exercise oxygen cost per unit body weight when dogs performed work ranging from 40 to 70% of maximal oxygen consumption in the morning (20 hours postprandial) as opposed to afternoon (2 hours postprandial). In addition, about 5% greater mechanical efficiency was noted in the afternoon runs. Meals in these experiments consisted of laboratory chow, which is high in protein and carbohydrate and low in fat. Rodahl *et al.* (1964) found that two of four human subjects in the postabsorptive state could not complete 360 minutes of light work (1.3–1.7 liters/minute). A third subject was totally exhausted upon completion of the work. Six subjects who were provided breakfast prior to, and lunch during, the work were able to complete the task with little difficulty. Blood glucose levels were severely depressed at the completion of work in the fasting subjects, while in the fed subjects blood glucose was maintained at normal levels throughout the exercise.

Dill *et al.* (1932) studied the effects of carbohydrate supplementation on endurance capacity. In their experiments with three dogs, endurance time for the same run was at least doubled with carbohydrate supplementation during the exercise. Their experiments with the "famous" dog Joe will serve as an illustration. Under the control conditions of cool ambient temperature and water provided *ad lib.*, Joe was able to perform work at the rate of 176 kpm/minute for slightly less than 2 hours. When sugar supplement was provided at 30-minute intervals, under the same conditions, Joe performed the same work for 17 hours, at which time the investigators terminated the experiment. During a third run, at the same work load, no supplement was provided until initial exhaustion at 4.5 hours. At this time sugar supplement was provided and Joe was able to continue work for an additional 1.5 hours. Again the investigators terminated the experiment, although they expected work could have continued for several additional hours. Exhaustion in these experiments was always characterized by hypoglycemia, while blood sugar levels were elevated during the supplementation. Young *et al.* (1959) found no significant difference in working capacity between carbohydrate-supplemented and nonsupplemented dogs. However, in these experiments no attempt was made to control heat storage or fluid balance, and it is likely that exhaustion in these animals was due to other than nutritive causes.

Christensen and Hansen (1939) supplemented exhausted subjects who exhibited hypoglycemia, and symptoms thereof, with oral glucose. Glucose supplementation alleviated the hypoglycemic symptoms, elevated blood glucose levels, and the subjects were able to continue working for an additional hour. A definite relationship between exhaustion and the availability of circulating glucose has not been established. In some instances of prolonged exercise resulting in definite symtomatic hypoglycemia, concomitant with exhaustion, both hypoglycemia and exhaustion have been prevented or alleviated by carbohydrate administration. Åstrand and Rodahl (1970) have suggested that exhaustion in these instances was related to the lack of substrate for central nervous tissue metabolism, which is restricted exclusively to carbohydrate. Presently, there is no evidence that maintaining blood glucose levels above the normal range will influence exhaustion during prolonged work. From a practical standpoint, the occurrence of hypoglycemia must be prevented when considering the attainment of maximal potential for performance. This requires special consideration for athletic events that are prolonged, usually take place several hours after a meal, and/or utilize dieting as a means of controlling weight. The maintenance of normal levels of blood glucose is also a consideration for normal working performance by individuals who are dieting or tend to skip meals.

There are different ways of maintaining blood glucose levels, and no method is best for all situations. Orent-Keiles and Hallman (1949) studied the relationship between breakfast composition and blood sugar levels. These authors observed that the intake of a high-carbohydrate meal resulted in a rapid rise of blood sugar followed by an equally rapid decline to levels below normal; the subjects experienced some symptoms of hypoglycemia. High-protein meals resulted in a gradual rise in blood sugar, which remained at an elevated level throughout the testing period. Thorn *et al.* (1943) have reported similar findings. These studies indicate that the ingestion of large quantities of carbohydrate, which are rapidly absorbed into the blood, results in a boluslike increase in blood sugar levels. The ensuing release of insulin from the pancreas is large, and a large quantity of insulin is present when carbohydrate absorption is complete, resulting in a clearance of additional sugar from the blood, driving blood sugar to subnormal levels. On the other hand, protein, which is an excellent secondary source of carbohydrate, is absorbed more slowly and converted to carbohydrate, resulting in a continuous addition of small quantities of sugar to the blood. Thus, the ensuing release of insulin is in graded proportion to the gradual increase of blood sugar and no hyperinsulin response occurs, allowing blood sugar levels to remain at slightly elevated levels for a long period of time. Although individuals engaged in normal daily activities, including heavy work, should probably avoid exclusively carbohydrate meals, athletes, for whom optimal performance is a necessity, would probably benefit more from carbohydrate supplementation throughout the time of performance. This is true because the conversion of protein to carbohydrate is an energy-requiring process, and it is important that as much as possible of the energy produced by an athlete goes toward the energy requirements of the performance. Thus, the periodic intake of carbohydrate will also maintain blood glucose levels above normal throughout the performance, in effect accomplishing the same ends as a protein-enriched meal without additional energy cost.

The previous discussion has concerned the acute effects of various fuels on performance. Longer-term dietary effects of various fuels on performance have also been studied. Several studies have reported increased mechanical efficiency resulting from high-carbohydrate diets. Krogh and Lindhard (1920) found an 11% increase, and Bierring (1932) an 8% increase, in the mechanical efficiency of subjects performing a work task when maintained on high-carbohydrate diets as opposed to subjects performing an identical task when maintained on high-fat diets. Gemmill (1942) recalculated the mechanical efficiencies in both of the previous studies and found the difference in work efficiency between high-carbohydrate and high-fat diets to be closer to 5%. In any case, even an increase in mechanical efficiency of this magnitude would be beneficial to an athlete performing at maximal capacity. Marsh and Murlin (1928) reported similar differences in the mechanical efficiency of a single subject maintained on a high-carbohydrate and high-fat diet. In addition, these authors found the mechanical efficiency of the subject to be 3% greater when he was maintained on a high-carbohydrate diet, as opposed to a normal mixed diet.

Christensen and Hansen (1939) studied the effects of dietary composition on the ability to perform prolonged, heavy work. Subjects maintained on a high-carbohydrate diet for several days could perform heavy work to exhaustion more than twice as long as subjects maintained on a high-fat diet for the same period of time. Respiratory quotients indicated that carbohydrates contributed less than 30% of the energy requirements throughout the exercise when subjects were on a high-fat diet, while when subjects were on a high-carbohydrate diet, the initial energy contribution by carbohydrate was greater than 70%, followed by a gradual decline to about 40% at exhaustion.

A more exact relationship between diet, carbohydrate metabolism, and work performance has been reported by a group of Swedish investigators in a series of studies. These investigators have developed and skillfully utilized a needle biopsy technique (Bergström, 1962; Hultman, 1967a) to determine glycogen content from serially obtained samples of muscle tissue. This technique has enabled them to evaluate and relate changes of muscle glycogen metabolism to various aspects of diet and heavy work. In studies in which subjects engaged in no heavy work, starvation for 5 days resulted in a moderate decrease in muscle glycogen stores. Over a 10-day period, in which the diet of the subjects was restricted exclusively to fat and protein, decreases in muscle glycogen similar to those observed during starvation were observed. An isocaloric diet, containing exclusively carbohydrates, resulted in a slight increase in muscle glycogen stores (Hultman, 1967b).

The first direct indication that muscle glycogen serves as a fuel source for energy metabolism during exercise was provided by Bergström and Hultman (1966a). In this study four subjects performed light work (300 kpm/minute) for 30 minutes. Pre- and postexercise muscle biopsies were obtained and the tissue analyzed for glycogen content. All subjects showed a significant decline of 29% in muscle glycogen after the exercise. Ahlborg *et al.* (1967) measured pre- and postexercise blood glucose and muscle glycogen concentrations in nine postabsorptive subjects. Work to exhaustion was performed at about 60% of W_{170} (mean: 710 kpm/minute). Postexercise concentrations of both blood glucose and muscle glycogen were significantly lower than preexercise resting values, and the glycogen stores of most of the subjects were almost totally depleted at exhaustion. Significant relationships were found between initial muscle glycogen concentration and total work time to exhaustion, and between initial muscle glycogen concentration and total energy developed during the exercise. At a later time the same procedure was carried out with two subjects receiving intravenous glucose administration. In spite of the fact that blood glucose concentration was elevated above 200 mg/100 ml, muscle glycogen was depleted to the same levels as during work without glucose administration. These investigators suggested that muscle glycogen is a limiting factor to work performance, even with the availability of more than adequate amounts of circulating glucose. Hermansen *et al.* (1967) studied trained and untrained subjects performing continuous and intermittent heavy exercise (mean: 76% of maximal oxygen consumption) to exhaustion. Muscle glycogen concentration, oxygen consumption, and RQ were determined before, at several intervals during, and after the exercise. Insignificant differences in the rate of muscle glycogen utilization between the trained and untrained subjects, and between the intermittent and continuous work, were observed. The exercise was characterized by a continuous fall in muscle glycogen concentration, and again exhaustion was accompanied by almost total depletion of muscle glycogen stores. Carbohydrate combustion, as calculated from oxygen consumption and RQ, was relatively constant throughout the exercise, while the rate of glycogen utilization declined as exercise progressed, reaching a very low rate during the final portion of the exercise. The authors speculated that during this final work period either another source of carbohydrate was made available to working muscle or previously inactive muscle tissue was brought into play. Correlation of performance time with initial muscle glycogen concentration was not possible due to the homogeneity of the latter.

The above studies suggest that the capacity to perform prolonged work may be influenced by the glycogen content of the working muscle. Therefore, if a means for increasing muscle glycogen content were available, the relationship between work capacity and muscle glycogen content could be clarified by study of a large range of muscle glycogen concentrations. In addition, if work capacity is a function of muscle glycogen content, then the means for improving this performance-related variable would also be available. Bergström and Hultman (1966b) have provided such a means. They employed one-legged exercise to exhaustion on a bicycle ergometer, with the nonexercised leg serving as a control. Following the exercise, subjects were maintained for 3 days on diets consisting almost exclusively of carbohydrate. Muscle biopsies were performed following the exercise and each morning of the subsequent 3 days, and glycogen concentration was determined. Following exercise, glycogen concentration from muscle of the control leg was at a normal level and exhibited a slight increase over the next 3 days. Glycogen content in the exercised leg was essentially depleted following the exercise but rapidly increased thereafter, attaining a level slightly greater than control after day 1 and a level about two times that of the control after day 3. In subjects maintained on diets containing almost exclusively fat and protein, following depletion by prolonged exercise, Hultman (1967b) found muscle glycogen concentration to be below the preexercise resting level even after 8 days. Thus, the muscle glycogen content could be varied over a broad range in the same subjects by controlling the diet following muscle glycogen depletion.

Bergström *et al.* (1967) then studied the interrelationship of diet, muscle glycogen, and physical performance. Each of their subjects was maintained at all of three different isocaloric diets: mixed, high fat and protein, and high carbohydrate. Subjects worked to exhaustion at 75% of maximal oxygen consumption after at least 3 days of maintenance on each of the diets. Work time to exhaustion was noted, and oxygen consumption and RQ were measured periodically during the exercise. Pre- and postexercise muscle glycogen content was also determined. Muscle glycogen was essentially depleted upon completion of the exercise after all three of the diets. The mean initial muscle glycogen concentrations following the mixed diet, the diet containing high fat and protein, and the high-carbohydrate diet were 1.75, 0.63, and 3.31 gm/100 gm wet muscle, respectively. The mean maximal working times were 113.6 minutes after the mixed diet, 56.9 minutes after the diet of high fat and protein, and 166.5 minutes after the high-carbohydrate diet. When data from all subjects, under all three dietary conditions, were compared, a linear correlation of 0.92 was found between work time to exhaustion and initial muscle glycogen content. A linear correlation of 0.92 was also found between carbohydrate combustion, as calculated from oxygen consumption and RQ, and muscle glycogen utilization during the exercise. These results clearly establish muscle glycogen stores as one of the variables on which optimal performance is dependent. These data also demonstrate that a high-carbohydrate diet, following depletion of glycogen from the muscle, results in increased muscle glycogen stores, thereby improving performance capacity.

A more practical demonstration of this relationship was provided by Karlsson and Saltin (1971). On two occasions (one being actual competition) subjects participated in a 30-km race, once after muscle glycogen depletion followed by a high-carbohydrate diet and once after a mixed diet. The average muscle glycogen concentration resulting from the high-carbohydrate diet was about twice that resulting from the mixed diet. Times for the 30 km were faster in all subjects following the high-carbohydrate diet than following the mixed diet; the mean difference was about 8 minutes. In addition, analysis of the split times for the races revealed that the pace during the early portion of both races was about the same and that a difference in pace between the two races was observable during the later portion of the races. This fall in running speed was associated with decreased levels of muscle glycogen.

From the preceding it is obvious that increasing muscle glycogen stores results in increased performance capacity, especially in endurance events. It is also obvious that muscle glycogen stores can be increased by dietary manipulation. In light of this, Åstrand (1968) has made some recommendations for proper preparation for athletic events longer than 30 minutes. He suggests depleting, by heavy exercise, the muscle glycogen stores in the same muscles that will be used in the event about a week prior to competition. This should be followed by a 3-day diet consisting primarily of fats and protein. Finally, large amounts of carbohydrate should be added to the diet during the 3–4 days immediately preceding competition. Two additional suggestions may also be added to these recommendations: first, to avoid heavy exercise during the days just before the event and, second, to take sugar supplementation during the course of the event.

IV. Vitamins

Along with excessive protein intake, vitamin supplementation is also a practice of athletes and other people seeking to improve the level of their performance. The question, again, is of what value, if any, is this vitamin supplementation. It is known that outright vitamin deficiencies impair physical performance. Indeed, fatigue and the inability to physically function are listed among the classical symptoms of most vitamin-deficiency states. A role in improving performance by supplementation has been suggested for the B-complex vitamins, especially thiamine (B_1), vitamin C, and vitamin E.

A. Vitamin B

The coenzyme activity of the B-complex vitamins forms an integral part of the respiratory chain in the metabolism of fats and carbohydrates. Because metabolism during muscular exercise is greatly increased, it is somewhat logical to assume that the requirements for B-complex vitamins are also increased. Bicknell and Prescott (1945) have estimated that the thiamine requirement (one could also assume the requirement for all B-complex vitamins) during severe exercise is about 15 times greater than at rest. This increase corresponds very well with the increase in metabolism during severe exercise, and one could assume the daily requirements for B vitamins to be a function of daily metabolism. The daily metabolism of athletes or individuals engaged in heavy work is two to three times greater than that of their more sedentary counterparts, and it is probable that their requirements for vitamin B are also increased to this extent.

Several studies (Archdeacon and Murlin, 1944; Foltz *et al.*, 1944; Johnson *et al.*, 1942) have shown that diets deficient in thiamine and low in B-complex vitamins, in conjunction with daily heavy exercise, lead to a relatively rapid onset of symptoms of thiamine deficiency. Williams *et al.* (1940) have further shown that thiamine-deficiency symptoms appeared much more rapidly in active subjects when compared with sedentary subjects maintained on the same low-thiamine diet. The time of onset of thiamine-deficiency symptoms in these studies ranged from about 1 to 8 weeks depending on the severity of thiamine restriction, which ranged from 0.05 to 0.38 mg/1000 kcal.

In a series of well-controlled experiments, Keys and associates (1943, 1944, 1945) also studied the relationship between thiamine intake and physical activity. No diminution of strength, endurance, speed, or coordination was noted in moderately active subjects (3000 kcal/day) maintained for 10–12 weeks on thiamine intakes between 0.23 and 0.96 mg/1000 kcal. Moderately active subjects (3300 kcal/day) receiving low B-complex vitamin intakes for 161 days also showed no decrements in work performance. No decrement in performance was noted in subjects maintained for 40 days on low B-complex vitamin intakes (0.16 mg thiamine/1000 kcal) with metabolic costs of up to 4800 kcal/day. Following 161 moderately active days on low B-complex vitamin intake (0.19 mg thiamine/1000 kcal), further restriction of B-complex intake (0.008 mg thiamine/1000 kcal) and increase of metabolic cost to 4000 kcal/day resulted in decreased physical performance after only 8 days. Previously vitamin-supplemented subjects experienced physical performance decrements after 13 days of the same severely restricted B-complex vitamin intake and increased daily metabolic cost. It was suggested that the status of B-complex vitamin stores prior to periods of vitamin deficiency, conjuncted with heavy work, influenced the rate at which deficiency symptoms (including decreased work performance) occurred.

The case for B-complex supplementation is hazy. Field studies have reported beneficial effects. Gounelle (1940) reported improved performance, as judged by order of finish in international competition, in cyclists given high supplementation of thiamine. McCormick (1940) found the same to be true for swimmers. Frankau (1943) found the performance time of shuttle running to be significantly improved with B-complex supplementation, while placebo administration did not show the same.

More controlled laboratory studies have reported no beneficial effects from B-complex supplementation. Simonson *et al.* (1942) and Keys and Henschel (1942) noted no improvement in endurance, efficiency, or strength with B-complex supplementation of subjects whose daily activity ranged from moderate to heavy. Henschel *et al.* (1944) noted no difference in the ability to perform in the heat between B-complex-supplemented subjects and placebo controls. Acclimatization and the ability to perform heavy work during periods of up to 1 week of heat exposure were also the same in both groups of subjects.

A relationship between thiamine requirements and daily metabolic activity is highly probable. Bourne (1948) and Vytchikova (1958) have recommended increases in daily thiamine intake for athletes and individuals engaged in heavy physical activity above the recommended 1.5–2.0 mg/day. However, both the caloric and protein intake of these individuals are also elevated to meet metabolic demands, and it is likely that the additional requirement for B-complex vitamins will be adequately met by the diet, protein being an excellent source of these constituents.

B. Vitamin C

Possible justification for vitamin C (ascorbic acid) supplementation also has some theoretical basis. Like the B-complex vitamins a role in energy metabolism has been ascribed to vitamin C, being placed in the electron transport chain between DPNH and one of the cytochromes (Staudinger *et al.,* 1961). Administration of ascorbic acid to *in vitro* preparations of blood resulted in a distinct shift of the oxygen dissociation curve to the right, the amount of shift being directly proportional to the ascorbic acid concentration (Horejsi, 1970). If present *in vivo,* this type of shift could facilitate oxygen unloading and increase the amount of oxygen available to the cell.

Vitamin C deficiency resulted in decreased work performance; the reported times of onset of reduced work performance were noted as 2 months (Johnson *et al.,* 1945), 3 months (Crandon *et al.,* 1940), and 4 months (Farmer, 1944) following the beginning of diets deficient in vitamin C. Keys (1943), in reviewing earlier studies, noted no improvement in work performance in a normal environment with vitamin C supplementation up to 270 mg/day and no improvement in the performance of hard work in the heat with supplementation up to 540 mg/day.

A renewed interest in vitamin C supplementation was brought about by the excellent showing of the Russian athletes at the Rome Olympics in 1960, which they attributed, in part, to elevated vitamin C intakes. Van Huss (1966) has reviewed the more recent studies (all of foreign origin) of vitamin C supplementation that show beneficial effects. According to Van Huss, Des Marais, a Canadian, showed that vitamin C-supplemented rats were able to continue running in a revolving drum for longer periods than controls. Prokop, of Vienna, supplemented vitamin C (100 mg/day) in athletes with normal serum ascorbic acid levels and found improvements in physical performance. Hoitink, a Dutch worker, showed all-out work performance to be greater immediately following 1–2 weeks of vitamin C supplementation (300 mg/day) than that prior to, or 1–2 weeks after, the supplementation period. Russian investigators have also supported vitamin C supplementation. Yakolev has suggested daily requirements ranging from 75 mg for the recovery period from speed or strength exercises to 300 mg for prolonged endurance exercises. Efremova has recommended daily intakes of 100 and 200 mg of vitamin C for nonathletes engaging in light and heavy work, respectively. Van Huss (1966), himself, evaluated the acute effects of both natural and synthetic vitamin C supplementation on work performance. Supplementation was given 2 hours prior to work performance tests of 10 minutes of running at a submaximal work load or an all-out run at near maximal work load. Strength, reaction time, and recovery measures were also obtained. Results from this study did not show any difference in the effects on performance of vitamin C and placebo (control) supplementation. Enhancement of the recovery process, i.e., a faster return to normal, was noted in the vitamin C-supplemented subjects. Taken as a whole, the more recent studies suggest that vitamin C supplementation may improve physical performance, while the older literature negates this contention. Further controlled studies of longer periods of supplementation and its effect on endurance work performance (prolonged time at a submaximal work load) are needed to clarify the role of vitamin C as an ergogenic aid.

C. Vitamin E

Cureton (1954) and Cureton and Pohndorf (1955) studied the effects of wheat germ oil supplementation, concomitant with hard physical training, on physical performance by middle-aged subjects. They found that subjects taking only wheat germ oil, without physical training, showed no improvement. Subjects taking wheat germ oil and receiving physical training showed significantly greater improvement on tests of treadmill running time and other performance parameters than did placebo controls undergoing physical training. However, Cureton and Pohndorf (1963) did not show any beneficial effects from wheat germ supplementation in similar experiments with younger subjects. Thomas (1957) supplemented athletes in training with vitamin E. Two groups of subjects were given vitamin E or placebo for 5 weeks, and then the administration of vitamin E or placebo was reversed in the groups for an additional 5 weeks. No differences in performance parameters between the two groups were noted in measurements made at 0, 5, and 10 weeks. The value of vitamin E (wheat germ products) as an aid to performance, is open to question and must await further investigation.

V. Summary

It has been previously concluded that a well-balanced diet is all that is necessary to insure optimal performance. Assuming that proper caloric balance is maintained, the evidence suggests that proper dietary manipulation can result in performance improvements.

It is doubtful that excessive protein intake or protein supplementation is of benefit to attaining an optimal nutritional level for performance. A need for increased protein intake during periods of positive nitrogen balance, as when prolonged heavy work is performed during athletic training, has been demonstrated. In addition, a phenomenon termed "sports anemia," which is characterized by decreased levels of blood hemoglobin and albumin during the initial days of heavy physical conditioning, has been observed and shown to be a function of relative protein deficiency. However, the proportion of protein in the average Western diet provides more than the normal protein requirements, and if this proportion is maintained during periods of increased caloric intake and requirements, any additional protein requirements will be more than adequately provided.

Under normal conditions the actual fuels for performance are restricted to a balance of fats and carbohydrates. The theoretical efficiency of oxygen utilization increases as the proportion of carbohydrate oxidized increases. A shift to carbohydrate utilization has been shown to occur during heavy exercise. This is a distinct advantage as it is at this work level, when the capacity to deliver oxygen is near the upper limit, that efficient utilization of oxygen becomes important to performance. Dietary manipulation has been demonstrated as one of the most important factors that influences the availability of carbohydrate as substrate for exercise. It has been demonstrated that, if carbohydrate is made available by simple ingestion, greater amounts of it are utilized as substrate for exercise metabolism. Carbohydrate supplementation has been shown to prevent or alleviate exhaustion associated with the hypoglycemia that often occurs during very prolonged work. Longer-term dietary studies have also indicated that increased carbohydrate intake enhances performance potential. Several studies have reported increased mechanical efficiency resulting from maintaining subjects on high-carbohydrate diets. Subjects maintained on high-carbohydrate diets could also perform heavy work to exhaustion much longer than subjects maintained on high-fat or mixed diets. A direct relationship between the initial muscle glycogen level and the ability to perform prolonged heavy work has been demonstrated, exhaustion being associated with almost total depletion of muscle glycogen stores. Increasing muscle glycogen stores has resulted in increased performance capacity, especially in endurance events. Muscle glycogen stores can be increased by dietary manipulation, and the following procedure is recommended for preparation for endurance events.

1. About a week prior to competition, the depletion, by heavy exercise, of the muscle glycogen stores in the same muscles that will be used in the event
2. Immediately following this a 3-day diet consisting of fats and protein
3. The addition of large amounts of carbohydrate to the diet during the 3–4 days just preceding competition
4. The avoidance of heavy exercise during the days just before the event
5. Sugar supplementation during the course of the event

Vitamin supplementation is a common practice among athletes. An increased need for B-complex vitamins has been demonstrated for athletes and others with greatly increased daily metabolic activity. However, as is the case with protein, it is likely that the additional requirement for B-complex vitamins is adequately met by the increased dietary intake. There is available subjective evidence that vitamin C supplementation enhances performance potential, and some support for this contention is available in the current scientific literature. Although definitive studies have yet to be performed, vitamin C supplementation probably offers the best possibility of a vitamin with ergogenic value. Proof of this awaits further investigation. Ergogenic benefits have also been suggested for vitamin E, but this conclusion seems highly questionable.

References

Ahlborg, B., Bergström, J., Ekelund, L.-G., and Hultman, E. (1967). *Acta Physiol. Scand.* **70**, 129.

Archdeacon, J. W., and Murlin, J. R. (1944). *J. Nutr.* **28**, 241.

Asprey, G. M., Alley, L. E., and Tuttle, W. W. (1963). *Res. Quart.* **34**, 267.

Asprey, G. M., Alley, L. E., and Tuttle, W. W. (1964). *Res. Quart.* **35**, 227.

Asprey, G. M., Alley, L. E., and Tuttle, W. W. (1965a). *Res. Quart.* **36**, 233.

Asprey, G. M., Alley, L. E., and Tuttle, W. W. (1965b). *J. Amer. Diet. Ass.* **47**, 198.

Asprey, G. M., Alley, L. E., and Tuttle, W. W. (1968). *Res. Quart.* **39**, 231.

Åstrand, P.-O. (1967). *In* "Nutrition and Physical Activity" (G. Blix, ed.), pp. 7–15. Almqvist & Wiksell, Stockholm.

Åstrand, P.-O. (1968). *Nutr. Today* **3**, 9.

Åstrand, P.-O., and Rodahl, K. (1970). "Textbook of Work Physiology." McGraw-Hill, New York.

Atwater, W. O., and Benedict, F. G. (1903). *U. S. Dep. Agr. Tech. Bull.* No. 136, 126–187.

Ball, J. R. (1962). *Res. Quart.* **33**, 163.

Bergström, J. (1962). *Scand. J. Clin. Lab. Invest. Suppl.* **14**, No. 68, 1–110.

Bergström, J., and Hultman, E. (1966a). *Scand. J. Clin. Lab. Invest.* **18**, 16.

Bergström, J., and Hultman, E. (1966b). *Nature* **210**, 309.

Bergström, J., Hermansen, L., Hultman, E., and Saltin, B. (1967). *Acta Physiol. Scand.* **71**, 140.

Bicknell, F., and Prescott, F. (1945). "The Vitamins in Medicine." Heineman, London.

Bierring, E. (1932). *Arbeitsphysiologie* **5**, 17.

Bock, A. V., Vancaulaert, C., Dill, D. B., Fölling, A., and Hurxthal, L. (1928). *J. Physiol.* **66**, 162.

Bourne, G. H. (1948). *Brit. J. Nutr.* **2**, 261.

Bourne, G. H. (1968). *In* "Exercise Physiology" (H. B. Falls, ed.), pp. 155–172. Academic Press, New York.

Cathcart, E. P., and Burnett, W. A. (1926). *Proc. Roy. Soc. London Soc.* **B99**, 405.

Christensen, E. H., and Hansen, O. (1939). *Scand. Arch. Physiol.* **81**, 160.

Coleman, M. C., Tuttle, W. W., and Daum, K. (1953). *J. Amer. Diet. Ass.* **29,** 239.
Crandon, J. H., Lund, C. C., and Dill, D. B. (1940). *N. Engl. J. Med.* **223,** 353.
Cureton, T. K. (1954). *Amer. J. Physiol.* **179,** 628.
Cureton, T. K., and Pohndorf, R. (1955). *Res. Quart.* **26,** 391.
Cureton, T. K., and Pohndorf, R. (1963). *Res. Quart.* **34,** 440.
Darling, R. C., Johnson, R. E., Pitts, G. C., Consolazio, F. C., and Robinson, P. F. (1944). *J. Nutr.* **28,** 273.
Daum, K., Tuttle, W. W., Martin, C., and Myers, L. (1950). *J. Amer. Diet. Ass.* **26,** 503.
Dill, D. B., Edwards, H. T., and Talbott, J. H. (1932). *J. Physiol.* **77,** 49.
Farmer, C. J. (1944). *Fed. Proc. Fed. Amer. Soc. Exp. Biol.* **3,** 179.
Foltz, E. C., Barborka, C. J., and Ivy, A. C. (1944). *Gastroenterology* **2,** 323.
Frankau, I. M. (1943). *Brit. Med. J.* **2,** 601.
Gemmill, C. L. (1942). *Physiol. Rev.* **22,** 32.
Gounelle, H. (1940). *Bull. Soc. Med. Hop. Paris* **56,** 225.
Haggard, H. W., and Greenberg, L. A. (1939). "Diet and Physical Efficiency." Yale Univ. Press, New Haven, Connecticut.
Havel, R. J., Naimark, A., and Borchgrevink, C. F. (1963). *J. Clin. Invest.* **42,** 1054.
Hedman, R. (1957). *Acta Physiol. Scand.* **40,** 305.
Henschel, A. F., Taylor, H. L., Mickelsen, O., Brozek, J. M., and Keys, A. (1944). *Fed. Proc. Fed. Amer. Soc. Exp. Biol.* **3,** 18.
Hermansen, L., Hultman, E., and Saltin, B. (1967). *Acta Physiol. Scand.* **71,** 129.
Horejsi, J. (1970). *In* "Red Cell Metabolism and Function" (G. J. Brewer, ed.), pp. 9–20. Plenum, New York.
Hultman, E. (1967a). *Scand. J. Clin. Lab. Invest. Suppl.* **94,** 1.
Hultman, E. (1967b). *In* "Physiology of Muscular Exercise" (C. B. Chapman, ed.), pp. 99–114. Amer. Heart Ass., New York.
Hutchinson, R. C. (1952). *Nutr. Abstr. Rev.* **22,** 283.
Johnson, R. E., Darling, R. C., Forbes, W. H., Brouha, E., Egana, E., and Graybiel, A. (1942). *J. Nutr.* **24,** 585.
Johnson, R. E., Darling, R. C., Sargent, F., and Robinson, P. (1945). *J. Nutr.* **29,** 155.
Karlsson, J., and Saltin, B. (1971). *J. Appl. Physiol.* **31,** 203.
Keys, A. (1943). *Fed. Proc. Fed. Amer. Soc. Exp. Biol.* **2,** 164.
Keys, A., and Henschel, A. F. (1942). *J. Nutr.* **23,** 259.
Keys, A., Henschel, A. F., Mickelsen, O., and Brozek, J. M. (1943). *J. Nutr.* **26,** 399.
Keys, A., Henschel, A. F., Mickelsen, O., Brozek, J. M., and Crawford, J. H. (1944). *J. Nutr.* **27,** 165.
Keys, A., Henschel, A. F., Taylor, H. L., Mickelsen, O., and Brozek, J. M. (1945). *Amer. J. Physiol.* **144,** 5.
Keys, A., Brozek, J., Henschel, A., Mickelsen, O., Taylor, H. L., and Simonson, E. (1950). "The Biology of Human Starvation." Univ. of Minnesota Press, Minneapolis.
Kraut, H. A., and Müller, E. A. (1946). *Science* **104,** 495.
Kraut, H., Müller, E. A., and Müller-Wecker, H. (1953). *Biochem. Z.* **324,** 280.
Krogh, A., and Lindhard, J. (1920). *Biochem. J.* **14,** 290.
McCormick, W. J. (1940). *Med. Rec.* **152,** 439.
Marsh, M. E., and Murlin, J. R. (1928). *J. Nutr.* **1,** 105.
Mayer, J., and Bullen, B. (1960). *Physiol. Rev.* **40,** 369.
Mayer, J., Roy, P., and Mitra, K. P. (1956). *Amer. J. Clin. Nutr.* **4,** 169.

Orent-Keiles, E., and Hallman, L. F. (1949). *U. S. Dep. Agr. Circ.* No. 827.
Pitts, G. C., Consolazio, F. C., and Johnson, R. E. (1944). *J. Nutr.* **27**, 497.
Rasch, P. J., and Pierson, W. R. (1962). *Amer. J. Clin. Nutr.* **11**, 530.
Rasch, P. J., Hamby, J. W., and Burns, H. J., Jr. (1969). *Med. Sci. Sports* **1**, 195.
Rodahl, K., Horvath, S. M., Birkhead, N. C., and Issekutz, B., Jr. (1962). *J. Appl. Physiol.* **17**, 763.
Rodahl, K., Miller, H. I., and Issekutz, B., Jr. (1964). *J. Appl. Physiol.* **19**, 489.
Simonson, E., Enzer, N., Baer, A., and Braun, R. (1942). *J. Ind. Hyg.* **24**, 83.
Staudinger, H., Krisch, K., and Loenhäuser, S. (1961). *Ann. N. Y. Acad. Sci.* **92**, 195.
Taylor, H. L., Buskirk, E. R., Brozek, J., Anderson, J. T., and Grande, F. (1957). *J. Appl. Physiol.* **10**, 421.
Thomas, P. (1957). Thesis, Univ. of Southern California, Los Angeles.
Thorn, G. W., Quimby, J. T., Clinton, M., Jr. (1943). *Ann. Intern. Med.* **18**, 913.
Tuttle, W. W., Wilson, M., and Daum, K. (1949). *J. Appl. Physiol.* **1**, 545.
Tuttle, W. W., Daum, K., Myers, L., and Martin, C. (1950). *J. Amer. Diet. Ass.* **26**, 332.
Tuttle, W. W., Daum, K., Imig, C. J., Martin, C., and Kisgen, R. (1951). *J. Amer. Diet. Ass.* **27**, 190.
Van Huss, W. D. (1966). *Nutr. Today* **1**, 20.
Van Itallie, T. (1968). *Nutr. Today* **3**, 2.
Von Pettenkofer, M., and Voit, C. (1866). *Z. Biol.* **2**, 459.
Vytchikova, M. A. (1958). *Chem. Abstr.* **52**, 14787.
Williams, R. D., Mason, H. L., Wilder, R. M., and Smith, B. F. (1940). *AMA Arch. Intern. Med.* **66**, 785.
Yamaji, R. (1951a). *J. Physiol. Soc. Jap.* **13**, 476.
Yamaji, R. (1951b). *J. Physiol. Soc. Jap.* **13**, 483.
Yoshimura, H. (1965). *In* "Proceedings, Symposia on Arctic Biology" (L. Vaughan, ed.), Vol. V, pp. 85–120. Fort Wainwright, Alaska.
Young, D. R., Iacovino, A., Erve, R., Mosher, R., and Spector, H. (1959). *J. Appl. Physiol.* **14**, 1013.

Chapter 13

Drugs and Hormones

Lawrence A. Golding

I. Introduction

Ever since the advent of athletic competition, man has sought the magic ingredient that would make the super athlete or would at least give him a winning edge over his opponent. The use of drugs, foods, and other substances for ergogenic purposes is as old as athletics itself. Athletes and coaches strive for maximal performance and are always willing to experiment with possible ergogenic aids.

When an individual breaks a record or performs extraordinarily well, one immediately examines his training regime or his diet to determine whether a unique training method or a new diet or drug enabled him to excel. Unfortunately, the proven and acceptable training methods are too often obscured by fads and fallacies associated with the use of so-called ergogenic aids. Because of these fads, hard work and scientific training procedures are too often abandoned. Almost every drug that is claimed to favorably affect any system of the body, especially the muscular, respiratory, or circulatory system, has at one time or another been suggested as an adjunct to a regular training program.

The dictionary defines ergogenic as something that "tends to increase work output, especially by eliminating fatigue symptoms." In this broad frame of reference, vitamins, carbohydrates, proteins, or any substance that is depleted during prolonged physical activity, or is necessary for normal health maintenance, might be considered ergogenic. However, in this chapter, I shall refer to ergogenic aids only as those substances that are not found in normal diets but are taken for the express purpose of improving performance. Vitamins can be included in this category only if taken in excessive amounts.

Any drug that pharmacologically aids the muscular, circulatory, or respiratory system is a potential ergogenic drug. Digitalis, Coramine, lecithin, and cocaine have been used in experiments on human performance because of their stimulating effects on these systems. Some alkaline preparations have been suggested as antifatigue substances because they may counteract the increased acidity of the blood during and after exercise. Most of these drugs have proven useless in aiding physical performance. Even adrenaline, a hormone known to prepare the body for action, when supplied exogenously does not improve physical performance.

Still the search goes on for some synthetic substance that will increase physical performance beyond the limits of traditional physical training. Drugs that have been proven worthless have been abandoned in favor of newer drugs with the fervent hope that, at last, *something* will take the athlete beyond his present capabilities.

Many substances have been tried as ergogenic aids. The philosophy of many athletes is that unless the substance is harmful, it might as well be tried; however, too often the contraindications of many of the drugs are unknown. Even drugs known to be dangerous are sometimes used if there is any indication that the drug will aid the athlete's performance. A search of the literature reveals many studies investigating the effect of drugs, hormones, diet supplements, and other substances on physical and mental performance. Some substances seem more popular than others either because their properties suggest that they should improve performance, or because studies have shown them to have some benefit. The following are among the many substances studied.

Adrenaline	Negative ionized air
Alcohol	Noradrenaline
Alkalies	Oxygen
Amphetamines	Phosphates
Aspartates	Protein
Caffeine	Sodium chloride

Cocaine	Steroids
Coramine	Sulfa drugs
Gelatin	Ultraviolet
Lecithin	Vitamins
Metrazol	Wheat germ oil

Many of these substances are actually categories of substances and can be further expanded. The amphetamines, for example, include four major types and each of these is more commonly referred to by its trade name—Benzedrine or Dexedrine.

Many substances have never been carefully studied; others have merited only one or two studies. The long list of possible ergogenic drugs can be reduced to very few, since there are only three or four drugs actually used by athletes today about which some controversy exists.

This chapter will discuss some of the more commonly used drugs: amphetamines, androgenic–anabolic steroids, and aspartates. The first part will deal with the amphetamines, which have been researched extensively, and the anabolic steroids, about which comparatively little has been written. Medical authorities have condemned the use of these drugs on ethical as well as medical grounds, with apparently little effect; their use is still widespread. It is not the purpose of the author to condone or condemn the use of drugs by athletes, but to report the results of available studies. The author has taken great care to present the research in a scientific and unbiased manner. However, philosophical and psychological implications are necessary and desirable when one discusses the emotionally packed issues involved in the use of amphetamines and anabolic steroids.

Every study has limitations. No study can be completely controlled, contain no false assumptions, or cover every eventuality. But any scientific evidence, even from a limited number of subjects or from a poorly controlled study, is better than testimonial information or "old wives' tales." We cannot be so close-minded that we refuse to accept the validity of studies that show beneficial effects from drugs, simply because we have a personal bias or because the results oppose convention. Open-mindedness must be maintained. The present-day coach, trainer, physician, and athlete are desperately seeking factual and scientific evidence concerning the use of drugs, and the following review will attempt to give that evidence.

A. Experimental Design for Drug Studies

The design of experiments varies, depending on (a) the number of subjects, (b) the experimental treatment, (c) statistical design, and

(d) the type of phenomena being investigated. In drug studies it is desirable to have a large number of subjects so that the statistical conclusions apply to the general population. However, many times because of the nature of the drugs being used, studies must be done with a limited number of subjects and must often be case studies.

In drug studies it is also desirable to follow a double-blind design. This means that a placebo is used and that neither the subject nor the researcher knows whether the subject being tested has taken the drug or the placebo on any particular test day. The placebo must look, taste, and smell like the drug being tested. It must also be an inert substance that cannot have any effect on the subject's performance or on any of the test results.

Because of informed consent requirements established by the federal government, human experimentation has become extremely difficult, and the double-blind procedure has become impossible to maintain. Subjects usually must be adults, and granting agencies are hesitant to approve studies using dangerous or questionable drugs, even though subjects agree to take the drugs.

A number of studies on anabolic steroids have been done by researchers who have known athletes who are using steroids or who plan on using them. They have contacted these athletes and asked them to be measured and tested prior to their taking the steroids and then have tested them again after they have used the drug. This system makes a double-blind procedure impossible; yet the opportunity to test individuals who plan on taking drugs is too good an opportunity to miss, simply because a double-blind procedure cannot be followed.

Studies investigating the effect of amphetamine require the use of a placebo since the phenomenon being studied is the psychological effect. The placebo is the only mechanism to ensure the control of psychological advantages or disadvantages.

As previously mentioned, if drug studies had to always follow accepted and desirable research designs, few studies would be undertaken and less information than we now have would be available. Objective measurements on individuals using drugs are better than testimonial information and wishful thinking of users.

II. Amphetamines

Dextroamphetamine sulfate is a powerful central nervous system stimulant that increases alertness, attentiveness, and the ability to do mental tasks. It is more popularly known for its ability to reduce or abolish the sense of fatigue and to depress appetite. Being a sympathomimetic drug, it is capable of causing vasoconstriction, increased blood pressure and heart rate, respiratory stimulation, smooth muscle relaxation in the bronchi, pupillary dilation, elevated blood sugar, and increased muscle tension. The ordinary therapeutic dosage used to achieve cortical stimulation is 5–10 mg.

Amphetamine is described as a white, odorless, crystalline powder that is slightly soluble in alcohol and freely soluble in water. A 5% solution in water has a pH of 5–6. It can be obtained legally only by prescription and is sold in tablets, ampules, and sustained-release capsules.

In this chapter, the term amphetamine will be used to refer to racemic amphetamine, the dextrorotatory isomer *d*-amphetamine, and methamphetamine. The amphetamines are available for use as the free bases and salts; most commonly these are amphetamine, *d*-amphetamine sulfate, and methamphetamine hydrochloride. These drugs are sold in drugstores under a variety of trade names. The amphetamines are often in combination with barbiturates to soften the effect on the central nervous system.

In the mid-1950's the alleged widespread use of amphetamine by athletes during competition was brought to the attention of the American Medical Association. In 1957 the AMA appointed a Committee on Amphetamine and Athletics. Questionnaires were sent to coaches, trainers, and athletes, requesting information on the use of amphetamine by athletes. When the questionnaires were returned and tabulated, less than 1% indicated any knowledge of the use of amphetamine during athletic performance. A similar survey was conducted by the American College of Sports Medicine in 1958. Thirty-five percent of the returned questionnaires indicated that amphetamine was being used by athletes during competition.

With so much interest and controversy being generated by the use of amphetamine, the Committee on Amphetamine and Athletics of the American Medical Association supported two major research projects to test the actual effect of amphetamine sulfate on performance. Smith and Beecher (1959) found that 14–21 mg of amphetamine sulfate per 70 kg of body weight administered 2–3 hours prior to running, swimming, and weight throwing improved performance in 75% of the cases tested. This study received considerable criticism due to its design, statistics, and lack of control. Karpovich (1959) administered 10–20 mg of amphetamine sulfate to subjects 30 minutes before performances in track running, swimming, and treadmill running. He found that 50 of the 54 subjects showed no change in performance with the drug. Three subjects showed improved performance, while one showed a decrement.

Other studies on the effect of amphetamine sulfate (Benzedrine) on performance include a study by Foltz *et al.* (1943), who measured performance by exhaustive rides on a bicycle ergometer. They found that 10–15 mg of amphetamine sulfate had no significant effect on the performance of four conditioned subjects. Haldi and Wynn (1959) tested the effect of amphetamine (Benzedrine) on swimming performance. They found that 5 mg of amphetamine administered orally 90 minutes before a 100-yd swim had no significant effect on the time of the swim.

On the basis of knowledge gained from the previous studies, Golding and Barnard (1963) conducted a study to investigate the effect of *d*-amphetamine sulfate on all-out treadmill running. Ten conditioned and ten unconditioned subjects were given 15 mg of *d*-amphetamine sulfate or a placebo (lactose) 2–3 hours before the tests. The first, or rested, run was used to study the effect of the drug on initial performance. The second, or fatigued, run was performed 12 minutes after the completion of the rested run. Because amphetamines are capable of reducing or abolishing the feeling of fatigue, it was felt that the second run was necessary in order to study the effect of amphetamine sulfate on performance in a fatigued subject. Each subject performed the test six times (three with amphetamine and three with the placebo). A double-blind procedure for administering the drug and placebo was used, and at least 1 day of rest was allowed between each test.

An analysis of the rested and fatigued runs performed by conditioned subjects showed that *d*-amphetamine sulfate had no significant effect on performance. The rested and fatigued runs performed by the unconditioned subjects were also analyzed. Again, the drug had no significant effect on the performance of these runs. An analysis of the mean drug and mean placebo measurements taken in the rested state showed that the drug significantly increased heart rate and blood pressure but had no effect on respiration rate. The recovery rate for blood pressure after the rested runs was retarded by amphetamine, but the drug had no significant effect on recovery heart or respiration rates. Following the fatigued runs, recovery rates for heart rate and blood pressure were retarded by the drug, while respiration rate was again unaffected.

After every test period each subject completed a questionnaire regarding his feelings of fatigue and his subjective evaluation of his performance. He was also asked whether he felt he had been administered amphetamine or a placebo prior to the test. Only one of the twenty subjects knew when he had taken the drug and when he had not.

Until recently, when it was added to the Bureau of Narcotics list of dangerous drugs, amphetamine was easily obtained. It was widely prescribed by physicians as an appetite depressant in diet control and obesity. However, since drug abuse has become a major problem, physicians are dispensing it with more caution. In normal doses, however, it has no serious detrimental side effects. Its ability to stimulate individuals and suppress subjective feelings of fatigue make it a tempting ergogenic drug.

The use of drugs to improve athletic performance is not confined to the United States. Dumas (1971), medical supervisor of the French National Physical Education Teachers College, indicated that, in spite of strict controls, the use of drugs by athletes is spreading rapidly. He described drug abuse among athletes as a "cancer in sports."

Surveys indicate that amphetamines and their derivatives are the drugs most commonly used. They are often accompanied by analgesics, sedatives, and barbiturates, which set up a cycle of stimulation and depression.

Andriver (1971) indicated that drugging suppresses the organism's alarm bell and could push the athlete beyond his capacities, with possible disastrous results. He noted that surveys and investigations have indicated that a number of fatalities have occurred in athletics because of drug abuse, and he emphasized that "heatstroke" of the type associated with absorption of amphetamine can precipitate cardiac failure. It is known that stimulants taken in large doses can induce a number of reactions ranging from excitation and insomnia to hallucinations and delirium. Amphetamines can also affect sensory perception, blood pressure, digestion, and cardiac rhythm.

Due to the publicity received by champion cyclists who allegedly take amphetamine more as the rule than the exception, Wyndham and his associates (1971) studied the effect of 10 mg of methamphetamine on oxygen consumption, heart rate, minute ventilation, and blood lactate levels in two champion cyclists working at rates between 2000–16,000 ft-lb/minute on a bicycle ergometer. No difference between the amphetamine and the placebo was noted for submaximal or maximal oxygen uptake, heart rate, or minute ventilation; blood lactic acid levels did change significantly. The two cyclists were able to continue to cycle at maximal effort for a longer period when on amphetamine. The study demonstrated that amphetamines do not increase the ability to do aerobic work, but the authors indicated that amphetamine helped the subjects to continue to exercise at high levels of work output for longer periods and enabled the cyclists to tolerate higher levels of anaerobic metabolism. Short-distance events may not present a danger to the athlete using amphetamine; however, events involving an hour or more of work could be dangerous because of a failure to recognize the danger signs of exertion and heat stress and to react to these warnings. The study was carefully controlled and the experimental design was good; however, two subjects are a very small number from which to draw conclusions. The study does give needed insight into the use of amphetamine in performance.

The French Antidoping Law of 1965 forbids the use of certain drugs by athletes in competition. Athletes suspected of drug use are examined by the faculty of the College of Medicine in Paris. The examination is based on two urine samples. A system of control and checks is outlined to guarantee honest accurate results. Since amphetamine is usually taken 2–3 hours prior to an event, it is easily detected in the blood or urine. The blood or urine is analyzed by thin-layer chromatography or electrophoresis. (Figure 1 represents a typical gas chromatogram of six amines.) However, usually only the winners of events are examined. They are disqualified if drugs are detected.

Athletes, however, are undaunted by fears and threats. The results of interviews with top athletes show that the desire to win is greater than either the fear of exposure or the possible harmful side effects of amphetamines. Too many athletes witness excellent performances by peers who take amphetamines and often credit the drug for these performances.

Since the use of amphetamine is so widespread, athletes tend to ignore any contraindications. Also, they are aware that large doses are administered to psychiatric patients with no apparent toxic effects. However, they seem to lose sight of the fact that abnormally high doses are administered under very stringent medical supervision. Some physicians seem to encourage the use of amphetamines by telling athletes that they are harmless in normal doses.

Agencies that control athletics are not concerned about the use of vitamins or other nutritional supplements, but they have become very concerned about the use of drugs. This concern and attempted control

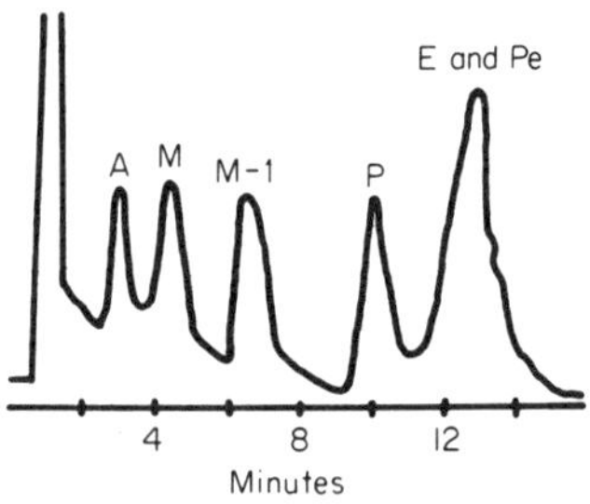

Fig. 1. Gas chromatogram of six amines (A, amphetamine; M, methamphetamine; M-1, mephentermine; P, phenylpropanolamine; E and Pe, ephedrine and pseudoephedrine).

by authorities tends to make the athletes believe that there must be a definite advantage to the use of these drugs to merit the controversy that their use generates. As the bodies that control athletics become more dogmatic in their disapproval of drugs and more persistent in their efforts to curb their use, the athletes have become more certain that drugs must affect performance advantageously. Otherwise, why all the fuss about something that has no effect on performance? One champion athlete explained that, if amphetamines were not helpful and if they did not aid performance, authorities would not be so "uptight" about their use. Athletes who take amphetamines to improve their performance do not consider themselves to be drug users in the same sense as people who take drugs merely to "turn on." They justify their use of drugs on a medicinal rather than emotional basis. It is interesting to note, however, that two out of four athletes interviewed indicated that they take amphetamines even when not competing because it helps in the performance of their daily tasks.

During the past few years, a great number of seminars, conferences, and articles have been presented on "doping" in athletics. The weight of evidence presented in experimental studies, as well as the clinical expertise of physicians, pharmacologists, and trainers, support the fact that amphetamines do not enhance physical performance and have no place in athletics. Experimental studies do not demonstrate increased physical performance, and the side effects of large doses of drugs can be harmful, especially during maximal performance.

Why then, in light of this evidence and knowledge, and in spite of stringent controls and regulations, is amphetamine still widely used? Amphetamine is a psychostimulant and produces an elevation in mood and a general feeling of being "pepped up." The athlete on amphetamine becomes keyed up for his event, which is desirable for optimal performance. He is mentally alert and, when observed objectively, appears to be emotionally ready to perform maximally. Mental attitude certainly can affect performance, and being mentally prepared for an activity or an event is desirable. Increased psychological preparedness appears to be the only rational justification for the continued use of amphetamine.

If psychological preparedness is the primary reason for an athlete's taking amphetamine, then evidence should be available to substantiate this pepping up of the individual's mental processes. Although an individual robbed of sleep is made alert by amphetamines, this is not the case in athletics. Athletes are seldom sleepy or tired prior to competition. Pierson and his co-workers (1961) studied the psychological effects of both amphetamine sulfate and a tranquilizer, meprobamate. The study involved subjective feelings as well as awareness of improvement in reaction time and movement time. Their study involved 26 adult male medical students who had been phenotyped for the study. This was done because it had been reported that somatotype was a consideration in determining reaction time and movement time. The subjects received a calcium carbonate placebo, 20 mg of amphetamine sulfate, or 800 mg of meprobamate in a double-blind design, 2 hours before testing. During the testing period, which lasted 15 minutes, an apparatus measured reaction time to a visual stimulus and movement time involving breaking a beam of light with the dominant hand. After the test, subjects were asked to explain whether they felt normal, tensive, or relaxed. Normal was assumed to mean that the subjects felt no physiological or psychological effects; tensive meant that the individual felt hyperexcited, aggressive, alert, or keyed up; and relaxed meant that the subject felt placid, relaxed, slow, sleepy, or lethargic. Since the subjects were medical students, it was felt that they would be better than average observers of these feelings. The statistical results indicated that the subjects could not identify which substance they had taken. Although the study showed that the subjects could not identify the amphetamine often enough to account for anything other than chance, it was, however, more readily identified than meprobamate. The subjective feelings of alertness or lethargy had no relation to speed of responses either in reaction or movement time, and body size had little relationship to the effect of meprobamate or amphetamine sulfate.

Since it is fairly well established that amphetamine does not improve or increase performance and that athletes taking amphetamines may do so to key themselves up for an event, this study is extremely important, because it indicates that, in a double-blind situation, subjects could not identify amphetamine. This study agrees with that of Golding and Barnard (1963), in which subjects given a questionnaire regarding whether they were on amphetamines or placebos were unable to distinguish the drug. These studies indicate that the psychological effect on athletes is entirely self-induced by their expecting to feel pepped up and ready to perform. In the light of this knowledge, more research needs to be undertaken to show the psychological benefits of expecting to feel good and its subsequent effect on performance.

Graham (1972) presented a method of minimizing motivational factors through the use of electromyography. The study investigated the effect of 15 mg of dextroamphetamine sulfate on the local muscular fatigue of the triceps brachii muscle during isometric and isotonic work. This was done by measuring, electromyographically, the integrated action potentials over 3-second time periods as the muscle contracted. The contractions were performed under varying loads and with the muscle in a rested or a fatigued condition. Maximal isometric strength, blood pressure, and heart rate were also measured.

The basic design of the study called for two groups of 18 subjects. One group performed an isometric exercise with the left triceps brachii and the other group performed an isotonic exercise with the same muscle. Each subject was tested once with a placebo, once with *d*-amphetamine, and once in a controlled condition with no capsule. The sequence of testing was rotated and all capsules were administered blind. The results indicated that 15 mg of amphetamine significantly decreased the integrated action potential of the triceps during isometric contractions in both the rested and the fatigued conditions. There was no significant effect on action potentials during isotonic exercise. Since it can be concluded that a decrease in the integrated action potential is associated with a reduction in the amount of muscular fatigue, it was shown that amphetamine sulfate did decrease fatigue during isometric contraction and that motivational factors were kept to a minimum.

Many individuals using amphetamines need a "downer" in order to sleep at night and so a cyclic pattern develops between "uppers" to enable the person to perform and "downers" to enable the individual to obtain needed sleep. This cyclic pattern is considered, by most psychiatrists, to be undesirable. The "upper," usually amphetamine, reacts differently when overcoming the effect of a barbiturate.

Air force fighter pilots required to take long missions lasting from 5 to 12 hours undergo some peculiar adjustments. They are required to go to sleep at an unusually early hour, get up early, and be on a long mission requiring the precision and skill involved in piloting, aerial refueling, and accurate accomplishment of their mission. Pharmacological support for inducing sleep as well as in-flight medication to combat fatigue are thought to be necessary. The demands motivated a study (McKenzie and Elliot, 1965) to investigate the effects of secobarbital and *d*-amphetamine on performance during a simulated air mission. The results on 48 subjects indicated that performance decrement occurred as a result of the use of secobarbital. Individuals receiving 200 mg of secobarbital at bedtime demonstrated a performance decrement 10 hours later at the beginning of a simulated flight and continued to show a decreased performance throughout the mission, which ended 12 hours later. The subjects receiving 5 mg of *d*-amphetamine showed an enhancement of performance and a lessening of fatigue. The importance of the study, however, was that those who received the amphetamine after the secobarbital, which had been administered the night before, also showed a decreased performance. Secobarbital apparently decreases the effect of *d*-amphetamine taken after barbiturate administration. The cyclic pattern prevents the amphetamine from having the effect it may have without the administration of barbiturates.

The news media and popular magazines carry numerous articles of athletes on drugs. In a three-part article in *Sports Illustrated,* Gilbert (1969) gives a blow-by-blow narrative of athlete after athlete using all manner of drugs. Names of top athletes along with their stories of drug taking for the purposes of improving performance, hastening recovery from fatigue, mastering pain, gaining weight and strength, and generally aiding the performance of their various athletic tasks are given in dramatic context.

Agencies that ban the use of drugs during athletic competition do so for a number of reasons. First, anything that may possibly affect the performance of an athlete must be available to every participant. Advantage gained by taking a drug that is not readily available to all is unfair. Hopefully, however, agencies forbid drugs mainly because they are concerned with the welfare of the athlete and are aware that indiscriminate use of drugs may produce deleterious effects.

The International Olympic Committee has announced that an athlete who is known to have used "dope" will be excluded from the Olympic Games. The surveys that were done 10 years ago showed that drug use was limited to only a few athletes. However, if those surveys were repeated today, the results would be vastly different; the figures would probably be reversed. The predominant attitude among authorities is that the solution to drug use by athletes is through understanding and education. However, the overly strong views of the "establishment" make it difficult for athletes to admit to the use of drugs. Too often the coach, trainer, or team physician plays the role of a disciplinarian instead of an understanding counselor, which makes the hope for drug control through athlete cooperation almost impossible.

Summary

From the results of surveys, interviews, and observation, amphetamine is the drug most widely used by athletes today. Amphetamine is a central nervous system stimulant known to abolish the sense of fatigue and to increase the fatigued individual's performance of tasks needing skill, dexterity, and concentration. In athletic-performance studies, the weight of evidence indicates that amphetamine does not improve physical performance. Most athletes do not perform when sleepy or fatigued and therefore should need nothing to abolish this kind of fatigue. The physiological effects of amphetamine can be dangerous in events requiring performance over a long period. The major reason for athletes taking amphetamine seems to be to get them "up" for their event: to key them up and make them psychologically ready for the contest. Athletes are highly motivated and, before contests, are often nervous and hyperirritable, and these conditions may well make restful sleep impossible, leading to the use of barbiturates to induce sleep. Studies indicate not only that the cycle of barbiturate to stimulant is undesirable, but that the stimulant does not act normally after a barbiturate. The moral, ethical and legal considerations are beyond the realm of this chapter. It is agreed by most team physicians, coaches, trainers, and sports-controlling bodies that the use of amphetamine is undesirable, harmful, and should be outlawed. The International Olympic Committee, the American Medical Association, and most athletic governing bodies have rules to disqualify athletes using amphetamines. Furthermore, research has indicated that amphetamine does not enhance physical performance.

III. Androgenic–Anabolic Steroids

The androgenic–anabolic steroids resemble the male sex hormones both chemically and functionally. Androgenic refers to masculinity; therefore, the androgenic hormones are those that affect male characteristics, especially secondary sex characteristics. Anabolic means to build up or construct, so that anabolism is the constructive or building process. Male, or androgenic, hormones are produced primarily by the testes, with testosterone being the principal androgen. The hormones also have an anabolic effect. The synthetic androgenic steroids have the same physiological effects as testosterone: (a) growth stimulation, (b) acceleration of bone maturation, (c) virilization, (d) possible weight gain.

The attempt to separate the anabolic from the androgenic effects has resulted in a variety of synthetic steroids. Until recently, the androgenic and anabolic steroids were nearly identical in their effects when given in equal doses. Pharmacologists, however, by manipulating the carbon atoms are attempting to increase the anabolic effect while decreasing the androgenic effect. In this manner the constructive effect of the hormone on metabolism and strength can occur without the androgenic effects. The modifications in the steroid structure may make the drug more suitable for experimentation. Medical authorities believe, however, that any drug sufficiently potent to alter the body's metabolism is sufficiently potent to have undesirable effects. A number of sources warn that prolonged administration of oral androgenic–anabolic steroids can result in an impairment of liver function. The problem of administering these drugs is further compounded because they affect the prepubital and postpubital user differently. Studies on the androgenic–anabolic steroids as they relate to physical performance are conflicting and confusing.

The androgenic–anabolic steroids are better known by their trade names rather than their generic names. Dianabol, a commonly used androgenic–anabolic steroid, is Ciba's trade name for methandrostenolone; likewise, Parke-Davis Company developed an anabolic steroid with the trade name Adroyd; Searle and Company has Nilevor; Organon, Inc., makes Maxibolen; and Winthrop Laboratories developed Winstrol. The action, use, and contraindications for the androgenic–anabolic steroids are about the same. Maxibolen, one of the newer drugs, can be used as an example. The action of Maxibolen (Organon, 1970) is primarily anabolic (protein saving). It promotes the body tissue building processes. By manipulating one of the carbon atoms, there is a reduction of the androgenic activity but an increase in the anabolic properties. Long-term chronic toxicity studies were undertaken using rats and dogs, and toxicity was observed only when the dosage reached 1600 mg/kg (van Waylen and Buyze, 1961). It is felt that since the normal clinical dose is less than 0.1 mg/kg a large margin of safety exists.

The indications for the drug use are in the management of any disorders characterized by protein depletion. Maxibolen has all the characteristics of anabolic agents including promotion of tissue building and weight gain, stimulation of appetite and a sense of well-being. It is also supposed to renew vigor and combat depression and weakness due to chronic illness or prolonged convalescence and is therefore useful in several ways. (a) It promotes weight gain. The drug is administered to patients who are underweight due to illness; the increase in appetite usually results in greater caloric intake and, if the diet is adequate, weight should increase. (b) Maxibolen may relieve the symptoms of osteoporosis. This is a reduction in bone mass unaccompanied by any change in chemical composition. It is found in malnutrition, rheumatoid arthritis and other conditions. It is often seen in older patients who report subjective improvement when using the drug, although this has been seldom supported by radiological examination. (c) Other conditions indicating possible use of Maxibolen are arthritis, geriatrics problems, chronic disease and convalescence, anemia, and occasionally in pediatric cases.

The precautions to be taken in the use of the steroid are many, especially with regard to the liver. It is definitely contraindicated for individuals with any liver impairment. Some patients without known liver disease may show BSP (bromsulphalein) retention and increased serum transaminase levels, which, however, reportedly return to normal after discontinuation of the drug. The drug may have a hypoglycemic effect and diabetic patients may have to adjust insulin requirements. Salt and water retention are also a possibility. Other adverse reactions to the anabolic steroids are inhibition of testicular functions, testicle atrophy, impotence, epididymitis and bladder irritability, nausea, excitation and sleeplessness, vomiting, diarrhea, decrease in the PBI (protein-bound iodine test of thyroid function), retention of sodium, chlorides, water, potassium, phosphates, and calcium.

The drug is obtainable only with a written prescription of a physician. The usual adult dosage is 5 mg/day, and intermittent therapy is recommended when the therapy is extended over a long period. The drug is usually taken in tablet form. Most of the anabolic–androgenic steroids manufactured by drug companies include warnings that the drug should not be taken by healthy persons in the quest for advantage in sports.

Anabolic steroids have been used in clinical medicine for many years. Liddle and Burke (1960) clinically compared the anabolic potencies of four commercially available steroids. Only metabolically stable subjects were employed and any who might require anabolic stimulation were excluded. Urinary nitrogen excretion was chosen as the parameter to determine anabolic activity. The study was carefully controlled and monitored. Dianabol was the most potent anabolic steroid tested and doses of 1.25 mg/day had an appreciable effect. There was no further significant weight gain beyond dosages of 2.5 mg, even up to dosages of 30 mg/day.

Other effects of the drug were that women developed acne, and the liver function test of BSP was influenced adversely with daily doses above 10 mg. Whether BSP retention is a significant test of liver function in steroid therapy is discussed at length by Kuzell and co-workers (1962), who studied 320 patients with various rheumatic diseases using methandrostenolone (Dianabol) for treatment. Their study showed successful management of various rheumatic disorders. Side effects were transitory, being easily controlled by reduction of dosage. Kuzell *et al.* also found similar results with dosages of 2.5 mg and 5.0 mg per day.

Lambert and Site (1961), using a double-blind type of design, studied the effect of Dianabol on weight gain of 26 hospital patients and 26 controls. Each patient received 5 mg twice a day. A control period of 4 weeks was used prior to drug therapy to determine the stability of their weights. Both groups then received either Dianabol or a placebo for a period of 7 weeks followed by a 3-week period when both groups received placebos. Finally, patients were followed for 15 additional weeks to determine any further weight changes. The study showed that the steroid-treated group had a significant weight gain. There were no side effects from the therapy.

Some studies with muscular dystrophy patients have indicated that anabolic steroids increase muscular strength; other studies have shown increases in body weight. If gains in weight and strength do result from anabolic steroid therapy, the steroids could be considered as ergogenic aids. If the increases in weight are due to water retention or an increase in adipose tissue, they would be of no value to the athlete. If, however, the weight gain favorably affects lean body mass, anabolic steroids would be of interest to weight lifters, wrestlers, weight-event athletes, and football players. As will be seen later in this section, empirical and testimonial evidence for weight and strength gains are extensive. Controlled studies, however, are not as plentiful and can be briefly summarized as follows. Four studies (Fowler, 1965; Samuels *et al.*, 1942; Casner *et al.*, 1971; Fahey and Brown, 1972) do not show any evidence that the use of anabolic steroids increases weight and strength. Six other studies (Johnson and O'Shea, 1969; O'Shea and Winkler, 1970; Maul and Hagerman, 1971; Bowers and Reardon, 1971; Johnson *et al.*, 1972; Ariel, 1972) conclude that weight and strength are increased. The majority of physicians, trainers, and coaches do not support the use of anabolic steroids, and controlling athletic bodies are legislating against their use.

Fowler *et al.* (1965) studied 47 healthy men ranging in age from 18 to 25 years. Ten were conditioned athletes and the rest were untrained students. The untrained men were assigned at random to one of four treatment groups: (a) those who received a placebo, (b) those who received androstenolene, (c) those who received the placebo and exercised, and (d) those who received androstenolene and exercised. The ten trained athletes were divided into two groups; five received placebos and five received androstenolene. The subjects on the drug received 20 mg of androstenolene per day. The study lasted 16 weeks. The subjects assigned to the exercise groups were enrolled in a physical conditioning program that met 5 days a week for 30 minutes a day. Both physical strength and physical working capacity were measured before and after the exercise program. The only significant increases were in the groups receiving exercise, but there were no significant differences between the placebo and the androstenolene-supplemented subjects. According to this study, there appears to be no evidence that anabolic steroids increase strength in young men and, hence, no justification for the use of anabolic drugs by athletes.

Samuels *et al.* (1942) studied the effect of methyltestosterone on the grip strength of young men. The study was limited to four subjects. The results showed no evidence of changes in grip strength through the use of the drug.

Casner *et al.* (1971) studied the effects of stanozolol, a commonly used clinical anabolic steroid, on the body weight, body composition, and strength of normal young men. Twenty-seven men were randomly divided into four groups: one group for steroid therapy, one group for steroid therapy and supervised progressive weight training, one group for placebo, and the fourth group for a placebo and weight training. The parameters measured included specific gravity, total body water, body weight, and muscular strength. The double-blind study lasted 56 days, and the drug dosage consisted of 2 mg of stanozolol taken three times per day on days 1–21 and days 28–49. Dietary records were kept on all subjects. No side effects associated with the drug therapy were reported, although no blood chemistry was done.

The analysis of the data showed that the only significant difference among the four groups was found in a change in body weight. Both groups taking the anabolic steroids gained significantly more weight than the placebo groups. A further analysis of the data indicated that the increase in weight may have been due to fluid retention as opposed to an increase in muscle mass. The authors concluded that, based on their research, there was no justification for the use of anabolic steroids. The study was well controlled, and the steroid dosage followed the pattern reported by athletes using steroids. The changes due to the weight training were not significantly different between the drug and placebo groups.

Fahey and Brown (1972) studied 28 male subjects between the ages of 19 and 32. They were divided into two groups matched on lean body weight and strength. Body composition, maximal oxygen uptake, and isotonic and isometric strength of the upper and lower extremities were measured. The training program consisted of 10 weeks of intensive weight training three times per week. One group received intermuscular injections of deca-Durabolin R (1.0 mg/kg body weight) at weeks 2, 5, and 8. The placebo, which was sterile saline, was administered similarly on a double-blind basis. Body weight and maximal oxygen uptake were unchanged in both groups after training. Although strength and lean body mass increased in both groups, there were no significant differences between the groups. Due to the informed consent requirements, the double-blind nature of the study had to be disclosed. The authors concluded that deca-Durabolin in normal doses does not significantly affect weight, lean body mass, strength, or maximal oxygen uptake.

Johnson and O'Shea (1969), using 12 subjects, showed that administering 5 mg of Dianabol twice daily during a 3-week weight-training class caused significant gains in weight, strength, and several anthropometrical measurements. They also reported an increased oxygen uptake.

In another study, O'Shea and Winkler (1970) reported that anabolic steroid treatment in three competitive swimmers and three weight lifters increased strength significantly during an 11-week training program, although there was no evidence that the steroid treatment improved swimming speed.

Recently, Maul and Hagerman (1971) completed a pilot study using anabolic steroids on five weight trainers, three of whom took 5 mg of Dianabol per day. They used a dosage pattern of 3 weeks on the drug and 1 week off, which is a pattern commonly used by weight men. The remaining two subjects served as controls. The study lasted 12 weeks, and the experimental subjects were tested on all parameters at the beginning of each "off" week. The control group was tested only at the beginning and the end of the 12 weeks. As evidenced by the data, the steroid group showed marked improvements in weight gain, total body girth, and isometric strength. Oxygen consumption measured during a standard submaximal ride on the bicycle ergometer seemed to vary among the individuals of both groups, some improving slightly, others showing a decrement. Heart rates for three of the subjects did increase markedly, which might indicate a slight trend toward a higher energy cost for the ride. Isometric strength results were difficult to assess; the steroid group improved slightly, while the controls decreased slightly. The data were treated by multiple-comparison analysis and tendencies were found to be significant. The authors reported their results as case studies since the small number of subjects raised the statistical rejection value to very high levels.

There appeared to be no significant changes in blood chemistry as a result of steroid administration. The Ca^{2+} level dropped slightly for the steroid groups and the Cl^{-} level went up a little, but not significantly. Liver clearance tests showed a normal trend, indicating that there was apparently no acute hepatic disturbance. Creatine phosphokinase (CPK) activity was significantly elevated in subjects of both groups for pre- and posttests and tended to be highly variable. The authors were careful to examine the blood at least 48 hours after the subject's last strenuous workout, since vigorous muscle activity tends to elevate CPK levels. The raised CPK levels were probably a result of the severity of the subjects' strength workouts.

Although the authors of this study used a small number of subjects and the dosage of steroids was small, the data are interesting and significant. The study was carefully controlled and the data reliable. Individual results were quite phenomenal, with one subject gaining 27 lb with accompanying increases in strength that could not have occurred by chance.

Bowers and Reardon (1971) studied the effect of an anabolic steroid on strength and anthropometrical measurements. Eighteen male subjects, matched by size, strength, and age, were given 30 gm of a 90% protein supplement each day during the study. The nine experimental subjects were given, in addition to the supplement, 10 mg of Dianabol daily for the last 21 days of the 5-week study. The nine controls were given a placebo in addition to the supplement.

The subjects were tested, put on a 5-week training program, which consisted of the bench press, squat, curl, and tricep extension, and then retested. Strength was measured by the bench press and squat tests. The anthropometric measurements included weight, bicep girth, chest circumference, waist girth, thigh circumference, and forearm circumference. Three skin-fold measurements were taken, and percent body fat and maximal oxygen uptake were measured. Significant improvements in the bench press, squat, and bicep and forearm girths occurred in the experimental group. The authors concluded that the results of this study indicate that anabolic steroids may have a positive effect on the acquisition of strength and muscular development, although no beneficial effect was observed on maximal oxygen uptake.

Ariel (1972) investigated the effect of Dianabol on the nervous system by measuring the various reflex components of the knee jerk reflex and on the skeletal muscle contractile force by testing maximal weight lifting. Using six male subjects aged 18–22 years, the study lasted 15 weeks. The time was divided as follows: first through eighth week, training period; eighth through eleventh week, placebo period (when all six subjects received a placebo); and twelfth through fifteenth week, three of the subjects were given 10 mg of Dianabol orally in a double-blind setting. The results indicated that the experimental group was stronger during the anabolic period. Also, the rate of progress was higher. The anabolic steroid had a significant effect on the components of the knee jerk reflex. The author concluded that the anabolic steroid acted favorably on the central nervous system and on the biochemical processes involved in the knee jerk reflex as well as in contraction of skeletal muscles.

Johnson and co-workers (1972) studied the effect of Dianabol on 31 male subjects between the ages of 18 and 31 years. The study consisted of a 4-week pretest period when subjects became familiar with the weight-training program and developed strength fitness, and when all testing was administered. Blood tests to evaluate liver function and a sperm count to determine fertility were also given as a precautionary measure. Subjects were tested on maximal oxygen uptake, dynamic strength (one repetition on bench press and squat), static strength (measured with cable tension tests), girth measurements, and skin-fold measures. Subjects were randomly placed in the treatment–placebo groups and the remaining subjects formed the control group. Dianabol or placebo was administered in a double-blind procedure. In addition, all subjects were given 20 gm of 92% protein powder daily to supplement their diet. The training period consisted of 1 hour three times per week for 3 weeks, and work was near maximum.

The results of the study showed that the anabolic steroid group increased significantly in dynamic and static strength, in weight, and in five of eight circumference measurements. The authors concluded that, when accompanied by a high-protein diet and severe muscular stress, anabolic steroids increase weight, strength, and muscle size. This study was well controlled and, although short in duration, showed positive results with the use of steroids. No detrimental side effects were reported, and blood tests did not show liver involvement.

Hagerman conducted interviews with athletes at the World Pentathlon Games in 1966, at the Olympic Games in Mexico City in 1968, and at various other athletic events. He compiled the case histories of individuals using steroids and believes that these accounts are reliable due to the nature of the interview and the anonymity of the athlete. The following are three examples:

1. A university shot-putter and discus thrower administered deca-Durabolin injections to himself four times per week, using 25 mg per injection. The average recommended dosage is 25–50 mg/week. This athlete used deca-Durabolin because of claims of no resultant liver damage. He reported significant weight gain and improvement in performance.

2. A Pentathlon competitor used 24 mg of Winstrol per day for 4 months. He reported an increase in weight, increase in lean body mass, marked improvement in swimming times, and a decrease in running times.

3. Two athletes, an Olympic shot-putter and a discus thrower, used Dianabol sporadically for 2 years. The longest continuous use was for 6 months, the pattern being 3 weeks on the drug and 1 week off. The shot-putter's weight over a 2-year period went from 225 to 280 lb, and his best shot-put performance of over 66 ft occurred during this period. The discus thrower went from 220 to 268 lb in less than 6 months. The

distance of his throws increased from the low 180's to 207 ft. The daily dosage for each individual ranged from two to eight times more than the recommended dosages.

Other interviews with similar results were conducted but are not reported because they are repetitive and too numerous. Secondary sources, that is, individuals telling of other athletes' experiences or changes on steroids, were readily obtainable but are not reported because of their possible unreliability.

Golding (1970, 1971) conducted similar interviews with champion athletes in various parts of the United States and Canada and found widespread use of anabolic steroids. Weight lifters and weight-event men in track appear to be the greatest users. Persons in individual events are more prone to use steroids than individuals in team activities, although a number of football players reported using steroids. At first athletes were reluctant to discuss drug use; however, after a rapport had been established, they were quite willing to discuss the drugs and their reactions. They needed to be reassured that the interview was strictly scientific, that no value judgments would be made, and that their anonymity would be safeguarded. Athletes themselves are anxious to know what research has discovered about the drugs they are taking. None of the athletes interviewed was found to be on any of the common street drugs. The drugs were used solely in conjunction with the athlete's performance and desire for excellence. Some case histories follow.

1. A university shot-putter used Dianabol just prior to indoor track season. He started in January and took a 5-mg Dianabol tablet each day for 50 days. He followed this procedure for 4 of the 8 years he had been competing. He was never out of training, as he worked out all year. Each episode on Dianabol brought about an increase in strength. A crude testing program was self-administered and in 1 month showed an increase in a clean and jerk from 335 to 365 lb and in a squat from 425 to 520 lb. When asked whether his decision to take the drug for 50 days was arbitrary, or one that he found gave him optimal benefits, he replied that he could obtain only 50 tablets each year.

2. A university shot-putter and hammer thrower used Dianabol twice a year, one series of tablets off season and one series just prior to the beginning of track season. He took one 5-mg Dianabol tablet daily for 3 weeks, skipped the fourth week, and repeated this pattern twice more. He spent 18 weeks a year taking Dianabol for 4 years, with no noticeable deleterious side effects. He was concerned with possible liver damage and had three liver function tests administered to satisfy himself that there was no liver impairment. He obtained the Dianabol in Europe

and brought back enough for himself and two fellow athletes. He observed weight increases and increases in strength evidenced by unusual gains in bench press, squat press, and arm curl.

3. A university football player signed by a professional team was desirous of gaining weight and improving strength in order to improve his chances for a successful professional career. He had had some experience with Dianabol during his junior year in college but had taken it only sporadically during the course of summer training for the fall football season. He discontinued the drug, not only because he was already an excellent performer, but also because he was concerned about the ethics involved and the fear of discovery. His uncertainty about his ability to compete successfully in the pros renewed his desire to take steroids. He read extensively and attempted to research anabolic steroid use. He did not find any of the articles referred to in this chapter, although he read much in the non-research-oriented magazines. He is presently on a 3-month regime of 5 mg of Dianabol per day.

Most users of steroids feel that beneficial effects in strength occur only when accompanied by heavy workouts—usually weight training, which tends to complicate findings, since this increase in training may account for some observed strength gains.

It is apparent that the use of anabolic steroids is extremely common, especially among weight men. Individuals are naïve to believe that athletes would not resort to these measures in their search for excellence. We are living in a drug culture and the sporting world is not immune. Drug taking is not considered immoral, unsportsmanlike, or dangerous by youth. Drug procurement is apparently easy, and athletes desiring drugs have little difficulty obtaining them. Many athletes admit that physicians supply them with anabolic steroids and, although they recommended normal dosages, they do little to prevent the individual from increasing the dosage at will (Golding, 1970, 1971).

National and international authorities are trying to control the use of the anabolic steroids in amateur athletes. However, the International Olympic Committee admits that the methods of testing for steroids cannot match the situations that arise. Guidelines for a campaign against "doping" were established at the Winter Games in Grenoble, France, in 1968 and the Mexico Games in 1968. Strong measures were planned for the Winter Games in Sapporo, Japan, in 1972 and at the Munich Games in 1972.

A. Beckett (1971, unpublished information), interviewed at the 30th International Congress of Pharmaceutical Sciences, said that scientists were examining a test battery for detection and control of drugs, especially the anabolic steroids, and that a control system would be introduced under which a license would be granted to an athlete before he could compete in his chosen sport. The main problem associated with the detection of anabolic steroids is that they are usually taken out of season, and any weight and strength buildup takes place well before the event. Therefore, any drug detection program initiated during the season would show no trace of the drug, even though the athlete may have gained considerable advantage over other competitors.

One of the suggestions under consideration for stemming the use of steroids by athletes is that officials keep systematic records of the weight of all potential Olympic athletes, particularly discus throwers and shot-putters. If there is a sudden change in weight in the months that precede the event, the officials will be entitled to request a check of blood and urine. This system of testing and record keeping is being proposed by the International Olympic Committee and will be carried out by the organizing committee for each sport under the supervision of medical committees set up by the 26 international federations. The International Olympic Committee will act as a high court in the event of a protest against disqualification. The International Olympic Committee's purpose is to create an atmosphere against drug abuse. Education is the answer in trying to make the athletes aware of the dangers associated with drug use. Drugs derived from illegal sources vary in purity, may be dangerous to health, and can be potential killers.

Summary

The use of anabolic steroids by athletes is widespread. Research on the effects of anabolic steroids on body weight, muscular strength, and muscle size is confusing and conflicting. The medical literature indicating possible liver impairment with the use of anabolic steroids further concerns athletes, trainers, coaches, and team physicians. Finally, ethical and legal considerations make the problem of anabolic steroid use one with impossible dimensions.

Four major investigations report that anabolic steroids do not help weight and strength development and indicate that the anabolic steroids have no place in athletics. They point out that weight gain may possibly be fat accumulation or water retention, and not lean muscle mass. Six other equally well designed studies report significant improvements in weight, strength, and muscle size. These studies report no significant side effects of drug therapy and suggest that gains occur when the strength workouts are near maximum and when accompanied by a high-protein diet.

The International Olympic Committee and other sporting control bodies are against the use of anabolic steroids by athletes, and regulations have been established to disqualify participants who are known to use steroids. With increased restriction on the use of human subjects in experimentation, well-controlled studies involving anabolic steroids are difficult to conduct. Investigators, attending physicians, and subjects are hesitant to undertake many of the experimental studies that may supply answers regarding steroid use. Only the less toxic or relatively accepted drugs are used in most research studies. The controls being suggested by the International Olympic Committee are a step in the right direction; however, the chances of their success with anabolic steroids are extremely slim.

IV. Aspartic Acid Salts

Potassium and magnesium aspartates have been used clinically in the treatment of fatigue. The basis for their use involves the ability of the urea cycle to clear ammonia from the blood. Blood ammonia normally results from three principal sources: (a) foods containing ammonia compounds, (b) metabolism within the cell, and (c) actively contracting skeletal muscles. It is a well-documented fact that blood ammonia levels are elevated following physical activity. Increased blood ammonia is thought to be one of the reasons for fatigue. The elevated blood ammonia concentrations are returned to normal values through the urea cycle, which converts the excess ammonia to urea, which is then eliminated from the body. The urea cycle, however, may not be able to clear all the ammonia, and it is postulated that aspartic acid (see Fig. 2) is the rate-limiting step (therefore possibly the weakest link in the urea cycle) in the conversion of ammonia to urea. It is thought that increasing the aspartic acid concentration through exogenous sources of aspartic acid salts would strengthen the urea cycle so as to allow for a more functional conversion process. The elevated blood ammonia concentration could then be more rapidly converted to urea, thus preventing substantial elevation in blood ammonia levels following exercise. The decrease in blood ammonia would thus partially prevent the manifestation of fatigue.

Laborit *et al.* (1957) studied the effects of the combined K and Mg

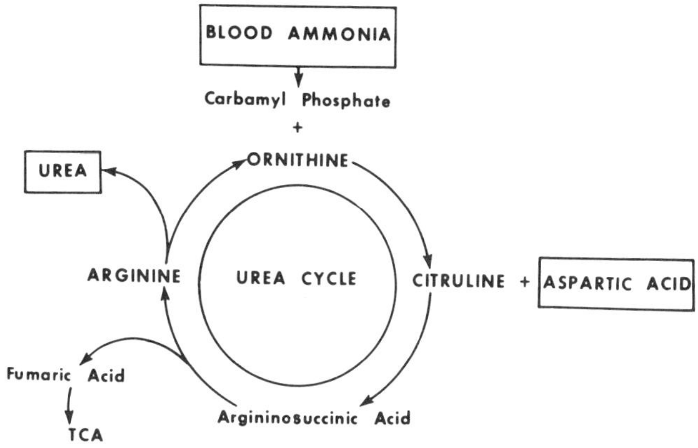

Fig. 2. The urea cycle.

aspartates on groups of white rats subjected to a standard swim test. It was found that the duration of the exercise after drug administration was significantly prolonged over that achieved with controls. After a standard rest period of 2½ hours, the animals were again given the swim test, and the aspartate-treated animals again swam longer than the other groups. Plasma ammonia levels were measured in the groups of rats subjected to the swim test. The ammonia levels of the control group increased; however, this increase was not seen in the group pretested with the potassium and magnesium aspartates.

In another study, Laborit *et al.* (1958) used 16 dogs, who breathed a mixture of 90% oxygen and 10% CO_2. These animals were given the combined salts of aspartic acid. Immediately after administration of the drug, plasma and expired CO_2 tension decreased and plasma urea concentration increased. This evidence supported the hypothesis that blood ammonia was being successfully converted to urea.

The administration of K and Mg aspartates to athletes reportedly had a positive effect on neuromuscular irritability, a significant reduction in existing fatigue, and supposedly a significant prophylactic effect against the induction of fatigue (Wyeth Laboratories, 1961). Most of the studies relied on the subjective judgment of subjects as to feelings of fatigue, and placebos were not always used. These and other studies have reported that aspartate therapy improves recovery from fatigue rapidly.

Consolazio *et al.* (1964) conducted a well-controlled experimental study on the effect of aspartic acid salts on the physical performance of men. Twelve healthy young men were matched on body weight and randomly assigned to an aspartate group or a placebo group. Subjects were not told to which group they had been assigned. The 9-week study consisted of 2 weeks of control and training, 5 weeks of either aspartate or placebo therapy accompanied by physical training, and 2 weeks of recovery. Either a placebo or 500 mg of potassium and magnesium salts of aspartic acid was taken orally twice daily. The physical training consisted of running 30 minutes on a motor-driven treadmill 5 days a week.

The results showed that there were no significant differences between the control and aspartate groups in (a) oxygen consumption, carbon dioxide production, oxygen debt, or RQ requirements; (b) recovery after an "all-out" run; (c) maximal breathing capacity or timed vital capacity. The authors concluded that there was no convincing evidence of the beneficial effects of aspartate therapy in humans in delaying the onset of fatigue.

Ahlborg *et al.* (1968) investigated the effect of potassium and magnesium aspartates on the capacity for prolonged exercise in man. This study is important because it also used human subjects rather than animals. Six men were selected from 300 healthy young men who had been tested on their ability to perform prolonged exercise to exhaustion. The physical fitness levels of these men were judged to be average. A pilot study was done on each subject to determine the work load on the bicycle ergometer that would result in exhaustion after about 90 minutes. The PWC_{170} test (physical working capacity at a heart rate of 170 determined by an electrocardiogram) was used as the test work load. The room temperature on the test days was between 21° and 23°C. The test was given on four consecutive days. On test days 1, 2, and 4, a placebo was given, and on the third test day, 1.75 gm of potassium–magnesium aspartate was given, followed by a similar dose every 6 hours prior to the test. The tests were administered at 1:00 P.M. each day. No standard diet was prescribed, although all foods ingested were reported. Since a high-carbohydrate diet tends to increase ability to do prolonged work, care was taken that only normal amounts of carbohydrates were ingested. During the tests, heart rate and respiration rate were recorded every second and tenth minute, and water was administered as needed.

The results showed that there was no significant difference between the amount of work accomplished on days 1, 2, and 4. However, on day 3, following aspartate administration, the amount of work accomplished was significantly improved. The mean work time increased from 85 minutes on days 1, 2, and 4 to 128 minutes on day 3. This 50% increase in work capacity is highly significant. The mean work performed on days 1, 2, and 4 was 93,500 kpm compared to 140,800 kpm on day 3, also a very significant improvement. This study indicates that the maximal capacity for prolonged exercise after administration of potassium–magnesium aspartate can be significantly increased.

It was hypothesized that a 50% longer work period at the same work load after administration of potassium–magnesium aspartate was due to a decreased rate of glycogen utilization and that the energy for a greater part of the work was supplied by fat. Other studies do not support the theory that potassium–magnesium aspartate improves muscle efficiency so as to require less energy for more work. No blood ammonias or ureas were measured.

One of the primary reasons for exhaustion in animals is the accumulation of ammonia resulting from deamination of adenylic acid to inosinic acid in the actively contractng skeletal muscle during strenuous exercise. Any substance that will prevent an increase in blood ammonia can possibly prevent the onset of fatigue.

L-Ornithine and L-aspartate are well-known intermediaries of the urea cycle essential to the incorporation of ammonia into urea. The effect of L-ornithine and L-aspartate mixture in lowering blood ammonia in rats has been demonstrated (Salvatore and Bocchini, 1961). It was shown that the combination of L-ornithine and L-aspartate was more effective in converting blood urea than was L-aspartate alone. The administration of L-ornithine and L-aspartate partially prevents an increase in blood ammonia by increasing the conversion of ammonia to urea.

In 1970, Cutinelli *et al.*, using 550 male albino rats, injected L-ornithine–L-aspartate (OA) one-half hour before the start of a strenuous swimming test. It was found, however, that in order to raise blood ammonia levels the rats had to be weighted to increase the amount of physical work, and the water temperature lowered considerably. Prior to the OA therapy, the animals displayed no protection against increased blood ammonia. Under the exercising conditions, the OA demonstrated a protective ability by lowering blood ammonia levels. In an attempt to demonstrate further protective ability of the OA, other blood parameters were studied. Levels of AMP, ADP, ATP, GTP, and GOT were observed: AMP, ADP, and ATP increased during the stress of exercise; however, only ATP was lowered by the OA administration. This could be explained as the utilization of creatine for resynthesis of creatine phosphate. The GTP level was also lowered by the administration of OA, suggesting a maintenance of the normal cellular membrane integrity under severe stress.

The authors concluded that the decrease of blood ammonia, ATP, creatine, and GTP in OA-treated animals demonstrates the efficiency of L-ornithine–L-aspartate administration in the treatment of severe physical exhaustion. Unfortunately, this study did not measure blood urea levels, which, if elevated, might support the theory that aspartate makes the urea cycle more efficient in handling increased amounts of blood ammonia and thereby eliminates the fatigue effects of ammonia accumulation.

Barnes *et al.* (1964) proposed another hypothesis for the enhancement of the urea cycle. Using rats as the experimental animal, they administered ammonium carbonate orally. It was proposed that, through the continuous stress on the OCA (urea) cycle by the exogenous ammonium, the enzymes of the cycle would be facilitated so as to allow for a more functional conversion process. Bjurstrom (1970), in a subsequent study, employed forced swimming on dogs and a similar ammonium carbonate regimen. He divided the dogs into three groups. Group 1 was physically trained; Group 2 was administered an ammonium carbonate regime; and, in Group 3, drug administration was accompanied by physical training. The results indicated that Group 3 swam significantly longer and had significantly lower blood ammonia levels than the other two groups. Unfortunately, neither of these studies measured the blood urea levels; therefore, the urea cycle facilitation theory could not be confirmed.

Similar studies in humans are difficult, since ammonium compounds are toxic and few, if any, are available commercially for human consumption. A few Swedish studies have reported using ammonium compounds in human studies, indicating that they may be available in Europe and that less caution is used in human experimentation.

Bjurstrom (1972) conducted a pilot study on blood ammonia and blood urea levels in humans before and after exercise on a bicycle ergometer. Blood ammonia increased substantially following exercise but was followed by little or no subsequent increase in blood urea nitrogen. These findings do not support the theory that conversion of blood ammonia to urea is the immediate fate of elevated blood ammonia nitrogen concentrations following exercise. It sometimes took as long as 90 minutes for blood urea levels to become elevated.

Bjurstrom and Golding (1972) are presently testing another possible theory relative to the body's ability to handle increased blood ammonia, and this approach is described below. Handler and Duda (1958) proposed that the conversion of glutamic acid to glutamine (glutamic acid and ammonia $\rightarrow$ glutamine) is the immediate fate of peripherally originating blood ammonia, not the incorporation of ammonia into urea through the urea cycle.

Ammonia resulting from skeletal muscle contraction combines with glutamic acid in the circulating peripheral blood, forming glutamine. The glutamine is subsequently deaminated in the liver or kidney, liberating ammonia in the urine as ammonium salts. The deamination of glutamine, however, appears to be a slow process with little or no increase in blood urea occurring until 60–90 minutes after the cessation of exercise, and even then only minimal elevations are observed. Research currently being conducted by Bjurstrom and Golding (1972) is concerned with evaluating pre- and postexercise concentrations of blood ammonia, glutamic acid, glutamine, urine urea, and blood urea. This work is being performed to specifically investigate the fate of elevated blood ammonia levels following exercise. Increases in glutamine without any concomitant increases in blood urea nitrogen or urine urea nitrogen immediately following exercise might well support the theory of Duda and Handler. Correlation between the reduction of glutamine and the increase in blood urea during recovery would somewhat negate the aspartate theory. If the glutamine hypothesis is true, glutamic acid may well be a better ergogenic aid than either ammonium compounds or aspartates.

SUMMARY

Not enough studies have been conducted on humans to merit any generalizations about the ergogenic effect of either the aspartates or the ammonium compounds. Most investigators have employed animals and the few studies with human subjects have had small samples. The previously reported postexercise blood ammonia and urea levels in man, as well as recent research findings from our laboratory, fail to support the exogeneous aspartate theory. Ammonium compounds, in this country, are still unavailable commercially, which makes human studies difficult. The administration of glutamic acid has not, as yet, been discussed in the literature. Aspartates, however, in normal doses are not harmful and present no serious contraindications, and further human experimentation should be undertaken.

V. Summary

The influence of amphetamines, anabolic steroids, and aspartates on physical performance has been reviewed in the present chapter. As with most alleged ergogenic aids, methodological considerations in the assessment of drugs and hormones are extremely important. Indeed, it is reasonable to suggest that much of the apparent disagreement in this area of inquiry frequently stems from differences in methodologies rather than actual effects. At any rate, it is quite clear that rigorous double-blind paradigms should be employed in the assessment of the ergogenic efficacy of drugs and hormones if at all possible. However, necessary informed consent practices sometimes rule out this possibility.

While the results of various surveys have disclosed that amphetamine is the drug most widely used by athletes, the available experimental evidence does not support this practice. With respect to the question of whether utilization of anabolic steroids facilitates muscular strength and body weight, the evidence seems to be equivocal. Aspartates have been found to improve physical performance in comparative studies involving rats and dogs. However, there is only limited evidence on the influence of aspartates on man's physical performance, and hence generalizations pertaining to man are not possible at this time.

References

Ahlborg, B., Ekelund, L. G., and Nilsson, C. G. (1968). *Acta Physiol. Scand.* **74**, 238–245.

American College of Sports Medicine (1958). *Report to the Committee to Study the Use of Drugs in Athletics,* April 1958.

Andriver, O. (1971). *Med. Trib.* **12**, 23.

Ariel, G. (1972). *Med. Sci. Sports* **4**, 54.

Barnes, R. H., Labadan, B. A., Myamoglu, B., and Bradfield, R. B. (1964). *Amer. J. Physiol.* **207**, 1242–1246.

Bjurstrom, L. A. (1970). Unpublished master's thesis, South Dakota State Univ., Brookings, South Dakota.

Bjurstrom, L. A., and Golding, L. A. (1972). Unpublished doctoral dissertation, Kent State Univ., Kent, Ohio.

Bjurstrom, L. A. (1972). Unpublished study, Kent State Univ., Kent, Ohio.

Bowers, R., and Reardon, J. F. (1971). Unpublished master's thesis, Bowling Green State Univ., Bowling Green, Ohio.

Casner, S. W., Early, R. G., and Carlson, B. R. (1971). *J. Sports Med. Phys. Fit.* **11**, 98–103.

Consolazio, C. F., Nelson, R. A., Matoush, L. O., and Isaac, G. J. (1964). *J. Appl. Physiol.* **19**, 257–261.

Cutinelli, L., Sorrentino, L., Tramonti, C., Salvatore, F., and Cedrangolo, F. (1970). *Arzneim.-Forsch.* **8**, 1064–1067.

Dumas, P. (1971). *Med. Trib.* **12**, 31.

Fahey, R., and Brown, H. (1972). *Med. Sci. Sports* **4**, 54.

Foltz, E. E., Ivy, A. C., and Barborka, C. J. (1943). *J. Lab. Clin. Med.* **28**, 601–603.

Fowler, W. H., Gardner, G. W., and Egstrom, G. H. (1965). *J. Appl. Physiol.* **20**, 1038–1040.

Gilbert, B. (1969). *Sports Illustrated,* Part I, **30**, No. 25, 64–72; Part II, **30**, No. 26, 30–42; Part III, **31**, No. 1, 30–35.

Golding, L. A., and Barnard, R. J. (1963). *J. Sports Med. Phys. Fit.* **3**, 221–224.

Golding, L. A. (1970, 1971). Personal interviews with championship-level athletes.

Graham, G. (1972). Unpublished doctoral dissertation, Kent State Univ., Kent, Ohio.

Hagerman, F. (1966, 1968). Personal interviews at the 1966 World Pentathlon Games and 1968 Olympic Games.

Haldi, J., and Wynn, W. (1959). *Res. Quart.* **17**, 96–101.

Handler, P., and Duda, G. D. (1958). *J. Biol. Chem.* **232**, 303–314.

Johnson, L. C., and O'Shea, J. P. (1969). *Science* **18**, 957–959.

Johnson, L. C., Fisher, G., Sylvester, L. J., and Hofheins, C. C. (1972). *Med. Sci. Sports* **4**, 43–45.
Karpovich, P. V. (1959). *J. Amer. Med. Ass.* **170**, 558–561.
Kuzell, W. C., Glover, R. P., Bruns, D. L., and Gibbs, J. O. (1962). *Geriatrics* **17**, 428–441.
Laborit, H., Moynier, R., Trzebski, A., Guilo, G., and Baron, C. (1957). *C. R. Soc. Biol.* **151**, 1383–1386.
Laborit, H., Orrenovitch, L., and Leguen, F. (1958). *C. R. Soc. Biol.* **152**, 1359–1360.
Lambert, P. A., and Site, H. (1961). *Presse Med.* **69**, 1638.
Liddle, G. W., and Burke, H. A. (1960). *Helv. Med. Acta* **27**, 504–513.
McKenzie, R. E., and Elliot, L. L. (1965). *Aerosp. Med.* **36**, 774–779.
Maul, C., and Hagerman, F. (1971). Unpublished master's thesis, Ohio Univ., Athens.
Organon, Inc., West Orange, New Jersey. (1970). Drug description.
O'Shea, J. P., and Winkler, W. (1970). *Nutr. Rep. Int.* **2**, 351–361.
Pierson, W. R., Rasch, P. J., Brubaker, M. L. (1961). *Med. Sport* **1**, 61–66.
Salvatore, F., and Bocchini, V. (1961). *Nature* **191**, 705.
Samuels, L. T., Henschel, A. F., and Keys, A. (1942). *J. Clin. Endocrinol.* **2**, 649–654.
Smith, G. M., and Beecher, H. K. (1959). *J. Amer. Med. Ass.* **170**, 542–557.
van Waylen, R. G. A., and Buyze, G. (1961). *Acta Endocrinol. (Copenhagen)* **58**, 1.
Wyeth Laboratories (1961). Circular 2318.
Wyndham, C. H., Rogers, G. G., Benade, A. J. S., and Strydom, N. B. (1971). *S. Afr. Med. J.* **45**, 247–252.

Author Index

Numbers in italics refer to the pages on which the complete references are listed.

C

M

N

O

P

T

U

V

Subject Index

B

C

N

DATE			
Mar 31 '76			
RETURNED JUN 29 1988			
NO 22 '99			